AF333784

Medical Management of Rheumatic Musculoskeletal and Connective Tissue Diseases

Medical Management of Rheumatic Musculoskeletal and Connective Tissue Diseases

Jan Dequeker
University Hospitals
Leuven, Belgium

Gabriel Panayi
Guy's Hospital
London, England

Theodore Pincus
Vanderbilt University School of Medicine
Nashville, Tennessee

Rodney Grahame
Guy's Hospital
London, England

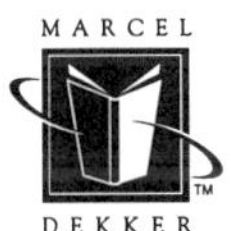

MARCEL DEKKER, INC.   NEW YORK · BASEL · HONG KONG

Library of Congress Cataloging-in-Publication Data

Medical management of rheumatic musculoskeletal and connective tissue
    diseases / Jan Dequeker ... [et al.].
          p. cm. -- (Clinical guides to medical management)
    Includes index.
    ISBN 0-8247-9847-3 (hardcover : alk. paper)
    1. Connective tissues--Diseases. 2. Arthritis. 3. Rheumatism.
I. Dequeker, Jan. II. Series.
    [DNLM: 1. Rheumatic Diseases. 2. Connective Tissue Diseases.
3. Diagnosis, Differential. 4. Vasculitis. 5. Bone Diseases.
WE 544 M489 1997]
RC924.M43   1997
616.7--dc21
DNLM/DLC
for Library of Congress   97-22374
                                                                     CIP

The publisher offers discounts on this book when ordered in bulk quantities. For
more information, write to Special Sales/Professional Marketing at the address
below.

This book is printed on acid-free paper.

Copyright © 1997 by MARCEL DEKKER, INC. All Rights Reserved.

Neither this book nor any part may be reproduced or transmitted in any form or
by any means, electronic or mechanical, including photocopying, microfilming,
and recording, or by any information storage and retrieval system, without
permission in writing from the publisher.

MARCEL DEKKER, INC.
270 Madison Avenue, New York, New York 10016
http://www.dekker.com

Current printing (last digit):
10 9 8 7 6 5 4 3 2 1

PRINTED IN THE UNITED STATES OF AMERICA

Preface

Musculoskeletal diseases, such as osteoarthritis, rheumatoid arthritis, systemic lupus erythematosus, gout, spondylitis, osteoporosis, soft tissue rheumatism, and regional musculoskeletal pain syndromes, collectively affect more than one-third of all adults in developed countries. The prevalence of musculoskeletal diseases will increase because of the increasing average age of the world's population. How well future physicians (primary care and specialist) manage musculoskeletal diseases will be an important factor affecting quality of life and health care costs.

Although there are many good textbooks on rheumatology, most of them focus mainly on inflammatory rheumatic diseases. We have lacked a core book that covers the management of musculoskeletal diseases and is useful for practicing clinicians and students. Many physicians come into contact with musculoskeletal symptoms and connective tissue diseases without having much training in this field. Even when clinical information on rheumatology has been available, it has often been restricted to stereotypic descriptions of the end stages of diseases; for example, that gout is big-toe arthritis and tophi, rheumatoid arthritis is ulnar deviation and swan-neck deformity, and osteoarthritis is osteophyte formation.

The purpose of this book is to provide the essentials on musculoskeletal and connective tissue diseases, based on the knowledge of experienced teachers from the United States and Europe, so that a correct diagnosis and appropriate management can be established from the onset of the first symptoms. "Rheumatism" is not a disease but a diagnostic problem to be solved. Any of more than 200 different disease entities — benign, invalidating, acute, chronic, and even neoplastic diseases — can be behind a musculoskeletal complaint.

The book is organized in a logical and practical way, giving diagnostic and management concepts for the early phase of each disease, plus background information on the pathophysiology, epidemiology, and impact of the disease on the patient and society. The reader will be able to codify and identify quickly the essentials of each musculoskeletal disease by referring to the chapter outlines, tables, figures, and index.

Chapter 1 covers the skills involved in taking a patient's history and giving a physical examination. The approach may seem simplistic, but over-reliance on laboratory and radiographic testing has led to oversight of these basic diagnostic techniques. In the diagnosis of musculoskeletal diseases more than for any other diseases, a careful reading of the clinical signs and patient's history is essential and cannot be substituted by technology. Therefore, rheumatology may serve as a model in the clinical education of the physician in training.

Clinical thinking and problem solving skills are of particular importance to those working with systemic connective tissue diseases. Chapter 2 provides guidelines for problem oriented differential diagnosis. The physician who comes to the correct diagnosis by cluster analysis of symptoms, which need to be substantiated by only one or two technical tests, should find this greatly satisfying.

Other chapters cover general broad diagnostic-pathogenetic topics such as infectous diseases, polyarthritis, spondylarthropathy, multisystem diseases, crystal arthropathy, localized painful conditions, metabolic bone disesases, and hereditary connective tissue diseases. The final chapter is devoted to current intra- and periarticular injection techniques feasable in general medical practice.

The chapters on diseases are structured according to the following model:

Definition
Clinical features
    early manifestations
    late manifestations
Confirmation of the diagnosis: Investigations
Differential diagnosis
Epidemiology and historical data

Pathophysiology
Management
Atypical forms
Prognosis: Impact of the disease

Each chapter is constructed around the most prevalent disease entity in the particular disease category. The chapter starts with the definition of the disease, then moves on to the early and late clinical features, how to confirm the diagnosis, difficulties in diagnosis, incidence of disease, pathophysiology and management, atypical presentations, and finally, patient prognosis and the impact of the disease on society.

The book is richly illustrated with drawings, tables, and photographs to present readers with the many clinical features of rheumatism. New imaging techniques, when they are relevant for diagnosis, and more in-depth pathophysiological mechanisms for the major entities are included to help students understand the basic mechanisms behind a disease process.

We, and particularly the coordinator of the book, Prof. Dr. Jan Dequeker, president of ILAR (International League of Associations for Rheumatology), together with Prof. Dr. Rodney Grahame, president of the Standing Committee on Education and Publiation, in the name of the regional leagues PANLAR (Pan-American League of Associations for Rheumatology), AFLAR (African League Against Rheumatism), APLAR (Asian Pacific League of Associations for Rheumatology), and EULAR (European League Against Rheumatism), want to ensure that physicians learn the principles of comprehensive care of musculoskeletal and connective tissue diseases and do not give up on rheumatic patients before implementing the effective and appropriate diagnostic and management measures that can be learned from this book.

The creation of this book required the help of a number of dedicated people. We must thank our expert collaborators in particular: for critically reading and correcting our manuscripts, Jo Verwilghen, René Westhovens, and Chester W. Fink; for providing excellent images, Pierre Schotsmans et al. (Pfizer, Belgium); for X-ray pictures, J. Malghem and Peter Brys; for permission to reproduce their publication on injection techniques, Roche-Syntex Belgium; for pictures of intraarticular injections, Guy Isaacs; and for secretarial assistance, Josette Cartois and Annemieke Vandereijcken.

Jan Dequeker
Gabriel Panayi
Theodore Pincus
Rodney Grahame

Contents

1

History and Physical Examination of a Patient with a Rheumatic Problem

1 HISTORY

Details about the patient's musculoskeletal symptoms, obtainable only from the interview, are priceless in understanding the patient's illness. These details (1) define characteristics of the complaints as the patient feels them, (2) suggest whether anatomically definable involvement is likely or not, and (3) permit evaluation of the patient's cooperation, motivation, and goals. Thus informed, the clinician may more readily achieve the objectives of accurate diagnosis and appropriate management while dealing with the patient as a complete human being rather than merely as a case. Therefore, it is important that the physician take time when analyzing the chief complaint, previous therapy, past medical health, and review of the systems. In addition, family health and personal and social history must be obtained.

1.1 Chief Complaint

Most patients come to the rheumatology clinic because of pain, swelling, and stiffness of joints with or without limitation of motion.

1.1.1 Pain

The phenomenon of pain is complex and subjective and often extremely difficult to define, measure, and explain. However, four broad diagnostic categories of pain may be defined (Table 1.1).

Table 1.1 Pain Categories

Neurogenic pain
Inflammatory pain
Mechanical pain
Psychogenic pain

Neurogenic Pain. Neurogenic pain results from nerve compression. It is therefore characterized by a specific pain distribution area, often occurring at night, and may be elicited in a particular position. A typical example is carpal tunnel syndrome, caused by compression of the median nerve in the carpal tunnel, resulting in pain and paresthesia in the area of innervation of the medial nerve (Fig. 1.1).

Inflammatory Pain. Inflammatory pain results from inflammation, with edema and swelling of the synovial membrane, leading to pain at night and marked morning stiffness. A typical example of inflammatory pain is that seen in patients with rheumatoid arthritis.

The pain at night will wake the patient in the second part of the night and may result in sleep disturbances. Morning stiffness is noted as soon as the patient wakes and it persists for hours (Fig. 1.2). Pain and stiffness improve after moving around. In addition, rest during the day may cause recurrence of pain and stiffness and is sometimes referred to as "gelling."

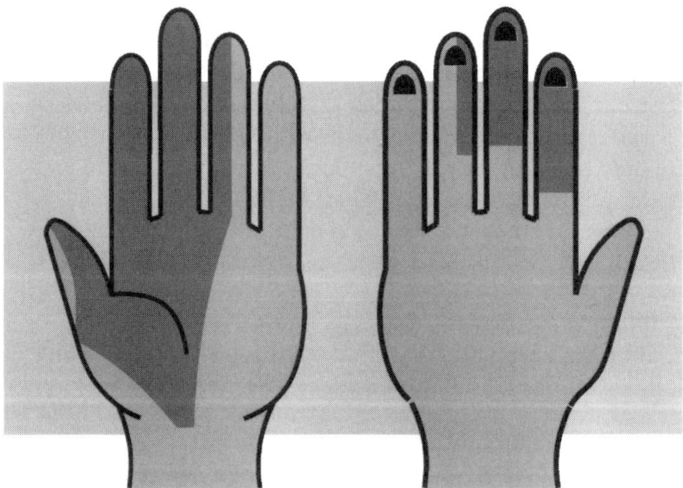

Figure 1.1 Pain distribution area in carpal tunnel syndrome.

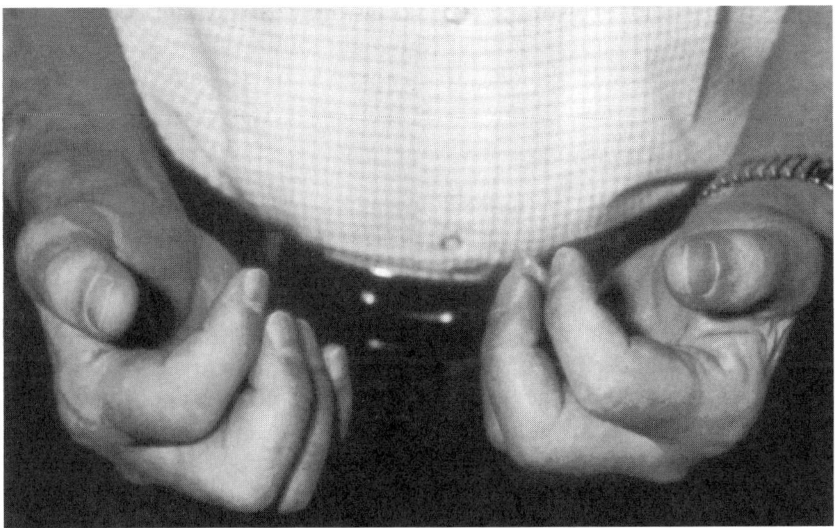

Figure 1.2   Morning stiffness in the hands.

The pain at night as well as the morning stiffness are caused by congestion of hypertrophic synovial tissue. Movement will mobilize this status of fluid or edema. In addition, antiinflammatory drugs will improve the stiffness. The duration of morning stiffness is a good indicator of the degree of inflammation, and this marker is useful in the evaluation of efficacy of treatment on follow-up.

Mechanical Pain.   Mechanical pain results from degeneration of articular and periarticular structures. This may be seen in osteoarthritis. The pain is characterized by a typical circadian rhythm, with progressive worsening during the daytime. At night and with rest the pain improves. Mobilization, however, will result in pain. Sometimes the patient complains at the initiation of movement, with a slight stiffness (minutes), and this is referred to as "starting pain."

Psychogenic Pain.   Psychogenic pain is associated with psychological problems, characterized by the absence of the circadian rhythm and morning stiffness. The pain lasts day and night, no improvement is seen with rest or movement, and may worsen in a stressful situation.

1.1.2 Swelling

Swelling is an important sign or complaint of a patient with rheumatic disease. Although assessment of swelling is certainly a function of the physical examination, valuable information can also be obtained from the interview or from comparison of the patient's history with physical examination. It is important to ask the patient about the onset of the swelling, i.e., whether it was acute or gradual or whether its course was intermittent or chronic.

1.1.3 Limitation of Motion

Limitation of motion is a frequent complaint of patients with rheumatic disorders. Patients express such limitation in the context of the difficulties they experience from restrictions on their activities during work and daily living. This information can be elicited by questions such as, "What ordinary daily activities can't you do for yourself?" If indeed there are restrictions of motion, the length of time they have been present should be determined with as much accuracy as possible. It is also important to determine whether the limitation of motion began abruptly (as indicated with tendon or muscle rupture) or gradually and intermittently before becoming chronic.

1.1.4 Stiffness

The word stiffness has different meanings to different patients. Some are connected with pain; others with fatigue, soreness, aching, tightness, swelling, restricted movement, or weakness. Stiffness should be differentiated from the more persistent pain or other symptoms of arthritis. Stiffness is usually defined as a discomfort or restriction perceived by the patient when attempting the first parts of easy movement of a joint after a period of inactivity. Stiffness usually develops after inactivity of one or more hours or after bed rest and sleep. When stiffness is severe it may improve slowly over several hours or not improve appreciably throughout the day. The absence of stiffness does not exclude the possibility of presence of systemic inflammatory rheumatic diseases such as rheumatoid arthritis, but such absence is uncommon.

1.1.5 Weakness

Weakness is loss of muscular strength. It may be a symptom of articular disease, myositis, other types of myopathies, or of neurologic conditions.

1.2 History of the Present Complaint

In the history of the present complaint one must focus on the type of onset, the location of the symptoms, and, last but not least, the number of joints involved. The type of onset may be acute or gradual. An acute onset is seen in acute rheumatic fever, gout, and septic arthritis. A gradual onset is more commonly seen in rheumatoid arthritis and osteoarthritis.

The location of the pain or the symptoms must be noted. Involvement of the axial skeleton as seen in ankylosing spondylitis or peripheral large and small joints as in rheumatoid arthritis should be noted. Of particular interest is the number and symmetry or asymmetry of the joint involvement.

In addition, the functional impact may provide information on the severity of the joint involvement. Important muscle dysfunction is seen in septic arthritis and gout.

It is useful to investigate the precipitating or aggravating circumstances of the rheumatic complaints. In systemic lupus erythematosus (SLE) a flare may be triggered by pregnancy, an infection, or sun exposure. Rheumatoid arthritis symptoms may improve during pregnancy and severe exacerbation may occur in the postpartum period. Exposure to drugs such as hydralazine and procainamide can induce SLE or other autoimmune diseases. A minimal trauma may cause a fracture in a person with osteoporosis. Unprotected intercourse may result in a sexually acquired reactive arthritis.

1.3 Background Information

A good description of the background onto which the complaints are grafted is often helpful in making the correct diagnosis. Certain rheumatic conditions occur more frequently in different age groups, in one sex or the other, and in certain families (Table 1.2).

1.3.1 Family History

A hereditary predisposition is known for a number of rheumatic diseases and should be looked for. A diagram of the family tree is a convenient way to report personal information regarding illnesses that might be related ethnically, psychologically, or environmentally to the patient's present illness. Rheumatologic disorders that occur in several members of the family

Table 1.2 Effect of Age and Sex on Incidence of Rheumatic Diseases

Age	♀	♂
Children	Acute rheumatic fever, Still's disease, postviral synovitis	
Young adults	Gonococcal arthritis	Reiter's syndrome
	SLE	Ankylosing spondylitis
Middle age	Rheumatoid arthritis	Osteoarthritis
	Osteoporosis	
Elderly	Polymyalgia rheumatica	

may have a genetic basis, but environmental factors should not be overlooked. Rheumatologic or other diseases that are likely to have occurred in other members of a rheumatic patient's family include rheumatoid arthritis, gout, psoriasis, colitis, infections, and predilection to degenerative joint diseases.

1.4 Past Medical History

After the history of the present illness is elicited, the next part of the interview is directed to the patient's past health. This part of the patient's history includes information of all previous major illnesses and injuries, especially those requiring medical attention or hospitalization. For patients with a rheumatic illness the past medical history can reveal previous conditions that are important to the present illnesses that were not appreciated as such by the patient, or symptoms that were diagnosed differently before. Uveitis, bursitis, and renal colic are examples of conditions that may be seen in certain rheumatic diseases. Other examples are gastrectomy induced osteomalacia, ovariectomy resulting in osteoporosis, diabetes mellitus for diabetic arthropathy and neuropathy.

1.5 Review of Systems

The history concludes with a review of systems. This is a final systematic check of other symptoms and minor illnesses that the patient may have had but has forgotten to mention.

2 PHYSICAL EXAMINATION

The general physical examination should be performed as for any other disease. A number of clinical features are of particular interest for rheumatic patients. The rheumatologic examination is an exercise in applied anatomy, with utilization of simple provocation or stress tests. Screening of the locomotor system should be included in any full general medical examination: many rheumatic diseases involve other systems and, conversely, many "general medical" conditions (particularly endocrine, metabolic, and neoplastic) affect locomotor structures.

2.1 General Appearance

As soon as the patient walks in the clinic, your physical examination starts. Look at the overall appearance; a diminished height may suggest scoliosis or osteoporosis; kyphosis and stiffness of the spine may imply spondylitis; obesity may suggest osteoarthritis; a duck-like gait may be the result of osteomalacia. The manner in which the patient walks and sits down may give you a good general idea about your patient's functional abilities.

The skin must be examined extensively as this may give extra clues to make the diagnosis. In Table 1.3 some examples of skin changes suggesting underlying rheumatic diseases are given.

Other organ involvement must be looked for. Pleuritis, pericarditis, valvular disease may be seen in autoimmune rheumatic diseases. Primary heart diseases or lung diseases can give rise to rheumatic complaints as seen in subacute bacterial endocarditis or pulmonary hypertrophic arthropathy.

Liver or spleen enlargement as well as adenopathy are aspects of all systemic diseases.

Table 1.3 Examples of Some Integumentary Changes Suggesting Underlying Rheumatic Disease

Lesion	Disease
Alopecia	Systemic lupus erthematosus (SLE)
Nail pitting	Psoriatic arthritis
Onycholysis	Psoriatic arthritis, Reiter's syndrome
Keratodermia blenorrhagica	Reiter's syndrome
Leg ulcers	Rheumatoid vasculitis, Felty's syndrome
Buccal or genital ulcers	SLE, Reiter's syndrome, Behçet's disease
Palpable purpura	Vasculitis
Nodules	RA, gout, amyloid, sarcoidosis, multicentric reticulohistiocytosis
Petechiae	SLE, idiopathic thrombocytopenic purpura
Raynaud's phenomenon	SLE, systemic sclerosis, limited cutaneous scleroderma
Nocturnal febrile macular rash	Juvenile rheumatoid arthritis, adult onset Still's disease
Erythema nodosum	Sarcoidosis, inflammatory bowel disease
Sun sensitivity malar rash	SLE
Rash over knuckles (Gottron's papules)	Dermatomyositis
Calcinosis	Dermatomyositis, systemic sclerosis, limited cutaneous scleroderma, apatite arthropathy
Hemorrhagic pustules	Gonococcal arthritis
Livedo reticularis	Antiphospholipid syndrome

2.2 Joint Examination

A systematic approach in inspecting and examining joints is the quickest and easiest way of obtaining valuable information. The examiner often begins with the joints of the upper extremity and proceeds to the joints of the trunk and lower extremity. Corresponding paired joints are compared systematically with each other and with normality and abnormality for that particular joint. Inspection and palpation supplement each other; they usually can be performed together and can be followed by evaluation of joint motion.

The patient should be as comfortable as possible since muscles and tendons overlying the joints must be as soft and relaxed as possible. The physician must examine the underlying joint adequately and obtain an accurate assessment of the status of the joint. Rough or forceful handling of inflamed joints may cause not only severe pain but also muscle spasm and loss of the patient's cooperation, so that further examination becomes difficult or unreliable.

Excessive muscle spasm and pain can usually be avoided by firm support of the area being examined and gentle handling of painful areas.

Examination of a painful joint requires moving it from the neutral to a relaxed position, with care taken to return the extremities slowly to a comfortable position before withdrawing the examiner's support. Quick motion should be avoided. When examining tendons, the examiner must be anatomically accurate and certain that the tendon, muscle, nerve, or other tissue is palpated. Simple explanation should be given to the patient of what is being done or is to be done; this is often necessary to obtain reliable observations.

All the joints should be examined even if the patient only complains about one. Figure 1.3 shows the 53 different joints that may be affected in rheumatic disease.

2.2.1 Physical Signs of Arthritis

Arthritis is a general term that describes the existence of disease within the joint itself. Synovitis, or inflammation of the synovial membrane from whatever cause, is therefore synonymous with arthritis. Either thickening of the synovial membrane or articular effusion is indicative of synovitis, and often both are present simultaneously in the same joint. The most common signs of articular synovitis are swelling, tenderness, and limitation of motion.

2.2.2 Joint Swelling

Swelling about the joint may be caused by intraarticular effusion, synovial thickening, periarticular soft tissue inflammation (such as bursitis or ten-

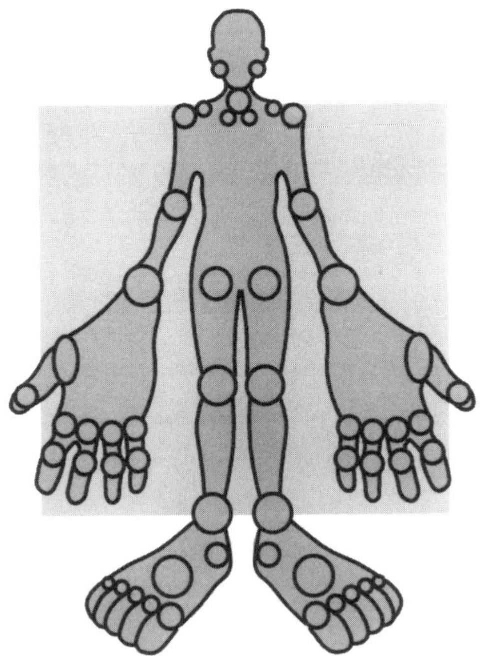

Figure 1.3 EULAR total tender joint index (53 joints).

donitis), or bony enlargement. These conditions need to be differentiated from one another (Table 1.4).

> *Periarticular soft tissue edema* is characterized by a diffuse edema with pitting that extends beyond the synovial joint.
> *Synovial thickening* may have a doughy or a boggy consistency on palpation. Familiarity with the anatomic disposition of the synovial membrane in various joints is important in differentiating soft tissue swelling due to synovitis from swelling of periarticular tissues.

Table 1.4 Joint Swelling

Periarticular soft tissue edema
Synovial thickening
Effusion in the joint (joint fluid)
Bony enlargement

Effusion in the joint (joint fluid) may be demonstrated by visible or palpable bulging of the joint capsule. In some joints the margin of the synovial membrane can be delineated on physical examination by compressing synovial fluid into one of the extreme limits of its reflection.

Bony enlargement is characterized by a hard proliferation of the joint border.

2.2.3 Joint Pain—Tenderness

The localization of tenderness (pain) by palpation should make it apparent as to whether the reaction is intraarticular or periarticular. Four types of pain can be differentiated in the physical examination (Table 1.5).

Elective pressure point pain is defined as pain elicited during examination by palpation of a particular part of the joint. Periarticular joint disease, rather than intraarticular abnormalities, causes this type of pain.

Diffuse, spontaneous joint pain is seen in an acute arthritis (septic arthritis or crystal-induced arthritis) whereby the joint is extremely painful and the patient holds it in the most comfortable position. When you attempt to palpate the joint the patient will withdraw or push your hands away.

Metacarpal/metatarsal squeeze pain is induced by tangential pressure over the joints of the hands and feet when laterally compressing the joint groups. A painful handshake is a good example of this type of pain. This clinical sign can be present before major swellings are manifest when the early inflammation is restricted to the edge of the cartilage.

Hyperflexion/hyperextension pain is elicited by movements of the joint, either extreme flexion or extreme extension. This type of pain is seen when inflammation of the synovium is present in the reflection area. This may also be a very early sign of inflammatory joint disease and arthritis, in particular of the knee and wrist.

Table 1.5 Joint Pain – Tenderness

Elective pressure pain
Diffuse spontaneous pain
Metacarpal/metatarsal squeeze pain
Hyperflexion/hyperextension pain

2.2.4 Joint Crepitus

Joint crepitus is a palpable grating or crackling sensation produced by motion. It indicates roughness or irregularity of the joint surface. Fine crepitus is provoked by the presence of granulation tissue or by eroded bone ends and can be felt, for example, in rheumatoid arthritis. The coarse crepitus is due to irregularity of cartilage surfaces usually caused by noninflammatory arthritis. Crepitus from within the joint should be distinguished from clicking joints generally indicating no pathology. Clicking sounds are caused by the flipping of ligaments or tendons over bony surfaces during motion or by induction of a vacuum.

2.2.5 Range of Motion

Limitation of motion may occur on either active or passive motion. In the former, motion is restricted when the patient attempts voluntary movement of a part. In the latter, motion is restricted when the examiner attempts movement of a part with the patient's muscles relaxed. When the active and passive range of motion are not equal, the passive range is usually greater and is thus a more reliable indication of the actual range of motion. Complete immobility of a joint is called ankylosis.

Generally, the movements are measured starting from a hypothetical zero point in which the person stands right up with arms and fingers extended on the body. The extended "anatomic position" of an extremity is thus counted as 0°. The joint mobility of an extremity has to be compared with the mobility of the contralateral one.

2.2.6 Muscle Testing

Muscle tests are used to determine the presence, extent, and degree of muscle weakness resulting from disease, injury, or disuse. Muscle function and joint function are closely related. The use of muscles is influenced by the status of joints moved by their muscles and vice versa. Because of the great variability of muscle strength among different people and the requirement of full cooperation of the patient during the testing, the accurate judging of muscle strength in the clinical setting can be difficult. Many systems have been described for grading muscle strength. One common and useful method employing numerals include 6 grades, 5 through 0. Grade 5 indicates 100% strength (normal) with complete range of motion against gravity and with full resistance. Grade 4 indicates good strength with complete range of motion against gravity with some resistance. Grade 3 indicates a fair strength with complete range of motion against gravity. Grade 2 indicates poor strength with complete range of motion with gravity eliminated. Grade 1 indicates minimum strength with evidence of slight muscle

Table 1.6 Screening History Rheumatic Complaints

Categorization of the pain — swelling or other complaint
Patient characteristics
Description disease onset and manifestations
General systems inquiry
Evolution of symptoms (over time)

contractibility (visible or by palpation) but no joint motion. Grade 0 indicates no evidence of contractibility.

When testing muscle strength, the part of the body being examined has to be positioned properly to eliminate the effect of gravity.

Some simple tests evaluating the functional capacity of the most important muscle groups are (1) the chair raising test (whereby the patient gets out of a chair without use of armrests, testing the quadriceps), (2) the sit-up test for the abdominal muscles, and (3) raising arms for the shoulder girdle.

3 SCREENING HISTORY AND PHYSICAL EXAMINATION

An exhaustive history and extensive examination for all conceivable rheumatologic abnormalities in every patient are time consuming and unnecessary. As with other systems, a brief history of rheumatic complaints (Table 1.6) and a brief screening procedure to pick up problems in defined regions (Table 1.7) are more appropriate. If an abnormality is detected a more

Table 1.7 Screening Physical Examination

General physical examination
    extraarticular manifestations
    mucocutaneous features
    organ involvement: heart, lung, intestine
Systematic joint examination
    joint swelling categorization
    joint pain categorization
    joint mobility
    muscle strength
Specific joint examination — screening examination
    Hand → elbow → shoulder
    Toes → knees → hip → vertebral column

detailed examination of affected regions (as described in the next section) can be undertaken to define the problem more precisely.

4 DETAILED JOINT EXAMINATION

A systematic method of examining joints is the quickest and easiest way of obtaining the available information (Table 1.8). The examiner often begins with the joints of the upper extremity and proceeds to the joints of the trunk and the lower extremity. Corresponding paired joints are compared systematically with each other and with respect to normality or abnormality for the particular joint. It is good to start this systematic examination with the hands because there you will find information of general interest for the rest of the skeleton (Fig. 1.4).

4.1 Hands

When examining the hands it is important to inspect and palpate but it is just as important to examine their basic function. The *pinch grip* (picking up a pin), the *key grip* (after taking or turning a key), the *hammer grip*

Table 1.8 Screening Locomotor System

1. Inspection of the patient walking
    toes-heel walk

2. Inspection of the standing patient
    from behind: lateral flexion — chest expansion — Trendelenburg
    from the side: touch toes (Schober) — cervical flexion
    from in front: cervical rotation — hands behind head — tender joints

3. Inspection/examination of the patient lying on a couch
    3.1. hand inspection: dorsal aspects
                               palmar aspects
          examination: tight fist
                               metacarpal squeeze
    3.2. wrist: flexion — extension
    3.3. elbow: flexion — extension — pronation/supination radial head
    3.4. shoulder: elevation — abduction — internal rotation
    3.5. foot: inspection soles — dorsum — metatarsal squeeze
    3.6. knee: flexion — extension — laxity
              patella: ballotment test
              balloon sign
    3.7. hip: flexion — extension
              external — internal rotation
    3.8. sacroiliac joints: stress test

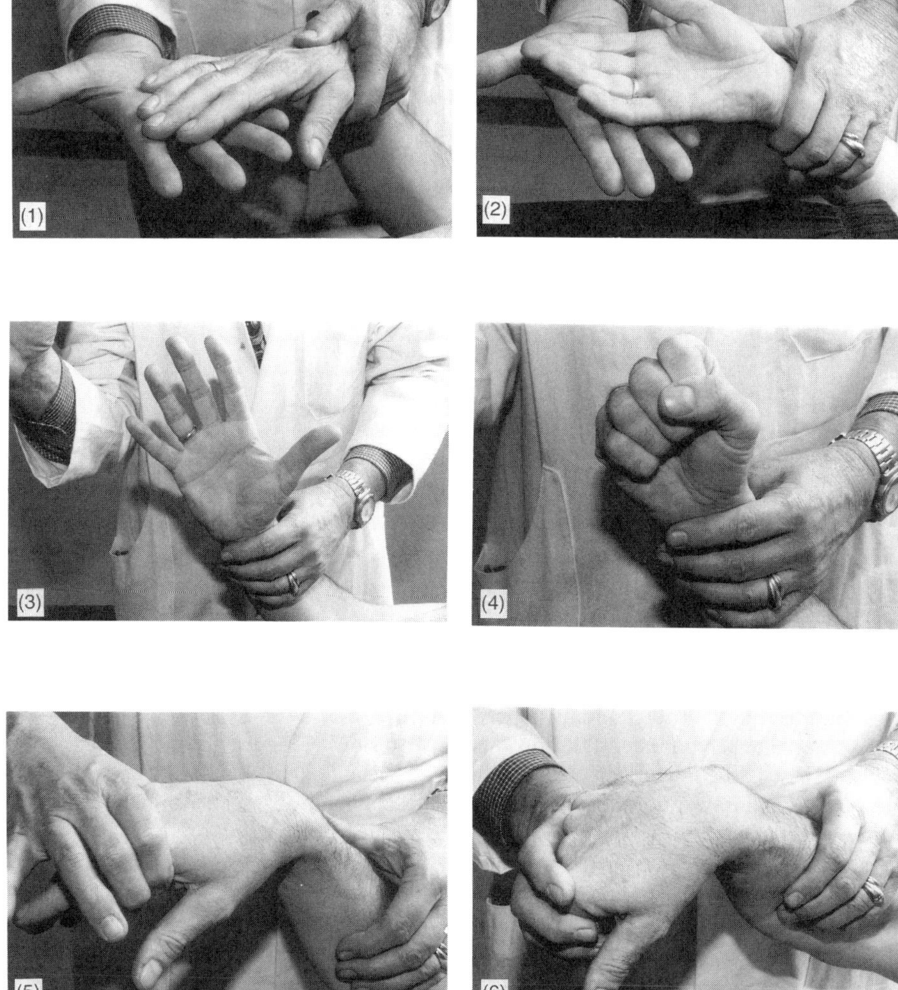

Figure 1.4a Sequences of routine systematic joint examination. (1,2) Hand inspection. Finger mobility: (3) extension; (4) fist; (5) metacarpal squeeze. Wrist: (6) with flexion. Wrist examination (7) extension. Elbow: (8) extension; (9) with flexion; (10) pronation–supination; (11) detection of subcutaneous nodules.

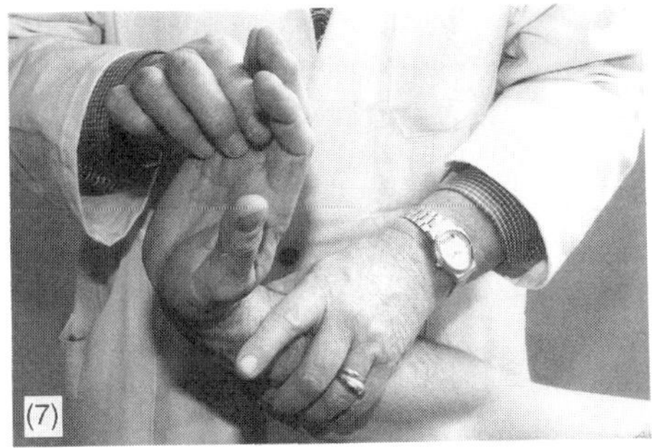

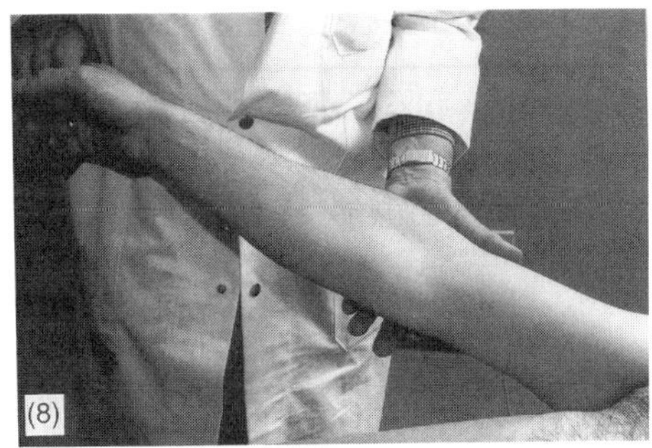

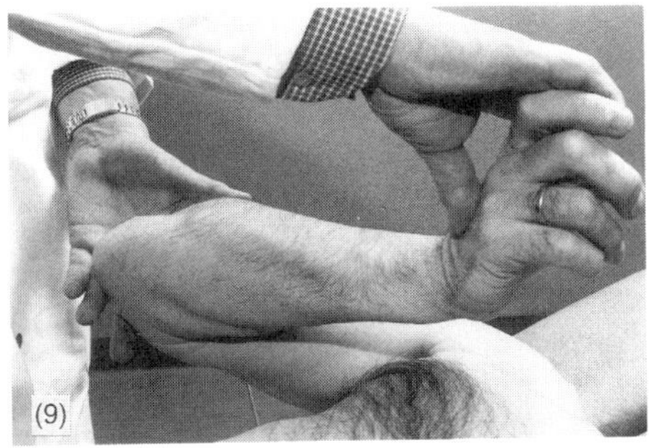

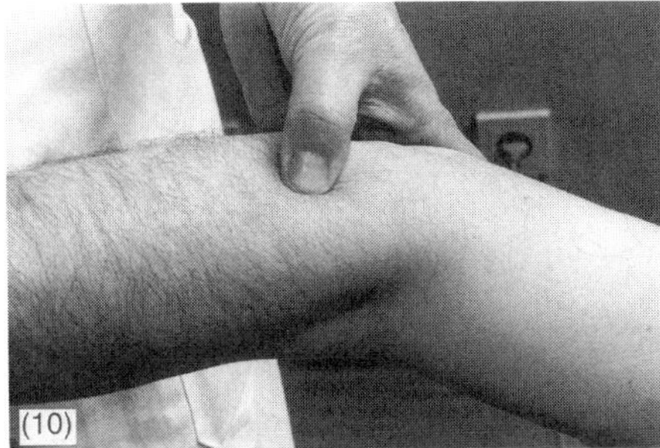

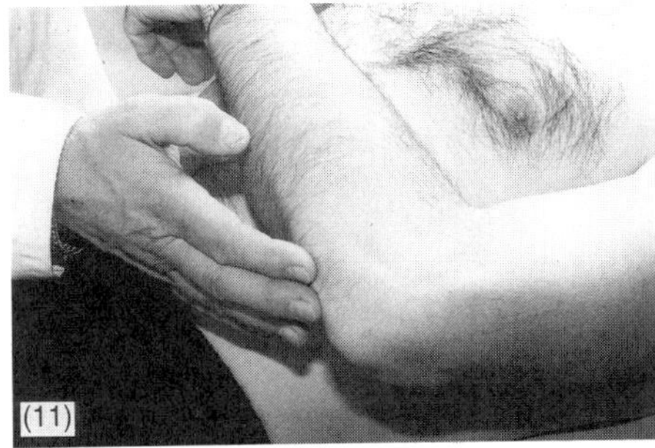

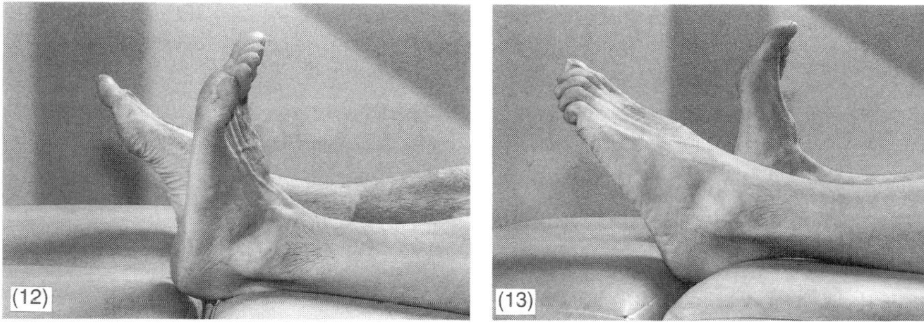

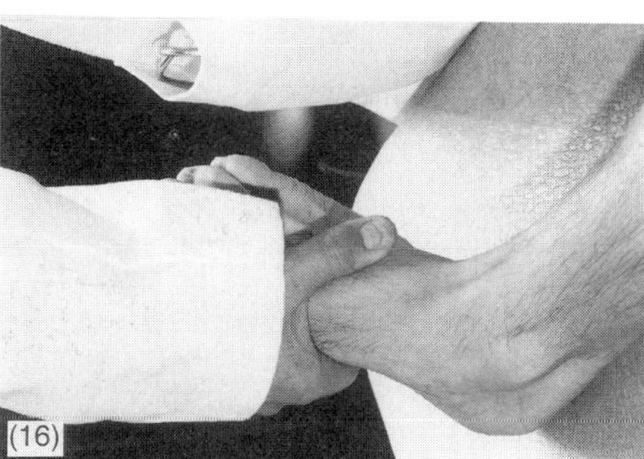

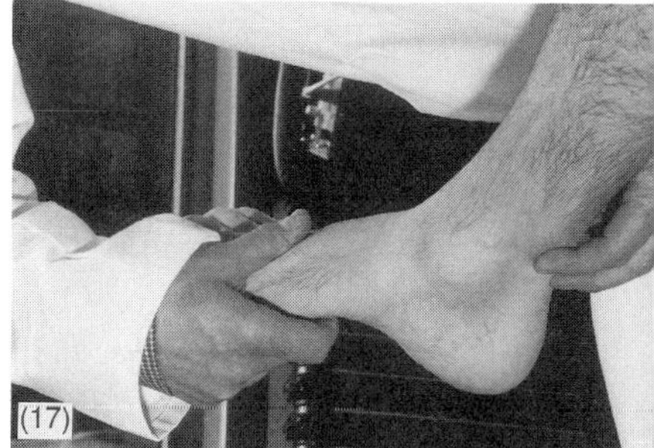

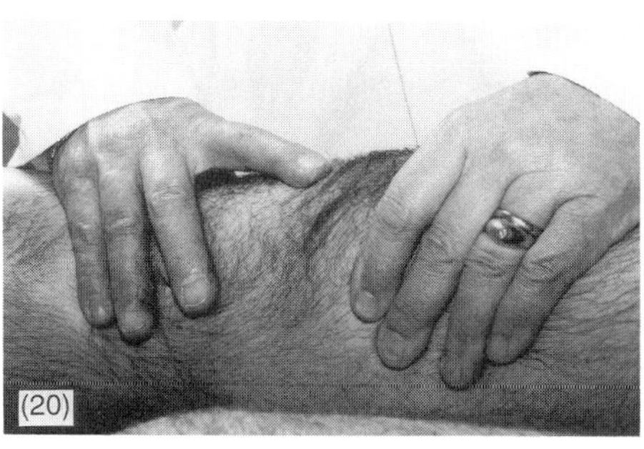

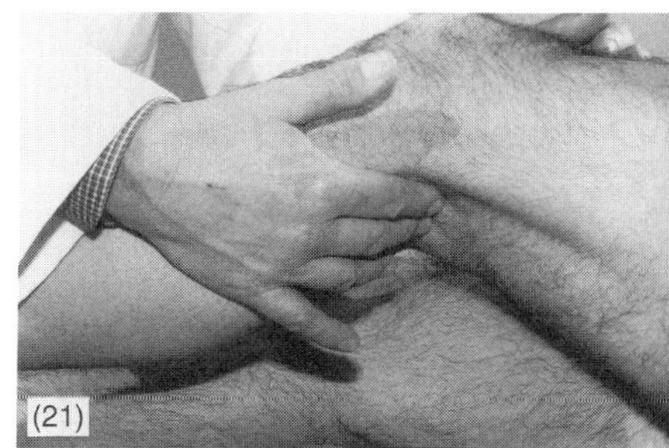

Figure 1.4b Sequences of routine systematic joint examination of lower limbs. Ankle mobility: (12) with flexion; (13) extension. Foot: (14) metatarsal squeeze; (15,16) mid-foot torsion; (17) ankle mobility. Knee: (18) inspection for skin deformity and muscle atrophy; (19) bulge sign; (20) ballotment of patella; (21) Baker cyst detection; (22) with flexion.

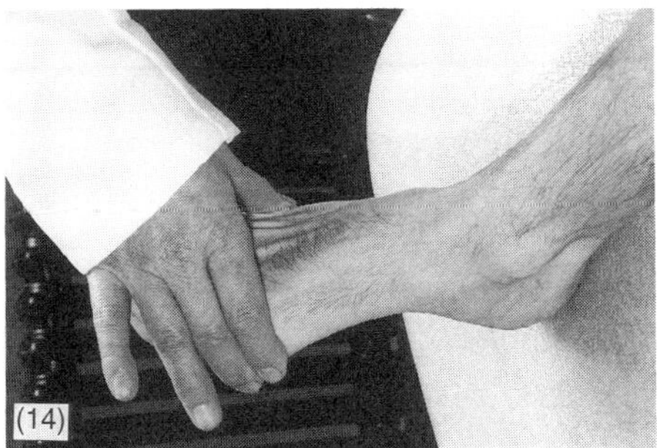

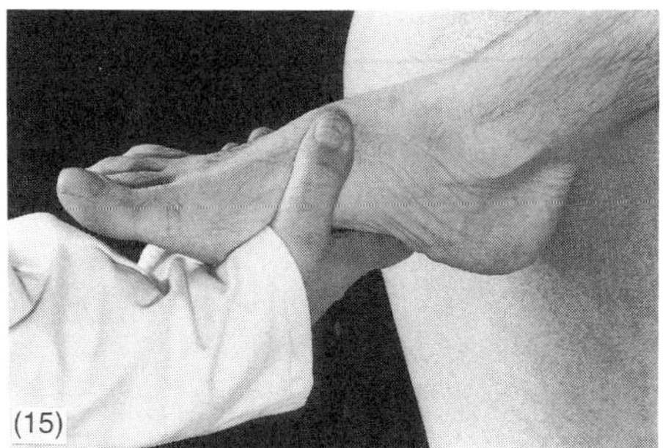

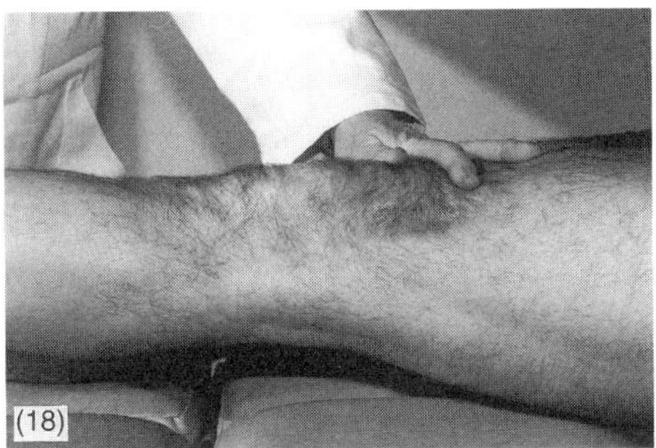

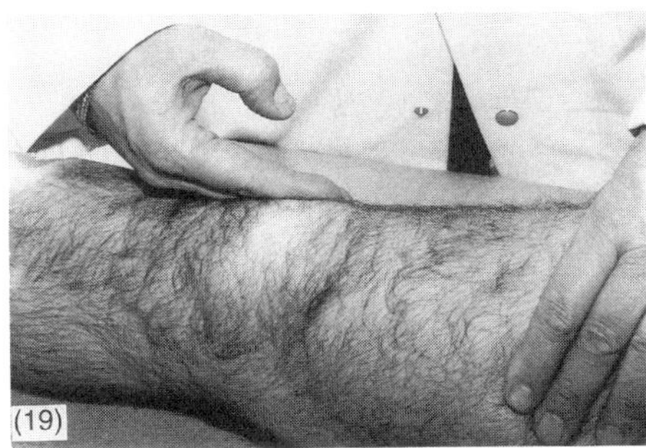

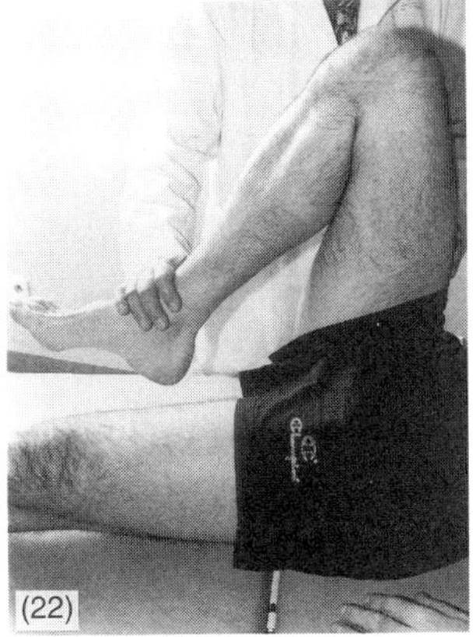

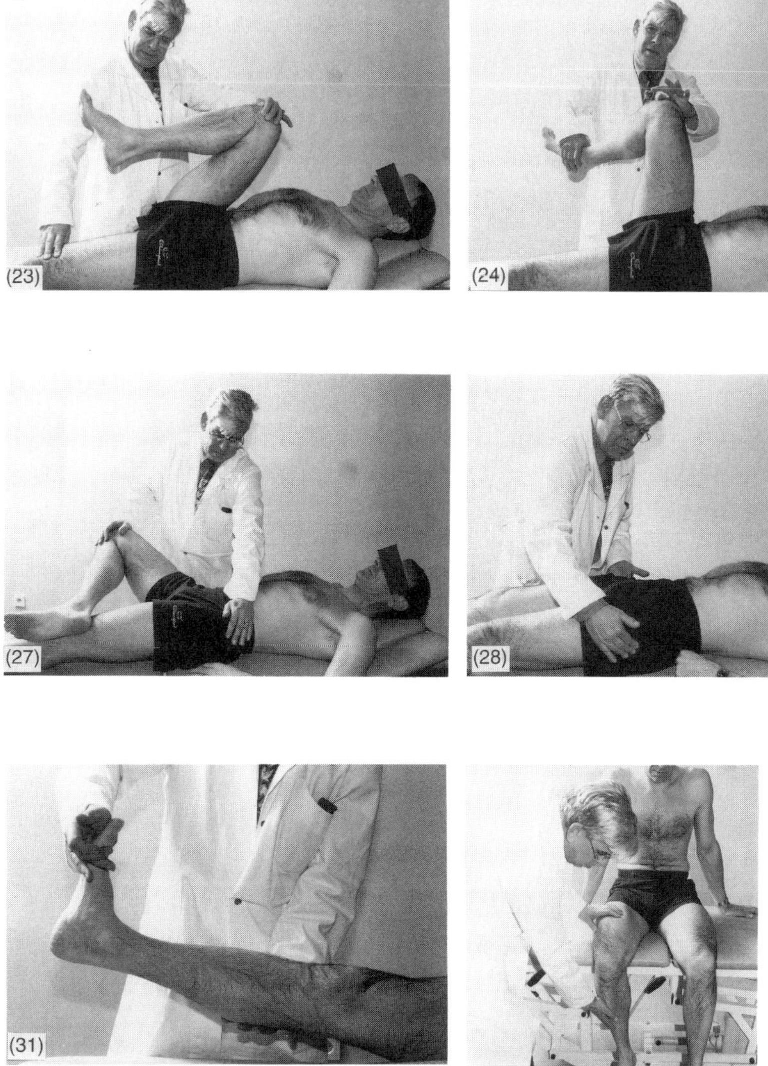

Figure 1.4c Sequences of routine systematic joint examination of hip girdle. Hip inspection: (23) with flexion; (24) medial rotation; (25) lateral rotation. (26) Sacroiliac joint test—forced abduction; (27) sacroiliac joint—Patrick sign; (28) palpation trochanteric area; (29) sacroiliac pressure test; (30) straight-leg-raising test—Lasègue sign; (31) forced Lasègue sign; (32) muscle power testing; (33) reverse Lasègue sign.

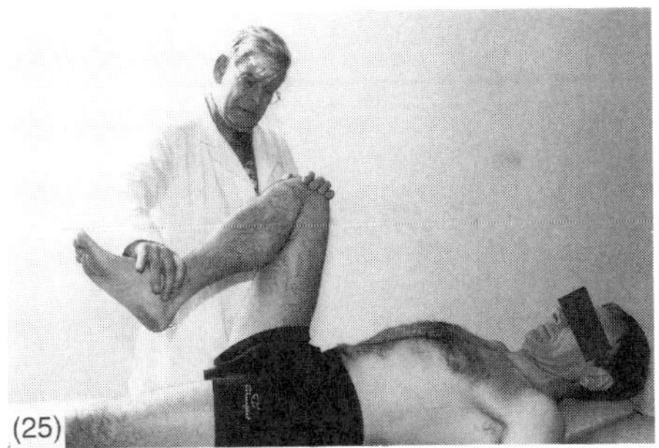

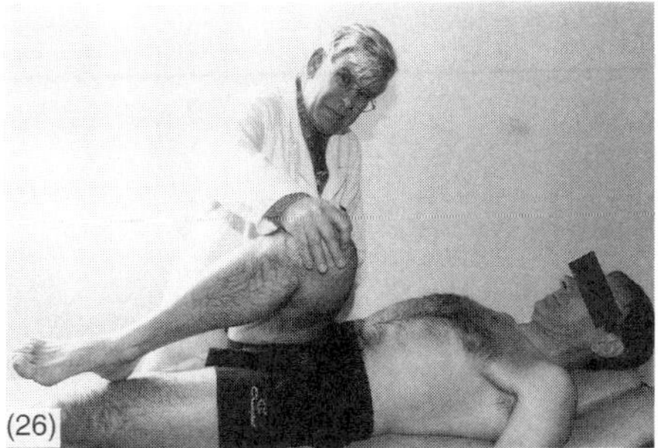

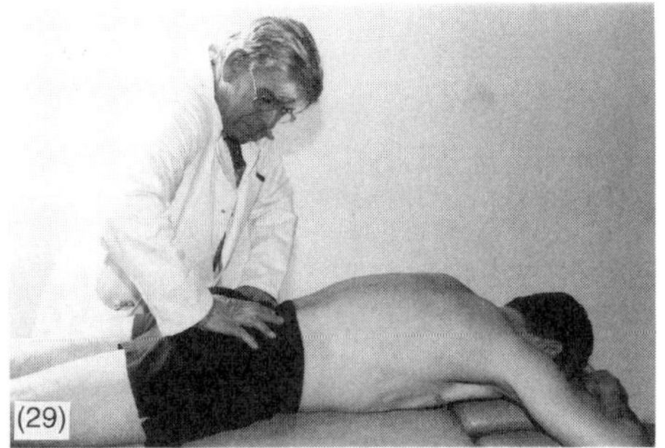

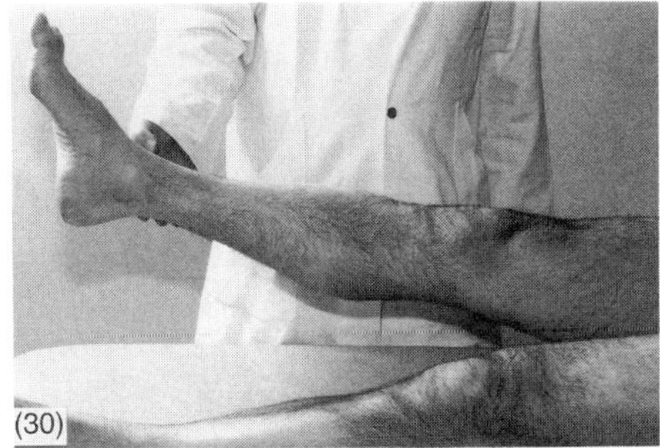

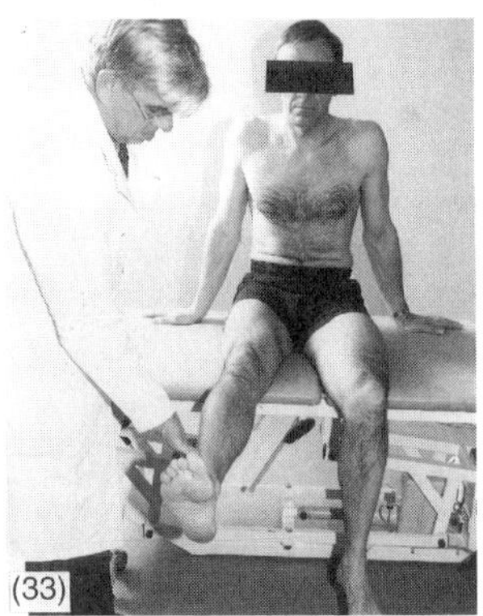

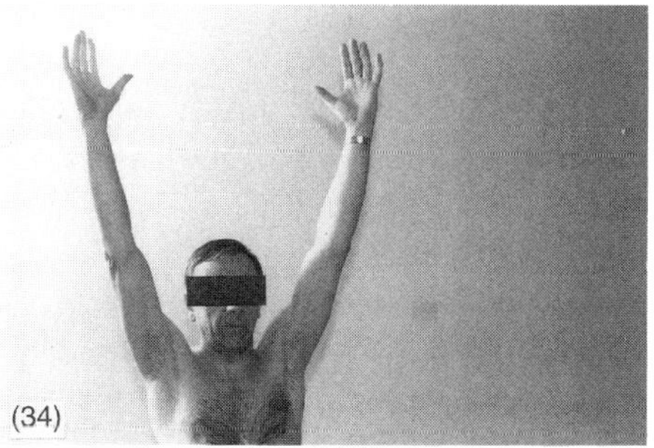
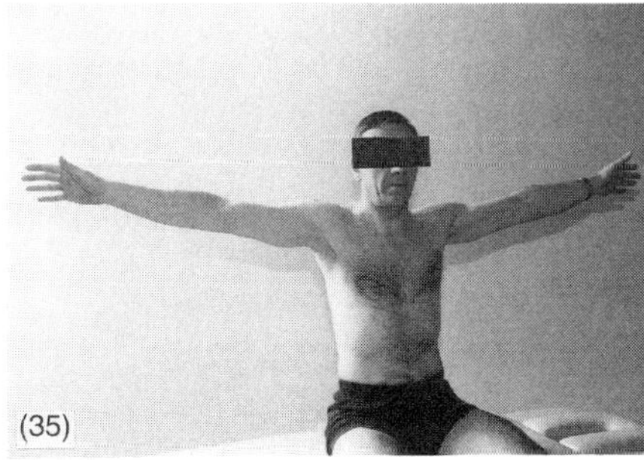

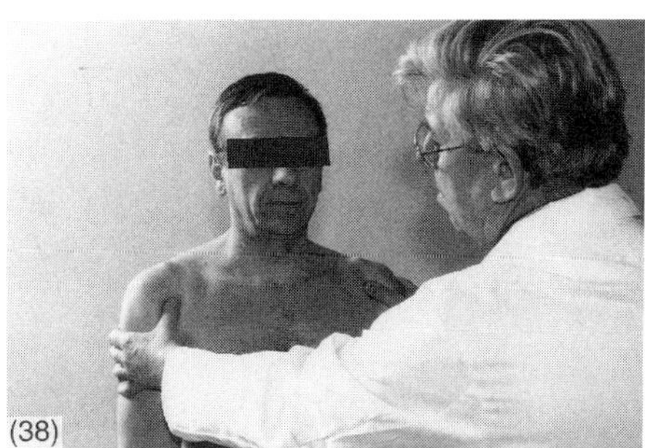
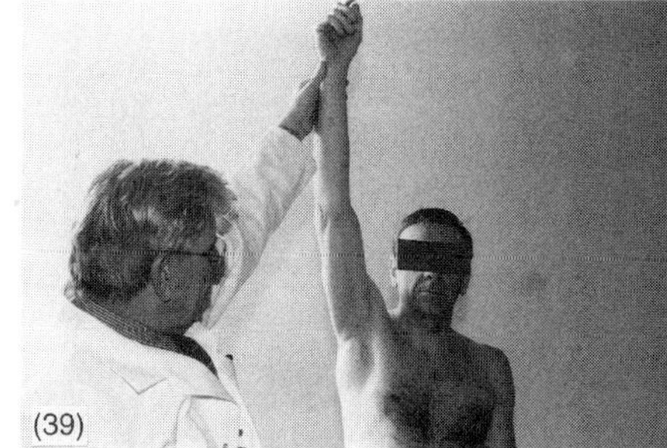

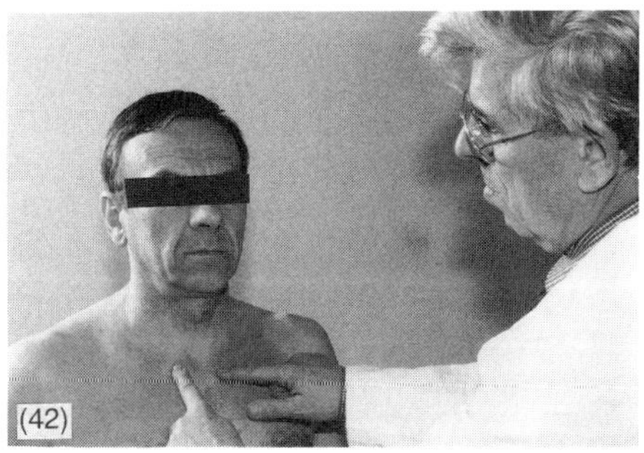
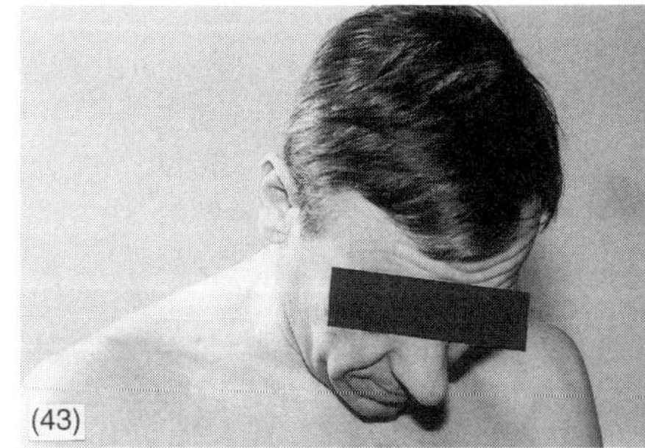

Figure 1.4d Sequence of routine systematic joint examination of shoulder-neck girdle. Shoulder: (34) active elevation; (35) active abduction; (36) backward internal rotation; (37) active elevation with backward flexion; (38) palpation of shoulder region.

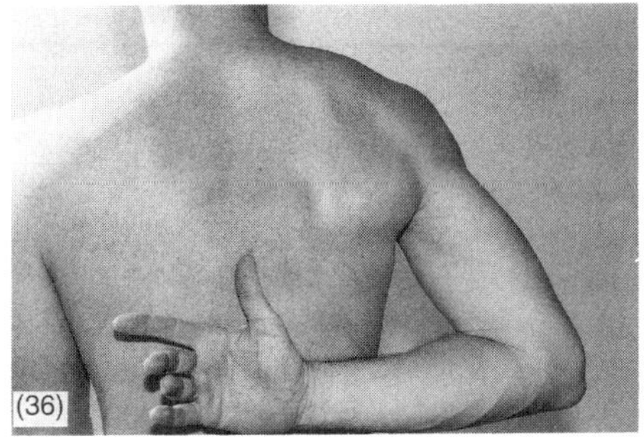
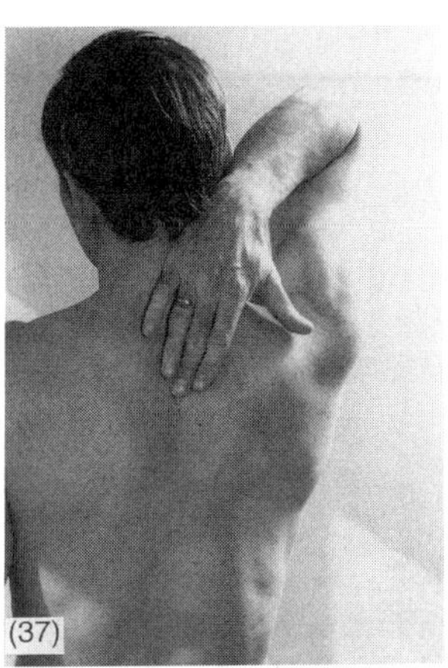
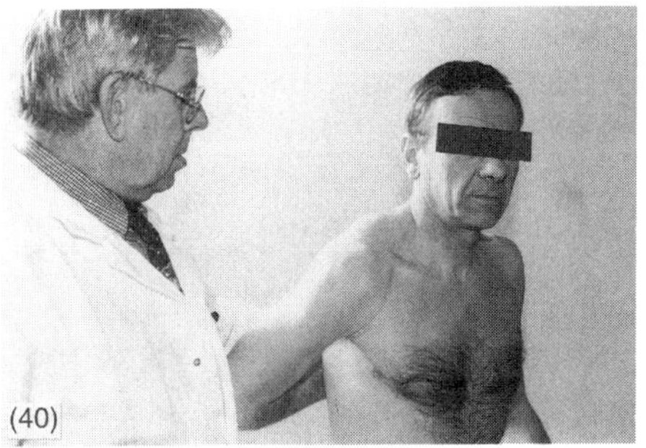
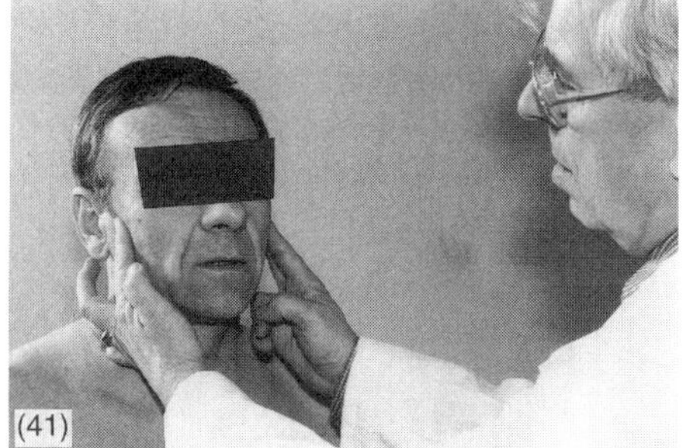
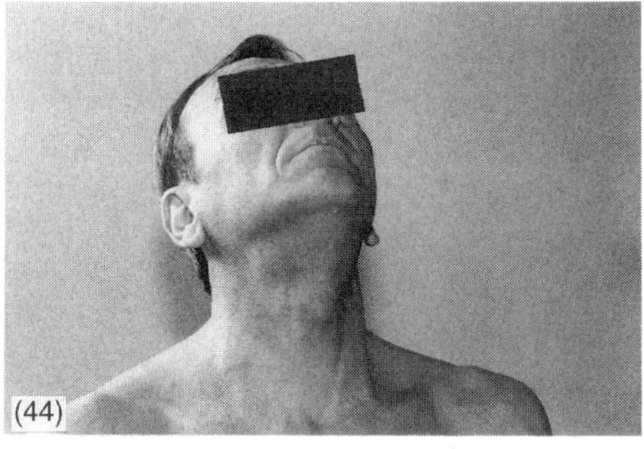
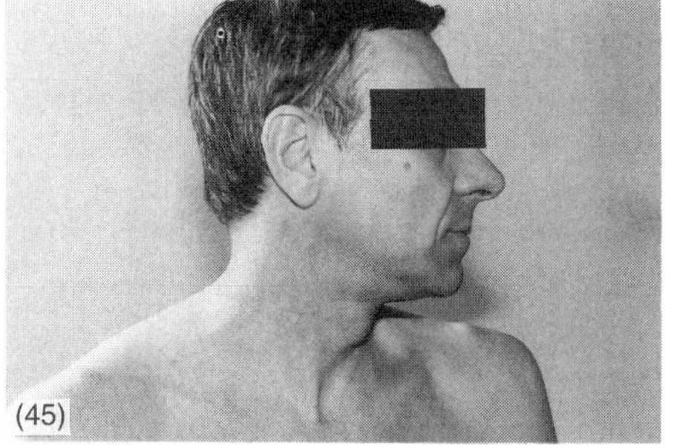

Figure 1.4d Continued. (39) Passive elevation; (40) passive internal rotation. (41) Palpation of temporomandibular joints; (42) examination sterno-clavicular joints. Cervical spine inspection: (43) with flexion; (44) extension; (45) rotation.

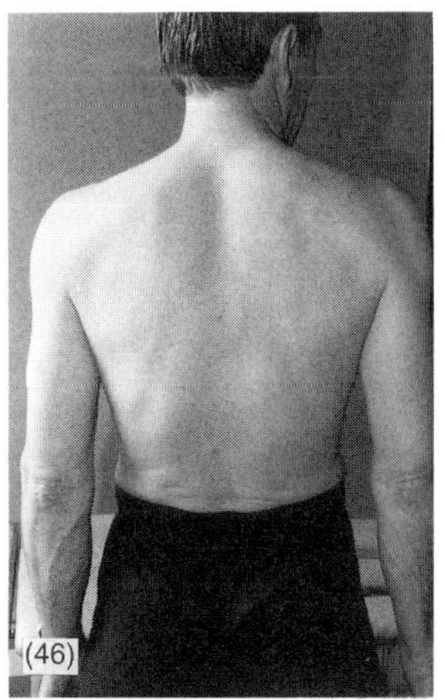

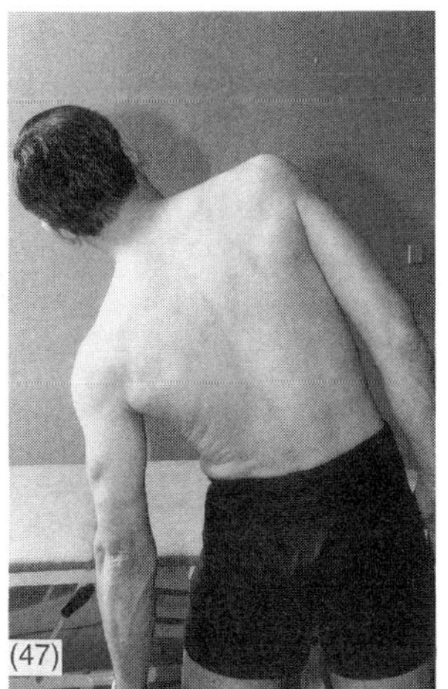

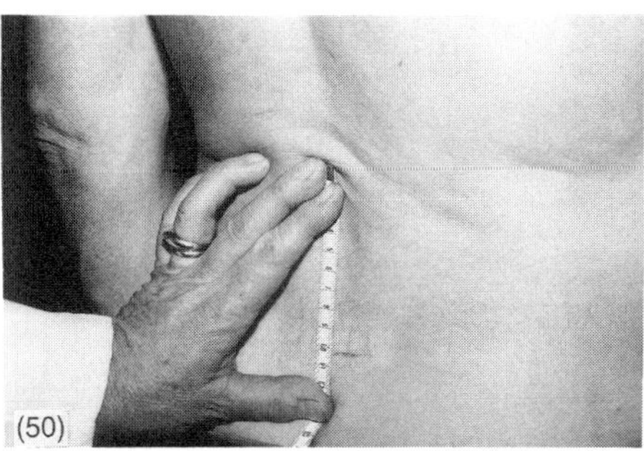

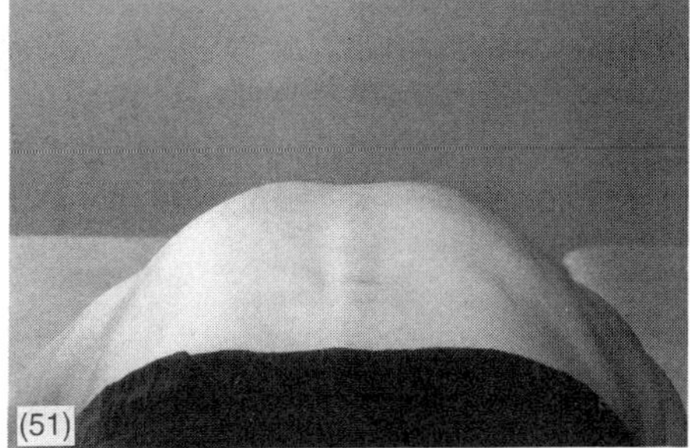

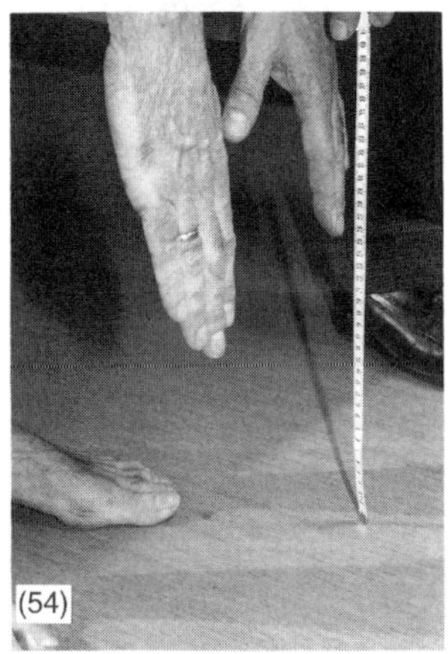

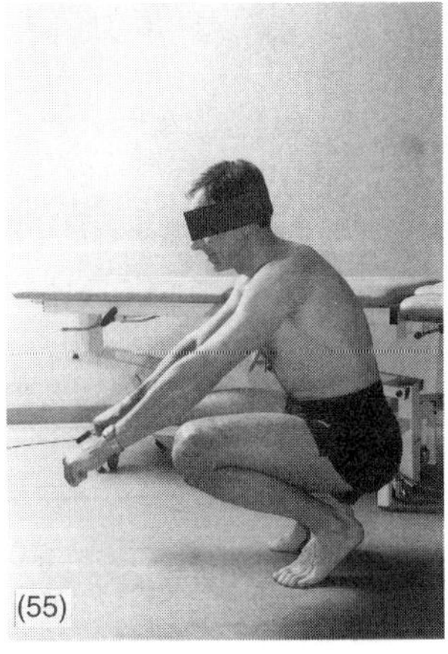

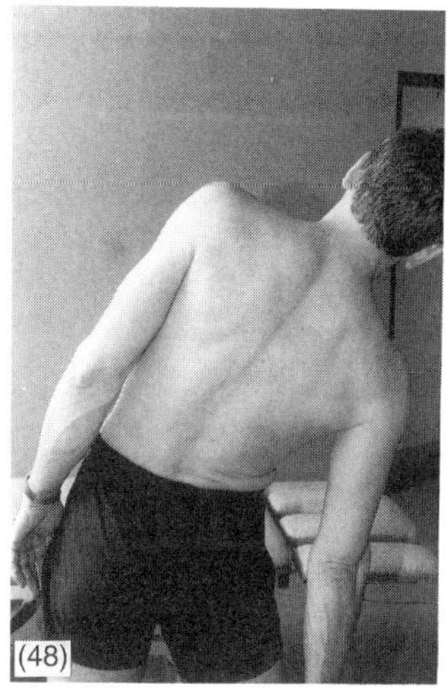
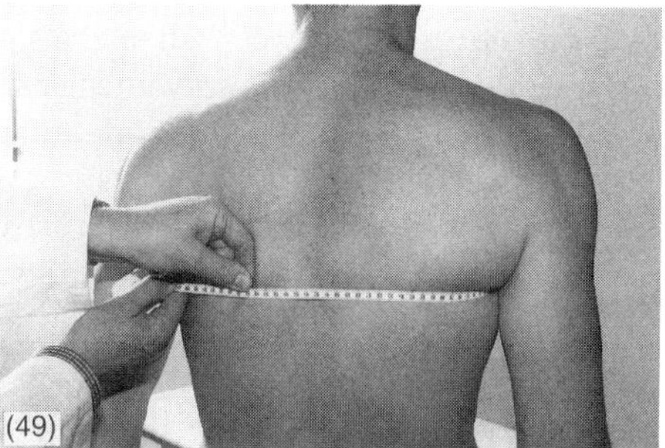
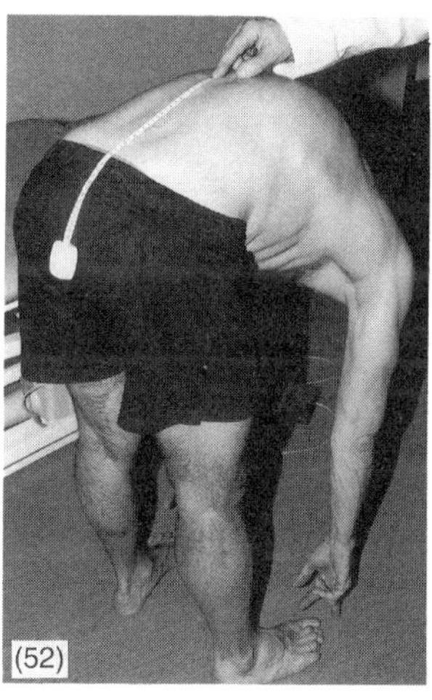
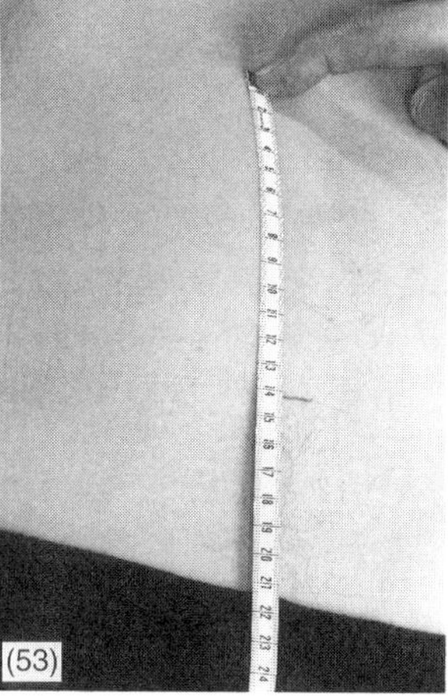

Figure 1.4e Sequence of routine systematic joint examination of dorso-lumbar spine. (46) Spine inspection; (47) lateral bending — left; (48) lateral bending — right; (49) chest wall expansion test; (50) lumbar spine flexion test — Schober index measure points; (51) inspection of chest wall symmetry on bending; (52) Schober index bending test; (53) Schober index; (54) fingertip to ground distance; (55) squatting test.

(picking up a hammer), and the *pen grip* (as for writing) are the four basic grips. In the hand the movement of the thumb is essential to perform the four different kinds of grips. Therefore the movements of the thumb are very complex. Abduction, adduction, flexion, extension, opposition, and retention of position are the six different movements that the thumb can perform. Opposition is complete when the thumb tip reaches the base of the little finger. An incomplete movement can be evaluated by measuring the distance between the tip of the thumb and the little finger.

Flexion of each individual finger can be measured either separately or in combination. *Finger lock* is the minimal distance of the finger tip to the base of the first phalanx with flexion at the distal interphalangeal (DIP) and the proximal interphalangeal (PIP) joints. The *fist lock* is the minimal distance between the finger tips and the MCP movement line with flexion of the metacarpal-phalangeal (MCP) joints. Spreading of the fingers is the distance between two fingers or the total maximum distance between the index finger and the little finger. Hyperextension of the PIP joint with flexion of the DIP joint is called a *swan-neck* deformity. Flexion of the PIP and hyperextension of the DIP joint is called *Boutonnière* deformity. These latter two forms of deformities are a consequence of chronic arthritis of the fingers (Fig. 1.5).

While inspecting the hands it is also important to note the swelling of the MCP, PIP, and DIP joints, which may result from articular or periarticular causes. It may be of interest to measure the circumference of each

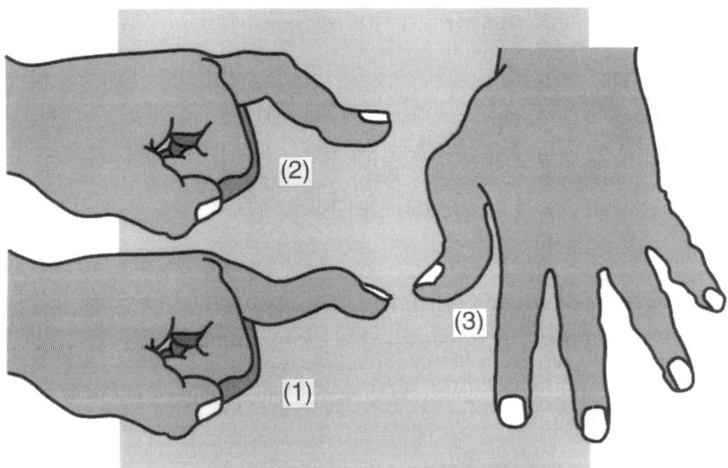

Figure 1.5 Combined deformities: (1) swan neck; (2) boutonnière; (3) Z-shaped deformity of thumb.

finger joint at the DIP and PIP level. The loss of normal knuckle wrinkle is indicative of soft tissue swelling and suggests synovitis. Synovial swelling will produce symmetric enlargement of the joint whereas extraarticular swellings may be diffuse and are often asymmetric, involving one side of a joint but not the other. Examination of the alignment of the fingers may reveal ulnar drift.

This results from stretching and eventual relaxation of the articular capsular ligaments secondary to synovial distention. This combined with muscle imbalance may cause the extensor tendon of the digit to slip off the MCP head on to the side of the joint.

Further helpful information is obtained from recognition of abnormalities of the terminal digits, including bony, soft tissue, and nail changes. Bone changes may be evident as osteophytic articular nodules. These may occur on the distal and proximal interphalangeal joints. When DIPs are involved they are described as *Heberden's* nodes, and when PIP joints are involved as *Bouchard's* nodes (Fig. 1.6). Telescopic shortening of the digits is produced by resorption of the end of the phalanx, is associated with wrinkling of the skin above the involved joints, and is called an opera-glass hand.

Soft tissue changes must be looked for during inspection. Synovial cysts on the dorsolateral side of the joints produce an extraarticular swelling on the dorsum of the hands (Fig. 1.7). Clubbing of the terminal phalanges is

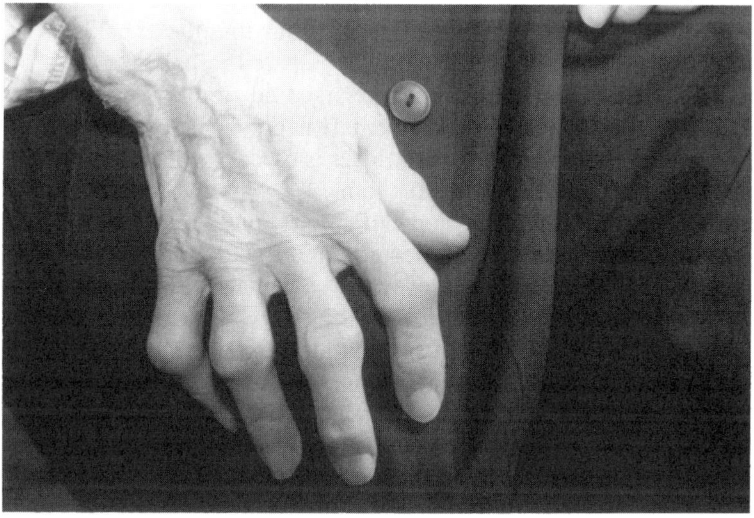

Figure 1.6   Heberden's and Bouchard's nodes.

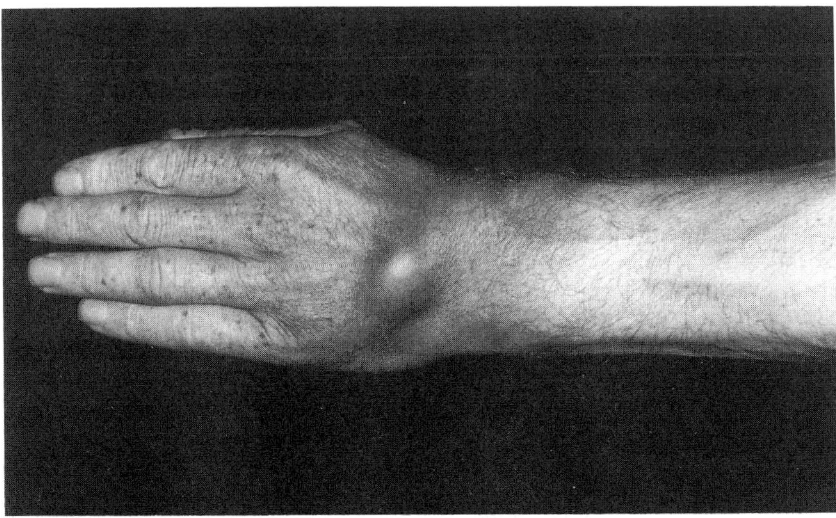

Figure 1.7 Wrist cyst.

also an example of soft tissue change. Nail changes include pitting, ridging, thickening, or discoloration. Changes in the skin includes pallor, redness, edema, atrophy, and ulcers.

Palpation of the MCP joints must be done by holding the particular joint in relaxed position of partial flexion. Use your thumbs to palpate the dorsal aspect of the joint while your fingers palpate the palmar aspect of the metacarpal head. Your remaining fingers should support the patient's hand. When palpating the PIP joint, your left hand supports the patient's hands while your right thumb and index finger is used to palpate simultaneously the medial and lateral aspect of the joint.

When palpating MCP, PIP, and DIP joints, one looks for synovial thickening or distension, tenderness, warmth, and fluctuation in three locations: the region of the joint space, over the proximal and over the distal phalanx of the joint examined. Normally, the synovial membrane cannot be palpated in the region of the joint space, but in the presence of synovial thickening the bony margins of the joint space are obscured by swelling.

4.2 Wrist

Movement of the wrist includes palmar flexion (flexion 80°), dorsiflexion (extension 90°), radial deviation (20°), and ulnar deviation (30°). A combination of these movements allows circumduction of the wrist. These movements require varying degrees of motion at both the radiocarpal and the midcarpal joints. Limited flexion and extension and slight rotation are permitted in the midcarpal joint. Pronation and supination of the hand and forearm occur primarily at the proximal and distal radio-ulnar articulations.

On inspection, swelling of the wrist may be found, which can either be localized or diffuse. Localized synovial swelling on the dorsum of the wrist may resemble and result from synovial outbulging of tendon sheaths or from outbulging from the synovial membrane lining the wrist joint.

Synovitis in the wrist is indicated by swelling or soft tissue fullness with or without tenderness and localized warmth, and is detected most reliably by palpation over the dorsum of the wrist. Because of overlying structures, accurate dorsal and palmar localization of the margins of the synovial reflections in the wrist may be difficult. True articular swelling of the wrist is often palpable just distal to the head of the ulna on the dorsolateral aspect of the wrist when the palm is turned down. Palpate the wrist firmly using two hands by placing both thumbs on the dorsum of the wrist and the second and third fingers on the palmar aspect of the wrist. The patient's wrist should be relaxed and in a straight position with the palm turned down. Move your thumbs above and palpate with the fingers below and from side to side over the depressed areas that lie over the region of the joint space just distal to the bony prominence of the radius and ulna. The close relationship between the tendon sheaths and the wrist joint often makes it difficult to differentiate localized tenosynovitis from articular synovitis at the level of the wrist. Swelling and tenderness localized to the region of the radius styloid process may result from stenosing tenosynovitis (de Quervain's tenosynovitis) in this area. Additional information can be obtained by palpating the wrist for cysts or nodules on bones or tendons and for changes in skin temperature or by provoking paresthesia in the median nerve region by tapping on the area of the nerve (Tinel's sign) or by hyperflexion of the wrist (Phalen's sign) (Fig. 1.8).

4.3 Elbow

The elbow, a hinge joint, consists of the humero-ulnar, the humero-radial, and the radio-ulnar joints. Flexion of the elbow ranges from 0 up to 160°. A few individuals normally lack 5–10° of extension and others may have 5–10° of hyperextension. The movement of flexion and extension occur in the humero-ulnar joint. The radio-ulnar joint allows the elbow to move in a 160° supination and pronation movement of the lower arm. Normally, there is a minimal valgus position (5°) between the upper arm and forearm. This angle may be larger, as seen in Turner's syndrome, after a fracture or in the hypermobility syndrome.

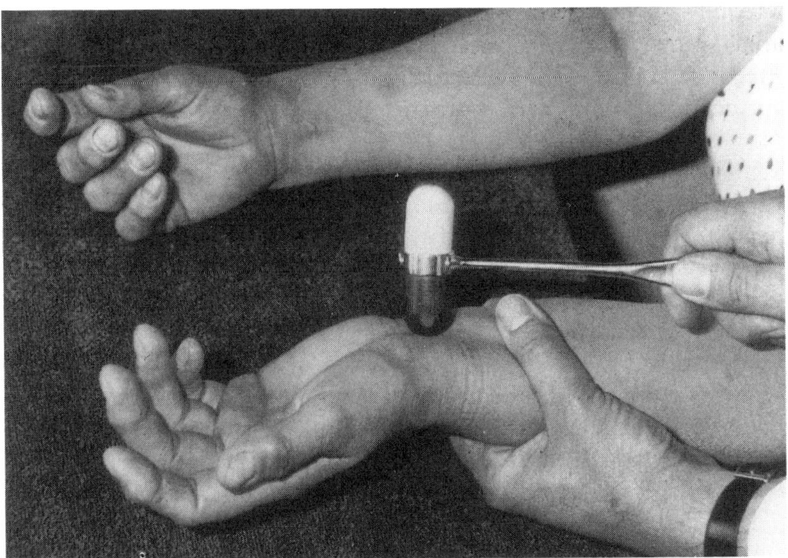

Figure 1.8 Tinel's sign.

Inspection of the elbows should be performed when the patient is sitting. Swelling and redness of the olecranon bursa are easily observed. Common sites for subcutaneous nodules are in the olecranon bursa and along the extensor surface of the ulna, distal to the olecranon. Psoriatic skin lesions may be present at the elbows. When there is an effusion or synovial thickening in the joint, the condition is usually first apparent as a bulge or fullness in the paraolecranon groove on each side of the olecranon process.

During palpation the elbow joint should be as relaxed as possible. When examining the left elbow, use your left hand to give firm support to the left forearm of the patient, and use your right thumb and fingers to palpate the joint. The right elbow is examined in the same fashion, except that you palpate with your left thumb and fingers and use your right hand to support the patient's forearm. The thumb is placed lateral to the paraolecranon groove; the forefinger or middle finger are both placed over the radial paraolecranon groove. These places are best palpated with the patient's elbow flexed about 70° from the position of complete extension and with the muscles relaxed. Pay particular attention to the medioparaolecranon groove as it is easier to detect synovial thickening or joint effusions on this side. Slowly extending the patient's arm while keeping your thumb and fingers on the paraolecranon grooves often helps in identifying synovitis.

The synovial membrane may bulge under palpating thumb or fingers as the forearm is extended. This maneuver also helps to distinguish tendons, muscles, fat pads, and ligaments from the synovial membrane in this area.

The olecranon bursa can be palpated easily for fluid, swelling, tenderness, local heat, consistency, loose bodies, and nodules. Other causes of nodules seen at the elbow are gouty tophi, nodules of acute rheumatic fever, calcinosis, reticular histiocytosis, and xanthomatosis. It is useful to note the precise place of the nodules as well as the color, local heat, size, number, consistency, mobility, and tenderness. The ulnar nerve groove can also be palpated for indication of thickening, irregularity, or tenderness. A frequent cause of pain in the elbow area is the so-called tennis elbow or lateral epicondylitis, where the pain on palpation is found just distal from the fixation (enthesis) of the common extensor tendon. Lifting a chair with the palm beneath the back of the chair gives no problems, but lifting with the palm downward elicits pain at the lateral epicondyle attachment.

The medial and lateral epicondyles of the humerus are common sites of inflammation, pain, or localized tenderness (medial — golfer's elbow, lateral — tennis elbow).

4.4 Shoulder

The shoulder is a complex joint, consisting not only of the glenohumeral joint but of the acromioclavicular joint, the sternoclavicular joint, the rotator cuff, the neighboring ligaments and bursae. The zero position of the shoulder is one in which the patient stands up with the arms hanging loosely alongside the body. Motion of the upper extremity on the trunk is normally a combination of movement of the shoulder girdle and the shoulder joint. The shoulder joint is capable of a wide variety of movements. It permits forward elevation (forward movement of the arm, in the sagittal plane, normally 0–180°), backward extension (dorsal flexion or backward movement of the arm in the sagittal plane, normally 0–160°), abduction (elevation of the arm from the side, 0–80°), adduction (lowering the arm to the side), rotation, and circumduction. Rotation of the shoulder can be measured in two positions, either with the arm alongside the body or with the arm in 90° abduction, both with the elbow flexed in 90°. In endorotation the forearm moves while in abduction downward. The fingertips normally can reach the lower scapula tip. In exorotation, the arm moves upward (Fig. 1.9 and 1.10).

Four simple maneuvers can be used as an introductory or screening procedure for evaluation of the range of motion of the shoulders (Table 1.9).

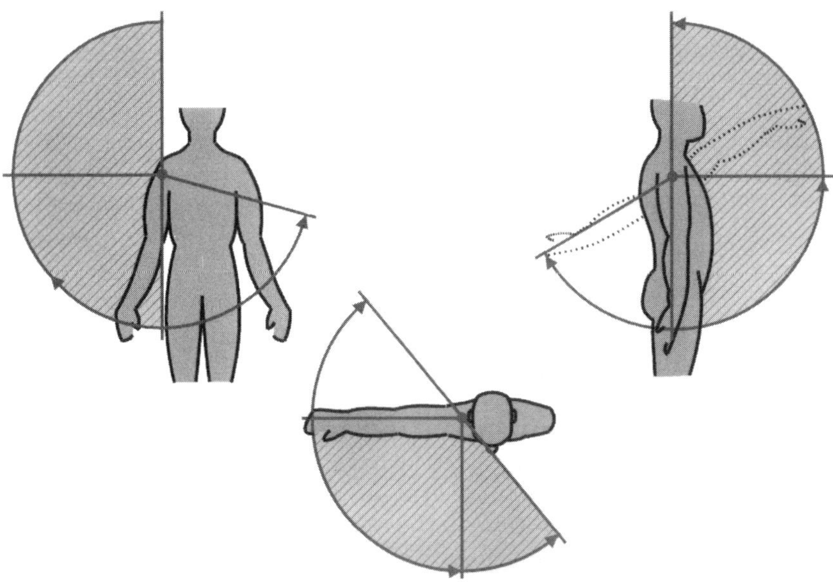

Figure 1.9 Horizontal and vertical movement of the arm.

Inspection of the shoulders is performed with the patient sitting or standing. Both shoulders are compared anteriorly and posteriorly for evidence of swelling and muscle wasting. Inequality or malposition of normal bony landmarks such as the clavicle, acromion, coracoid process or greater tuberosity of the humerus should be apparent by comparison of the two sides. A moderate amount of synovitis must be present in the glenohumeral joint to cause visible distention of the articular capsule. When present, the distention usually occurs over the anterior aspect of the joint.

Before the shoulder is examined by *palpation*, it is helpful to ask the patient to point out the area of maximal pain or tenderness by touching the involved shoulder with the hand of the uninvolved side. Pain originating in the shoulder joint must be demonstrable locally and reproducible by palpation or motion by the examiner so that the patient can localize tenderness in order to differentiate it from pain referred to the shoulder joint because of extraarticular and potentially serious diseases. Initially, the examiner can best evaluate abnormalities of the shoulder by positioning himself in front of the patient and by palpating both shoulders for evidence of swelling, tenderness, local heat, muscle spasm, and atrophy. The systematic examination of the shoulder includes palpation of the acromio-clavicular joint,

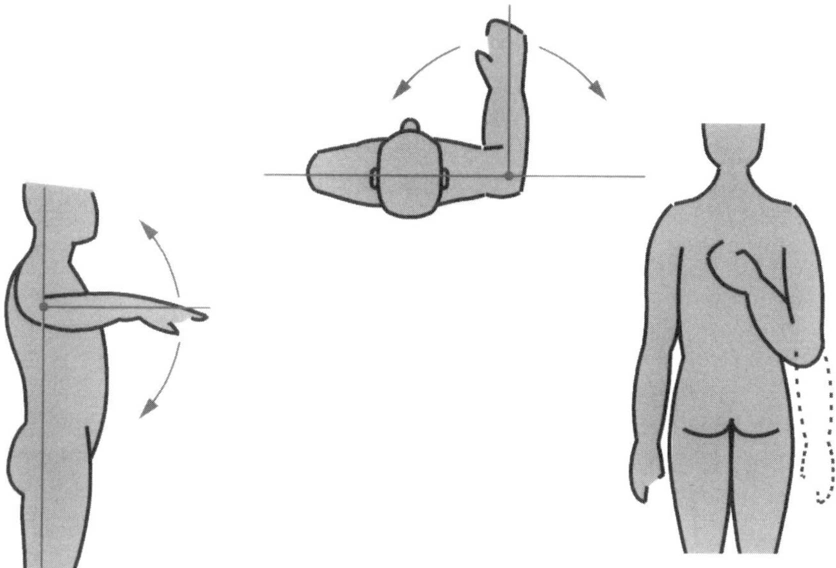

Figure 1.10   Rotation movements of the shoulder.

the rotator cuff, the region of the subacromial bursa, the bicipital groove, and the anterior, lateral, and posterior aspects of the glenohumeral joint and the articular capsule. The palpation of the axilla for adenopathies is also important.

The posterior portion of the rotator cuff (tendons of infraspinatus and teres minor muscles) is examined by asking the patient to abduct the arm across the chest and place the hand on the opposite shoulder. The

Table 1.9   Range-of-Motion Shoulder Test

1. The patient is asked to raise each extended arm upward in wide vertical arches (forward elevation) in an effort to touch the palmar surface of both hands together above the head.
2. The patient is asked to touch both hands on the top of his head with the elbows flexed and the upper extremities moving in a horizontal arc posteriorly.
3. The patient is asked to raise each extended arm above his head in a wide sideways arc in the coronal plane of the body (abduction).
4. The patient is asked to rotate his arm internally behind his back and place the back of this hand as high as possible between the scapulae.

examiner then stands in front of the patient and palpates the posterior surface of the humeral head by placing his thumb on the anterior aspect and his fingers on the posterior aspect of the patient's shoulder. The posterior portion of the rotator cuff moves beneath the examiner's fingers. The anterior portion of the cuff (subscapular tendon) is examined by placing the patient's arm in backward extension (drawn backward about 20° from the axillary line while the arm is still in abduction) and by palpating it anteriorly over the humeral head. The examiner then stands behind the patient and places his finger over the head of the humerus anteriorly while the patient internally rotates the arm by bringing his hand backward to the point between the scapulae. The superior portion of the rotator cuff (supraspinatus tendons) will be under the examiner's fingers and can be felt to move. During these maneuvers the examiner palpates for tenderness, swelling, firm nodular masses, or axial gaps (tears) in the cuff. Occasionally, the examiner can palpate the soft, tender swelling that may represent the remaining proximal part of a ruptured tendon attached to the humerus.

Inflammation or irritation of the subacromial bursa may result in palpable swelling, tenderness, and warmth of the upper portion of the arm in the region of the deltoid muscle and just distal to the acromion process. Inflammation of the synovial sheet or at the tendon of the long head of the biceps muscle produces pain in the region of the bicipital groove.

4.5 Hip

The hip is classified as a ball-and-socket joint formed by the articulation of the rounded head of the femur with a cup-shaped cavity of the acetabulum. It is a weight-bearing joint that combines a wide range of motion with great stability. The stability of the hip is due to the deep insertion of the head of the femur into the acetabulum, the strong fibrous articular capsule, and the powerful muscles.

The hip has a wide range of motion that permits flexion, extension, adduction, abduction, rotation, and circumduction.

The neutral position of the hip is the position in which the patient is lying down on a flat surface with the other hip in maximal flexion. In this position the lumbar lordosis is flattened out and a flexion contracture of the hip will become evident when the lower leg is lifted from the horizontal plane (*Thomas's test* for fixed flexion) (Fig. 1.11).

Extension of the hip is defined as the backward motion of the hip. This motion beyond the neutral position (0°) is sometimes referred to as hyperextension. To test the range of hyperextension, the patient must be in the prone position, with a pillow beneath his abdomen. The greatest degree of *flexion* of the hip is possible when the knee is also flexed. When hip

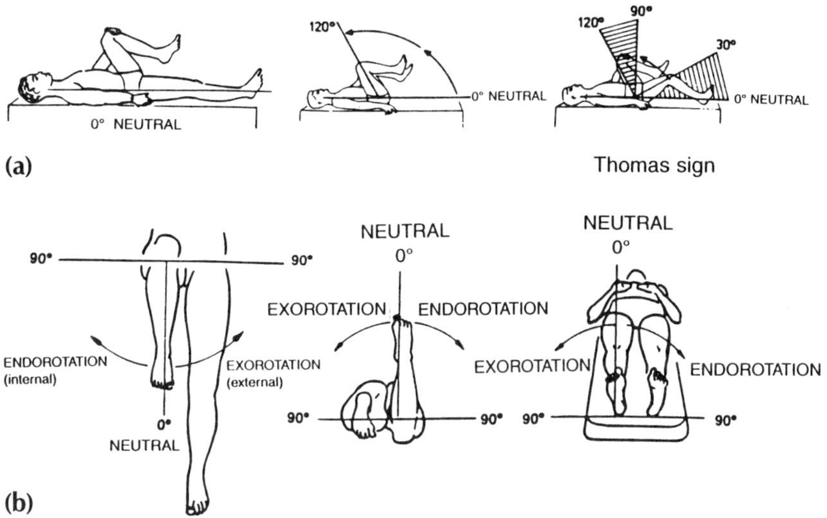

Figure 1.11 Hip mobility: (a) flexion, (b) rotation.

flexion is tested the examiner places his hand on the iliac crest to determine movement of the pelvis. Normally the thigh can be flexed about 120° from the neutral position.

Abduction and adduction are measured with both thighs and legs in extended position and parallel to each other while the patient is supine. Normally, when the leg and thigh are extended, the hips abduct about 40–45° from the neutral position. Motion of the pelvis may be detected in the course of unilateral testing of range of abduction by placing one hand on the iliac crest of the side opposite to the one being tested. Adduction with the leg straight is limited by the legs and thighs coming into contact with each other. However, when hip flexion is possible to permit crossing one leg over the other, the degree of adduction of the hip of the extremity on top can be measured. Adduction, then, usually is possible to about 20–30° from the neutral position. *Internal and external rotation* can be measured while the patient is supine with both hips and knees flexed, while the examiner swings the foot inward for measurement of external rotation of the hip and outward or laterally for measurement of the internal rotation of the hip. During this procedure the foot and thigh are moving in opposite direction. The hip normally rotates inward about 40° and outward about 45°.

A useful functional test of the hip is the squatting test. The patient is asked to squat by bringing hips and knees in flexion. If this test provokes pain or is limited then a lesion of hip or knee or both is likely.

Inspection includes evaluation of the patient's gait, apparent and actual length of legs, spinal curvatures, pelvic tilt, and scars of previous operations or trauma in the region of the hip. Inspection of the relationship of the femur to the pelvis is of particular importance in recognition of disease of the hip. In the presence of unilateral disease of the hip, the weight of the body in the upright position is often supported mainly on the healthy leg and in the prone position the leg of the involved part is usually placed in advance of the normal one because of flexion of the involved hip. This can be detected by having the patient stand erect and then alternate the body weight from one leg to the other. One side may be compared with the other by inquiring about the presence or absence of pain and noting disability or muscle spasm on each side in these positions. When there is an unstable or painful hip or when the abductors are weak, a positive Trendelenburg test can be found. Normally, when standing on one leg, the opposite side of the pelvis will rise up. In the presence of an unstable or painful hip the opposite side of the pelvis drops down. This is a positive Trendelenburg sign (Fig. 1.12).

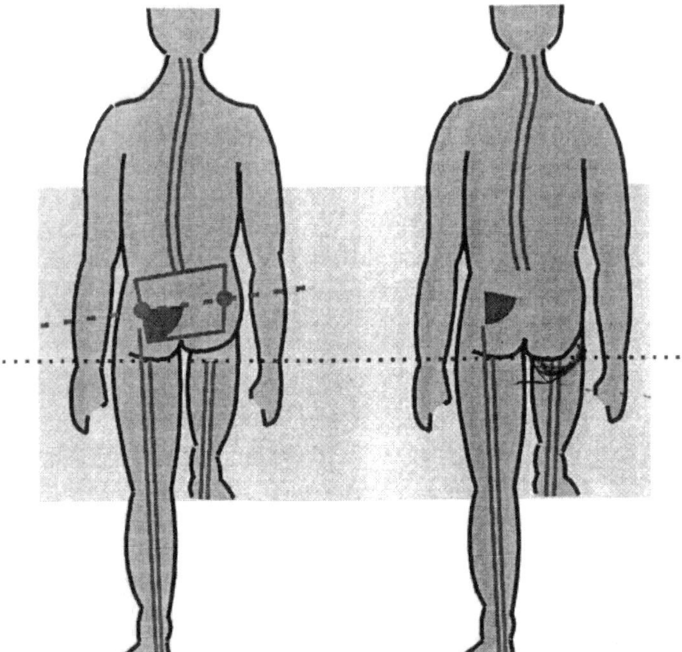

Figure 1.12 Trendelenburg test.

Hip flexion is one of the most common findings on inspection that suggest abnormality of the hip. The flex position relaxes the articular capsule of the hip, lessening pain, muscle spasm, and capsular distention.

The patient with a flexion deformity of the hip frequently assumes the characteristic position when lying supine on a flat surface. The spinal column is arched anteriorly in the lumbar region with production of lordosis and anterior pelvic tilt. Extension of the flexed hip usually aggravates the pain in the hip by pulling the iliofemoral ligaments tight over the anterior portion of the joint and thereby pressing the head of the femur firmly into the acetabulum. Flexion contracture of the hip is also indicated when the patient is lying prone and is unable to extend the hip fully or when the examiner is unable to lift the thigh into extension without simultaneously lifting the patient's pelvis.

Before examination by *palpation* is started, it is helpful to ask the patient to point out areas of pain or tenderness as carefully as possible. The examiner attempts to delineate the involved area more accurately by palpation while noting soft tissue swelling, tenderness, and deeper warmth where feasible. Synovial thickening or distention of the articular capsule usually cannot be palpated. Rarely, a large quantity of synovial fluid may produce palpable swelling over the anterior portion of the capsule in the region of the iliopectineal bursa if this communicates with the joint. It is difficult to differentiate involvement of the joint from tenderness of soft tissue structures overlying it. Occasionally, firm pressure behind and somewhat superior to the greater trochanter may cause tenderness if synovitis or effusions are present. Localized heat or warmth in the region of the hip usually indicates soft tissue inflammation rather than disease of the hip joint because of the joint's deep location. Disease of the hip may be suggested by pain in the region of the hip when the patient is supine and relaxed and the examiner percusses the heel with his hand or fist while the patient's leg is extended (*Anvil sign*). Palpation of the soft tissues surrounding the hip as the trochanteric bursa or the iliopectineal bursae may reveal pain or tenderness and may suggest tendinitis. Trochanteric bursitis causes localized swelling and tenderness over the greater trochanter of the femur. The pain is usually aggravated by active adduction and rotation of the hip carried out against resistance. Tenderness over the ischium may indicate ischialbursitis (*Weaver's bottom*) and is sometimes associated with swelling in this region.

Fullness and tenderness of the iliopectineal bursa can be detected by palpable swelling and tenderness in the area of the middle third of the inguinal ligament and lateral to the femoral pulse. The tenderness is aggravated by extension and is reduced or relieved by flexion of the hip.

4.6 Knees

The knee is the largest joint in the body. It should normally extend in a straight line (0°) and frequently can be hyperextended up to 15°. The degree of extension is determined by measuring the angle formed between the thigh and the leg. Normally, the angle of flexion ranges from 130° to 150°. A simple and useful though less precise way of comparing flexion of both knees is by contrasting the distance between the heel and the buttock when one or both knees are flexed as far as possible. Flexion contractures of the knee often complicate chronic involvement of this joint.

When inspecting the knee, you have to examine the patient while he is standing as well as lying down to disclose the valgus, varus, hyperextension, and flexion deformities (Fig. 1.13). Swelling of the knee joint may be more evident in a prone position. This is particularly so in the case of a Baker's cyst, developing at the posterior side of the knee. The knees generally are inspected best when the patient is relaxed and supine, with the knees extended as fully as possible. Synovitis of the knees is seen on inspection by distention and swelling of the suprapatellar pouch. The fullness of swelling commonly extends to about 5–6 cm above the superior border of the patella. Abnormal swelling in other locations adjacent to the knees should be differentiated from synovial thickening, effusion, or both. If the prepatellar bursa becomes distended, swelling develops on the anterior aspect of the knee between the patella and the overlying skin. Sharply demarcated

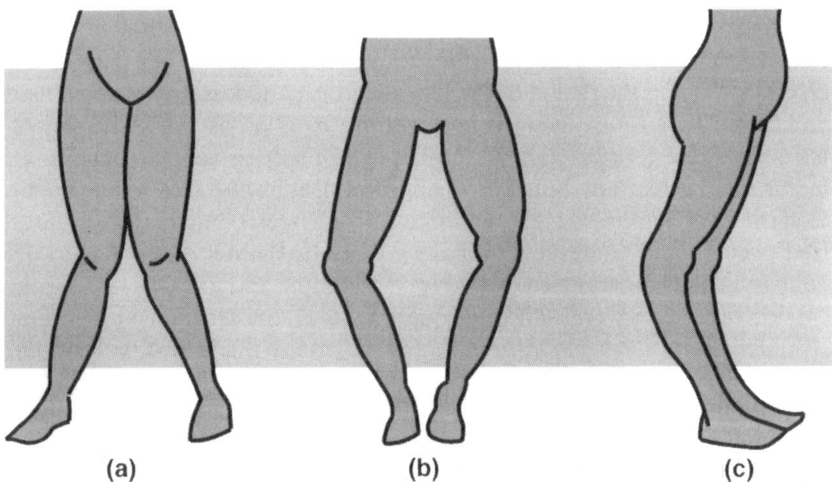

Figure 1.13 Deformities of the knee: (a) genu valgum, (b) genu varum, and (c) genu recurvatum.

margins usually indicate that the swelling is localized to the bursa. The anterior aspect of both sides should be observed carefully for evidence of atrophy of the quadriceps muscle. Atrophy in this muscle is a particularly significant finding because the quadriceps is the great extensor muscle of the knee and is essential for maintaining stability of this joint on weight bearing.

Whenever possible, it is best to palpate the knee with the patient supine and the knee extended. To palpate the suprapatellar part, the examiner's left hand should be placed lightly on the anterior aspect of the thigh about 10 cm above the superior border of the patella. The thumb is placed medially and the fingers are located laterally in a position that might be used to grasp the quadriceps muscle. With the thumb and fingers exerting mild to moderate pressure, the examiner carefully palpates the underlying tissue as the hand is moved gradually toward the knee joint in an attempt to locate the superior edge of the synovial reflexion of the suprapatellar pouch. Note the consistency, nodularity, thickness, warmth, and tenderness of the skin, subcutaneous tissue, and muscles. If fluid is present, it is often helpful if the examiner's right hand is used to push superiorly any synovial fluid from the lower reflections of the synovial cavity to distend the suprapatellar part further. Compressing the fluid in the extreme limits of the synovial reflexions over the region of the joint space causes the edge of the synovial membrane to become palpable as a bulge. The *ballotment of the patella* may be possible when effusion is present, but to be successful this requires a relatively large amount of joint fluid and is not a sensitive method for the detection of a small quantity of fluid in the knee. To perform the ballotment of the patella the suprapatellar part is compressed with the examiner's left hand and the patella is pushed sharply against the femur in an anterior-posterior direction with the fourth finger of the examiner's right hand (Fig. 1.14). Another maneuver that is most useful for the detection of minor degrees of effusion is referred to as the *bulge sign* (Fig. 1.4b). For this examination the knees are fully extended while the patient is in a supine position with the muscle relaxed; tapped pressure is applied both proximally and laterally by one of the examiner's hands to express the synovial fluid from the area. The examiner then taps the lateral edge of the knee with the other hand. A distinct fluid wave or bulge will soon appear on the medial aspect of the knee between the patella and the femur, even if a little fluid is present.

Next we examine the menisci and lateral ligaments. Tenderness localized at the medial or lateral aspects of the articular space suggests trauma or some other disorder of the meniscus. Other indications of injury to the meniscus include limitation of extension or locking, a snapping or popping sensation inside the joint, and local pain inside the knee toward the front of the joint or when extension is attempted. Instability of the knee involves the cruciate ligaments more frequently than the lateral ligaments. The

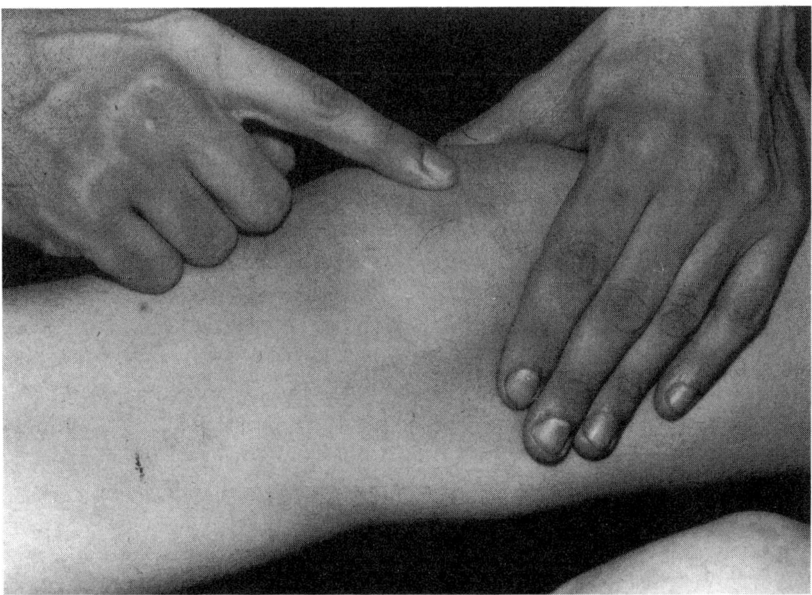

Figure 1.14   Patella ballotment.

ligaments may be tested in the following manner: With the patient supine and the knee in as close to 0° of extension as possible, the examiner fixes the femur with his left hand by grasping the lower anterio-lateral aspects around and under the knee, while grasping the ankle anteriorly with the right hand. Then he attempts to abduct and adduct the tibia on the femur in a rocking fashion. Normally, there is no motion. Increased mobility indicates relaxation of the medial or lateral ligament. To test cruciate ligaments, the examiner pulls the patient's flexed tibia toward himself and then pushes backward. Abnormally increased forward or backward excursion of the tibia on the femur indicates instability of cruciate ligaments (positive "drawer sign"). Destruction of the articular surface from a destructive arthritis of the joint also contributes to instability revealed by this maneuver.

Finally, examination of the patellofemoral joint should not be overlooked. In the elderly, pain and crepitatus of the patella is usually secondary to osteoarthritis. In young people it is usually secondary to chondromalacia patellae. When the patella can be moved over the medial and lateral condyles, there is luxation or subluxation of the patella.

4.7   Ankle and Foot

The foot and ankle are observed while the patient is standing, walking, and in a non-weight-bearing position. Both feet and ankles are compared from the front and back and from the sides for evidence of swelling and atrophy, deformities of the foot and toes, location of calluses, subcutaneous nodes, cutaneous changes, edema, and deformities of the nails.

Movement at the ankle (talotibial) joint is limited almost entirely to plantar flexion and dorsal extension. From the normal position of rest in which there is an angle of 90° between the leg and the foot, the ankle normally allows about 20° of dorsiflexion and about 45° of plantar flexion. Inversion and eversion of the foot occur mainly at the subtalar and other intertarsal articulations. Inversion of the foot (supination) exists when the sole of the foot is turned inward, and eversion exists when the sole of the foot is turned outward. From a normal position of rest, the subtalar joint normally permits about 20° of eversion and about 30° of inversion.

On inspection, mild swelling of the ankle joint may not be apparent but often can be detected by careful palpation. Synovitis of the intertarsal joints may occasionally cause an erythematous puffiness or fullness over the dorsum of the foot. Inflammation of the ligaments that hold the four parts of the foot together may result in weakening and laxity of the supporting ligament structures. When this occurs, the toes spread and the width of the forefoot is increased. Swelling and pain of the Achilles tendon and its insertion can be seen in patients with HLA B27–associated arthritis, but also in overuse injury (Fig. 1.15).

To palpate the ankle, the patient's foot is supported by the examiner's right hand. With the hand the examiner firmly compresses the posterior aspect of the articular capsule and synovial membrane to distend the articular capsule and synovial membrane anteriorly where they can be palpated by the fingers of the examiner's left hand, if synovitis is present. Then the Achilles tendon is examined. Palpable swelling and tenderness on the back of the heel may result from inflammation of superficial structures (subcutaneous bursa) or from inflammation of deeper structures (the Achilles tendon, the bursa between the calcaneus and the Achilles). Differentiation of these sites of involvement by palpation is important as a deeper bursal reaction often signifies inflammation secondary to synovitis. In rupture of the Achilles tendon a defect in the tendon may be palpable. Pain and tenderness under the anterior portion of the heel in the absence of any generalized disorder is frequently called plantar fasciitis. Next the intertarsal joints are palpated distal to the ankle between the examiner's thumbs on the dorsum of the foot and his fingers in the plantar surface of the foot. The midfoot torsion test is used for detection of lesions in this region. The metatarsophalangeal (MTP) joints are palpated between the examiner's thumb and forefingers. Squeeze pain or tangential pain of the metatarsophalangeal joint may be observed in cases of chronic synovitis, elicited by squeezing the metatarsal heads between thumb and fingers.

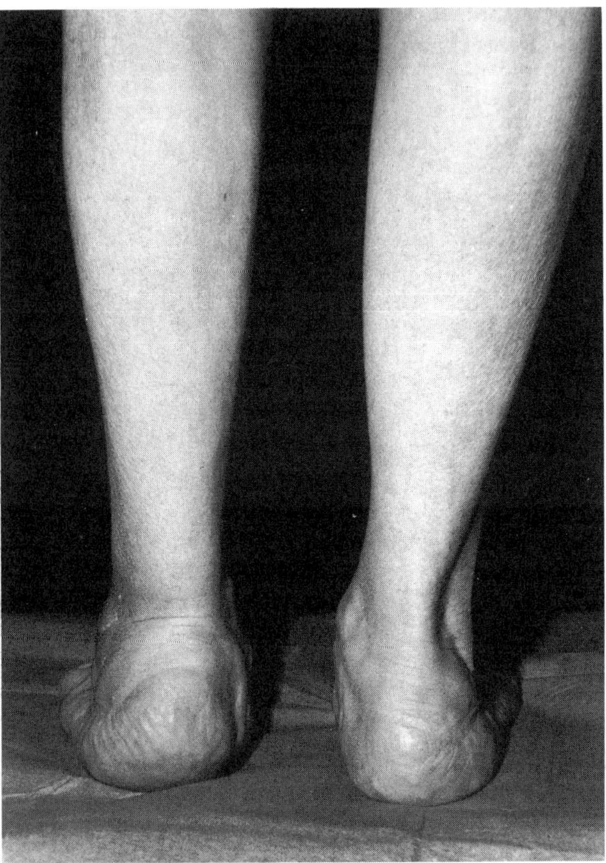

Figure 1.15 Inspection from behind, Achilles tendon.

4.8 Vertebral Column and Thorax

The vertebral column is the main support of the human body. The function is complex because it has to protect the nervous system in addition to keeping the body in equilibrium in the vertical position. The unique structure of the vertebral column allows flexibility of the trunk and helps to retain the upright posture by means of the coordinated action of muscles, ligaments, and bones. The vertebral column normally has four curves: two with anterior convexities and two with posterior convexities. The curves shaped on the vertebral column and the structure of the intervertebral discs help to absorb a substantial degree of shock or compression.

Inspection of the back should be made after the patient has removed all clothing. Then the patient is inspected from behind, from the side, and from the front. From behind it should be noted whether or not the spine is abnormally curved to one or the other side (scoliosis) or whether there is an exaggeration or flattening of the normal antero-posterior curves.

After inspection of the patient in standing position, we must examine the mobility of the spine. Flexion and extension takes place in the lumbar region; rotation in the thoracic region; and the rotation of the head between the atlas and the odontoid peg of C2. To examine flexion, the patient should bend forward and flex his or her head and neck as well as other segments of the vertebral column. With this motion, the lumbar lordotic curve will first flatten and then flex slightly. Normally, the flexed position when viewed from the side forms a smooth curve extending from the sacrum to the base of the skull. Flattening of the lordosis of the lumbar region while the patient bends forward indicates a normal motion in this portion of the spinal column. The degree of spinal flexion plus flexion of the hips is often recorded by measuring the distance from the fingertips to the floor. At the lumbar region, two marker lines, 10 cm apart, are made, starting from L5, with the patient in standing position (Fig. 1.16). On bending forward the lumbar lordosis is flattened out and the lines separate to 15 cm. The difference between the standing and bending positions is noted as the *Schober index*. The total spine mobility can be measured in the same way, whereby the distance between C1 and S2 is measured while standing erect and bending forwards. Normally, this distance will increase by 10 cm on bending.

The degree of extension of the vertebral column is determined by

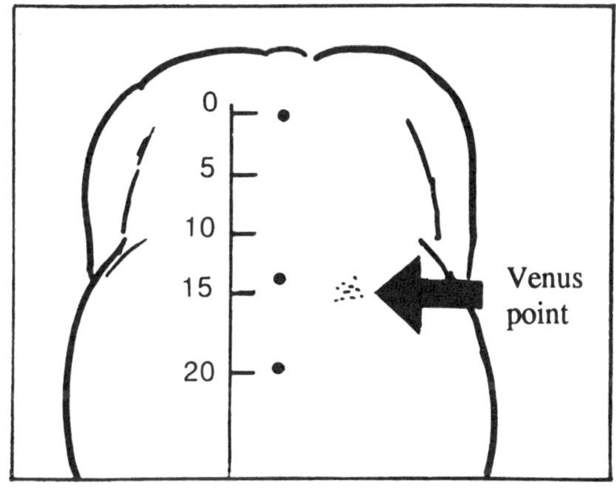

Figure 1.16   Schober test (10–15 cm): "Dimples of Venus."

having the patient bend backward. Stabilize the patient by placing a firm fist on the sacrum and, if necessary, help the patient to extend by pushing on the anterior side of the thorax. Extension usually increases the lordotic lumbar curve, straightens out the thoracic part of the vertebral column, and tilts the head backward.

Lateral motion of the spinal column is determined when the patient bends to one side and then the other. The normal spinal column has a smooth, lateral curve of about 50° from the upright position extending from the sacrum to the base of the skull. Normally the degree of lateral motion is equal on both sides (Fig. 1.17).

Rotation is evaluated when the patient rotates the trunk to one side and then to the other while the legs and pelvis are stabilized by the examiner's manual restraint. Rotation and hyperextension may reveal pain when the patient has degenerative disease of the interfacetal joints of the lumbar region.

Costovertebral motion is determined by measuring chest expansion during inspiration and expiration. Measurement of chest expansion with a nonelastic tape is easy and accurate. The nipple line in males or just above

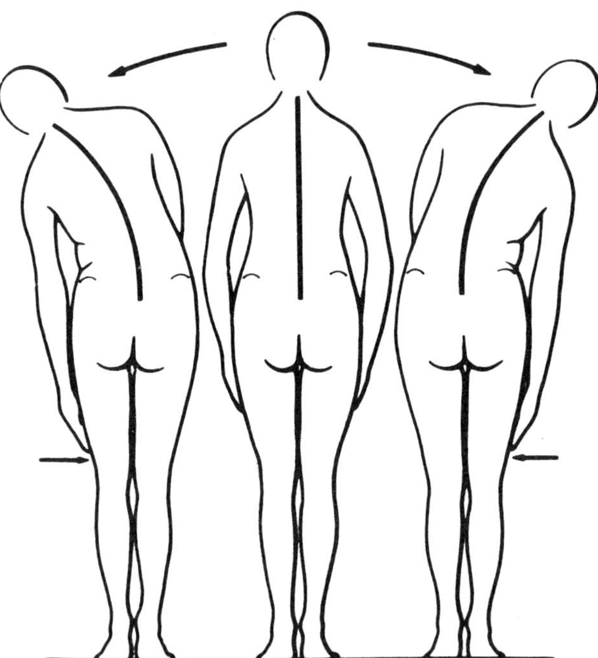

Figure 1.17 Lateral mobility.

it in females is a generally satisfactory and recommended standard for measurement of chest expansion. The degree of chest expansion, like other spinal motion, varies with age and general physical condition, but normally it is 10 cm in young adults (Fig. 1.18).

Palpation of the back should be performed while the patient is standing, lying prone, and sitting. When the patient stands and muscle spasm is present, palpation while the patient is prone is more satisfactory than that in any other position. In general, palpation is performed from the top downward. The posterior aspect of the vertebral column is palpated for evidence of abnormal prominence of any spinous process. A bony shelf or abnormal projection of one vertebra in relation to its adjacent vertebra suggests subluxation or spondylosis. The straight leg raising test is carried out by the examiner while the patient's legs are as relaxed as possible. The patient is in supine position. The examiner places one hand on the patient's heel and holds the foot firmly in dorsiflexion. While the examiner gradually elevates the thigh on the pelvis by moving the foot, his other hand is placed just above the patella of the side being tested. The limit of the angle of flexion is measured by the degrees in the angle formed between the surface

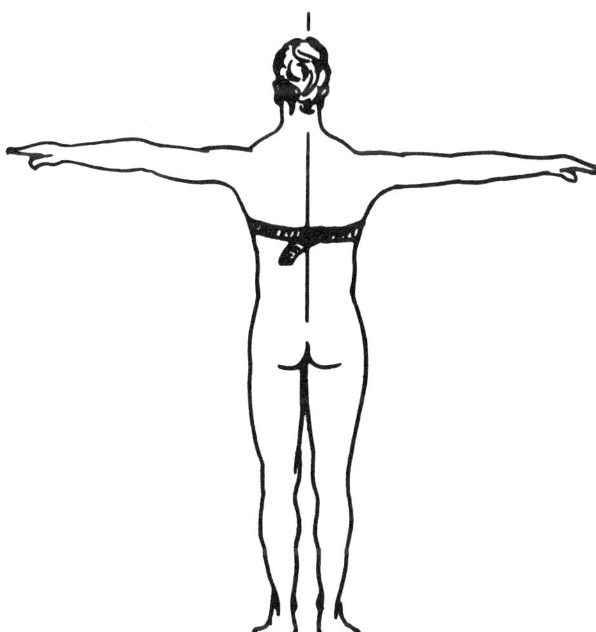

Figure 1.18 Chest expansion.

on which the patient is lying and the elevated lower extremity. Elevation of the lower extremity produces tension on the sciatic nerve and hamstring muscles, but normally each leg and thigh can be raised almost to a right angle without discomfort. When this examination induces pain in the region of the calves with a limitation of flexion at the hip from 20° onward, the test is considered positive and suggests nerve root irritation (Lasègue sign) (Fig. 1.19). The inverse Lasègue sign consists of extending both legs of the patient in front of him in a sitting position (Fig. 1.20). This can be further enforced by flexing the head and trunk and extending the arm in order to reach the toes. If one suspects the objectivity of the patient, then the "covered" Lasègue test (flip test) can be done with the patient sitting. Under the pretext of looking to the feet, we ask the patient to alternately extend both legs.

Neurologic examination, including the reflexes of the knee, the ankle reflex, and the strength of the first toe is necessary to examine patients with sciatic pain and to determine the exact location of nerve lesions.

Clinical examination of the spine should include testing the abdominal muscle strength. This can be done by asking the patient to sit up from supine position, without use of hands or arms. Weak abdominal muscles is the main reason for backache and lumbar hyperlordosis in middle-aged women.

4.9 Sacroiliac Joints

The evaluation of the sacroiliac joints is difficult and should be interpreted with caution. The five tests listed in Table 1.10 are useful for the detection

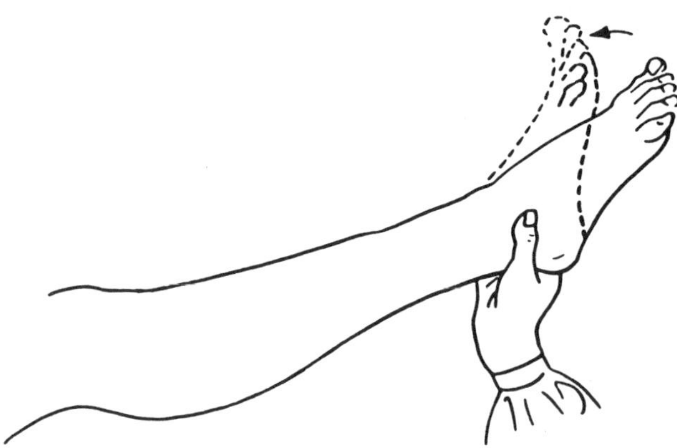

Figure 1.19 Lasègue and Bragard signs.

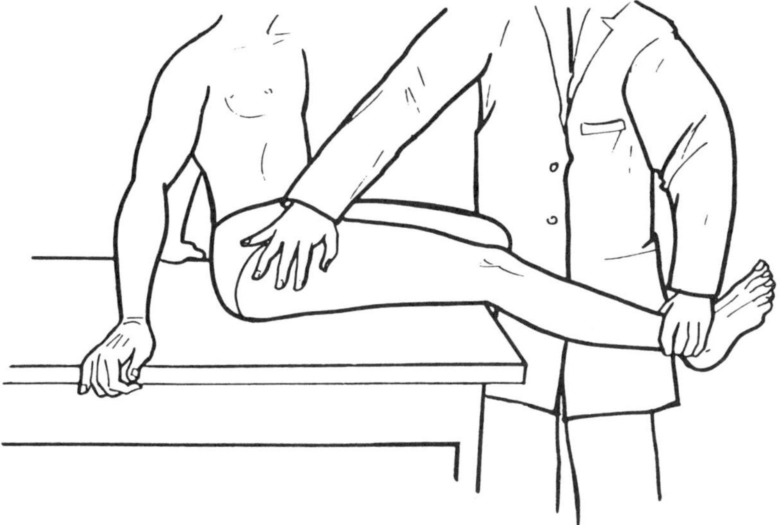

Figure 1.20   Inverse Lasègue.

of sacroiliitis. Only if the patient indicates pain in the sacroiliac joint or lateral radiation to the thigh should these tests be considered positive. These tests can also provoke pain when there is a disk or facet joint lesion, but the pain is then felt at different points in the back (Table 1.10, Fig. 1.21). The first and fifth tests are the most sensitive for detecting sacroiliitis. Trendelenburg's test can also be positive in sacroiliitis.

Table 1.10   Test Sacroiliac Joints

1. Pressure on the iliac crests toward the back and inward at the anterior superior spine on the iliac crest when the patient is lying on his back (Fig. 1.21).
2. Forced adduction with the lower leg in flexion with the patient lying supine.
3. Lateral compression of the pelvis with the patient lying on his lateral side.
4. Patrick sign: the heel is placed on the contralateral knee and the knee is pushed downward (Fig. 1.21). This test is also painful in hip disease.
5. Pressure on the lower parts of the back at the sacral region when the patient is in prone position.

Table 1.11   History and Physical Examination

Basis for
    correct diagnosis
    appropriate therapeutic plan
    database for follow-up

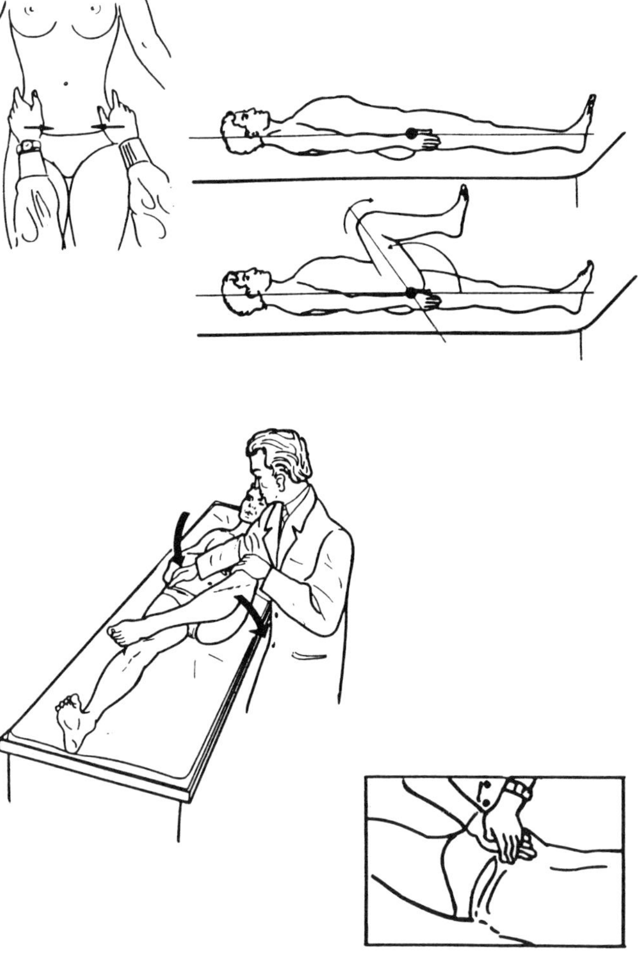

Figure 1.21   Examination of sacroiliac joints.

5 CONCLUSIONS

A thorough history and physical examination remain the cornerstones in the evaluation of patients with rheumatic problems. As many patients present with vague complaints or nonmusculoskeletal symptoms, these clinical skills are essential despite the recent advances in laboratory testing and radiologic imaging. Evaluation of articular and periarticular structures requires a special expertise that involves education and experience. In addition, careful attention to detail is essential in the proper evaluation, diagnosis, and management of rheumatic patients.

Clinical evaluation in rheumatology consists of the systematic collection of clinical material in a patient with a rheumatic complaint. This should lead to an oriented technical evaluation, a correct diagnosis, an appropriate therapeutic plan, and a database for follow-up (Table 11). Traditionally, clinical evaluation is divided into history taking and performance of a physical examination. The history and physical examination together provide most if not all information required for the diagnosis and management of patients with rheumatic problems. The skills for history taking and clinical examination are therefore of paramount importance.

2
Differential Diagnosis

1 DIAGNOSIS PROBLEM SOLVING STRATEGY

1.1 Introduction

A correct diagnosis is essential if therapy, prognosis, and prevention are to be carried out properly. A vague diagnosis of "rheumatism," a prescription for a pain killer based on a vague diagnosis, or a directive either that "there is nothing you can do for this" or "it will heal spontaneously" is undesirable. No diagnosis is more difficult for a patient to deal with than a diagnosis with a poor prognosis or a "probable diagnosis." A patient with pain will remain uncertain and will search until he or she finds someone who will make a diagnosis. With a diagnosis the patient can cope with pain more effectively and often even symptomatic therapy is no longer needed. The patient may end up without a diagnosis in the hands of someone who makes pseudodiagnoses and advises alternative or lucrative therapies.

The technical developments of the last decades give rise to an impression that a diagnosis in a patient with musculoskeletal symptoms now can be made infallibly with the help of laboratory tests, X rays, CT scans, magnetic resonance imaging (MRI) or scintigraphy and with invasive techniques such as arthroscopy and biopsy. However, all of these diagnostic tests often fail to establish to the correct diagnosis and may even give false-positive information suggesting a disease where none exists. For example, statistically 5% of normal individuals will have a positive antinuclear antibodies (ANA), elevated uric acid, or positive *Borrelia burgdorferi* test, but most of these people do not have systemic lupus erythematosus (SLE), gout, or Lyme disease. Furthermore, many abnormalities revealed by imaging techniques have nothing to do with the complaints of the patients. For the differential diagnosis, a careful history and physical examination remain the most important measures. The input of a good clinician will remain essential and irreplaceable.

Differential diagnosis is based on the integration of data obtained by history taking and physical examination in a synoptic list of identified problems, symptoms, abnormalities, or other relevant findings. This synoptic list contains the essential elements that build up a differential diagnosis. Carefully chosen additional investigations can then confirm the proposed working diagnosis or help exclude alternative diagnostic possibilities. Additional investigations may be useful and necessary in order to stage the disease, to judge the evolution, to delineate the local extension of the lesion, and to disclose lesions at a distance.

This approach to diagnosis is more cost-effective, intellectually satisfying, and medically accurate than blind investigations based on the hope that the diagnosis will emerge from these tests. The more tests ordered, the more false-positive results will be revealed. Accordingly, more needless tests and investigations will lead to more confusion and expense.

At present, the level of skills in history taking and in physical examination that are important for the practice of medicine is inadequate, and is replaced by an overreliance on tests.

1.2 Integration of History and Physical Examination

After history taking and physical examination it is worthwhile, even necessary, to summarize the clinical situation in a few words. The words used should be a translation of findings and symptoms in terms of medical concepts, preferably not yet in diagnostic terms. When the diagnosis is formulated too quickly there is the danger that the physician will be blinded by the provisional diagnosis to other possibilities that may be more accurate. This synopsis of information obtained by history taking and physical examination becomes more easily accomplished with more experience.

The first step in this process is to translate the individual items of the history, clinical examination, and earlier investigations into well-defined clinical concepts. This process of bringing together findings results in the formulation of the synoptic problem list. It will allow condensation of considerable information from a complex history into a comprehensive synopsis. This synopsis forms the basis for a limited number of considerations in differential diagnosis (diagnostic list) and results in a limited list of specific requests for technical investigations in order to confirm the diagnosis or stage of disease.

1.3 Producing the Synoptic Problem List

1.3.1 Demographic Profile of the Patient

The synoptic problem list begins with a description of the patient — gender, age, marital state, profession — which identifies the patient's place in society and provides important background information for the diagnosis. Most common rheumatic diseases occur more in women, e.g., rheumatoid arthritis, SLE, and osteoporosis; however, some diseases occur more often in men, e.g., ankylosing spondylitis, Reiter's disease, and gout. The frequency with which most rheumatic diseases occur also varies with age. Viral arthritis is seen more frequently in children; reactive arthritis and HLA B27–associated spondylarthropathy in young adults; and osteoarthritis, osteoporosis, chondrocalcinosis, polymyalgia rheumatica, and paraneoplastic syndromes almost exclusively in the elderly. Information on the family and on the patient's socioeconomic status and profession is important to have in order to estimate psychological consequences, social care, work load, work disability, professional environment, traumatism, and so forth.

1.3.2 Problem Identification

Chief Complaint. After the demographic profile, the synoptic problem list should specify first the chief complaint of the patient and not the past history problems. The main complaint of a musculoskeletal and connective tissue problem generally is pain, stiffness, and/or swelling, localized in or around a joint or muscles. It is now the art to convert the complaints and clinical findings into a diagnostic category. The first act of the physician is to place the chief complaint in one or four pain categories: neurogenic, inflammatory, mechanical, or psychogenic pain (see Chapter 1).

LOCALIZATION OF THE COMPLAINT. From the patient's description it is often easy for the physician to identify whether problems involve the joint, tendon, or muscle. Physical examination is necessary to confirm this impression. However, misleading exceptions are seen. Pain in the knee, for example, may be due to a lesion in the hip or a tendonitis at the great trochanter. Muscle pain in the neck may be the consequence of a shoulder lesion despite evidence of osteoarthritis of the cervical spine on X ray. In this case limitation of shoulder movements should alert the physician that the origin of the neck pain is probably the shoulder rather than the spine.

Pain in muscles and joints without abnormalities on physical examination should not be disregarded. Arthralgia may be the only expression of a systemic disease, such as SLE, periarteritis nodosa, or one of the main complaints of patients suffering from polymyalgia rheumatica or malignancy. Furthermore, patients with fibromyalgia may require as much attention from their physician as patients with inflammatory rheumatic diseases that may appear more likely to lead to disability and premature mortality.

DISTRIBUTION PATTERN. Some conditions are usually monoarticular (gout, septic arthritis); others oligoarticular (reactive arthritis) or polyarticular (rheumatoid arthritis, primary osteoarthritis). Therefore, in the synopsis it should be made clear if the complaint concerns a monoarticular, oligo(pauci)articular (four or fewer joints), or a polyarticular pattern.

The localization of the joint complaints in the upper or lower extremities, axial, symmetric or asymmetric, may provide information for the differential diagnosis. Involvement of the large joints of the lower extremities is often seen in reactive arthritis, Reiter's syndrome, and sarcoidosis. In chondrocalcinosis usually the knees and wrists are most often affected; in spondylitic syndromes shoulders, hip, and feet; in rheumatoid arthritis metacarpo(tarso)phalangeal joints and proximal interphalangeal joints of the hands and feet. Figure 2.1 shows the distribution pattern of the affected joints in a number of rheumatic diseases.

The duration of the complaints, the current changes at the present time, whether it is improving or progressing, the response to drugs already taken, and the functional consequences of the disease are also important. A clinical picture of short duration that is improving needs a different approach than one that has existed for months and is progressing. In acute monoarthritis, septic arthritis should be excluded immediately or crystalarthropathy diagnosed.

EXTRAARTICULAR FEATURES. The next points of the "synoptic problem" list are the findings from the history (past/present) and the findings on physical examination concerning extraarticular features (see general aspects of physical examination). Systematically during the history taking and physical examination, extraarticular manifestations should be sought especially in skin, mucosa, urogenital organs, gastrointestinal organs, and eyes.

PAST HISTORY. Further points in the problem list are those that are relevant for diagnosis, general health, adverse effect of drugs, and so forth. Relevant positive findings from the general history include weight loss or increase, hypertension, medication, heart failure, chronic obstructive lung disease (COLD), liver and kidney disease, alcohol and tobacco abuse, and so forth.

Also mentioned in the problem list are important diseases or events in

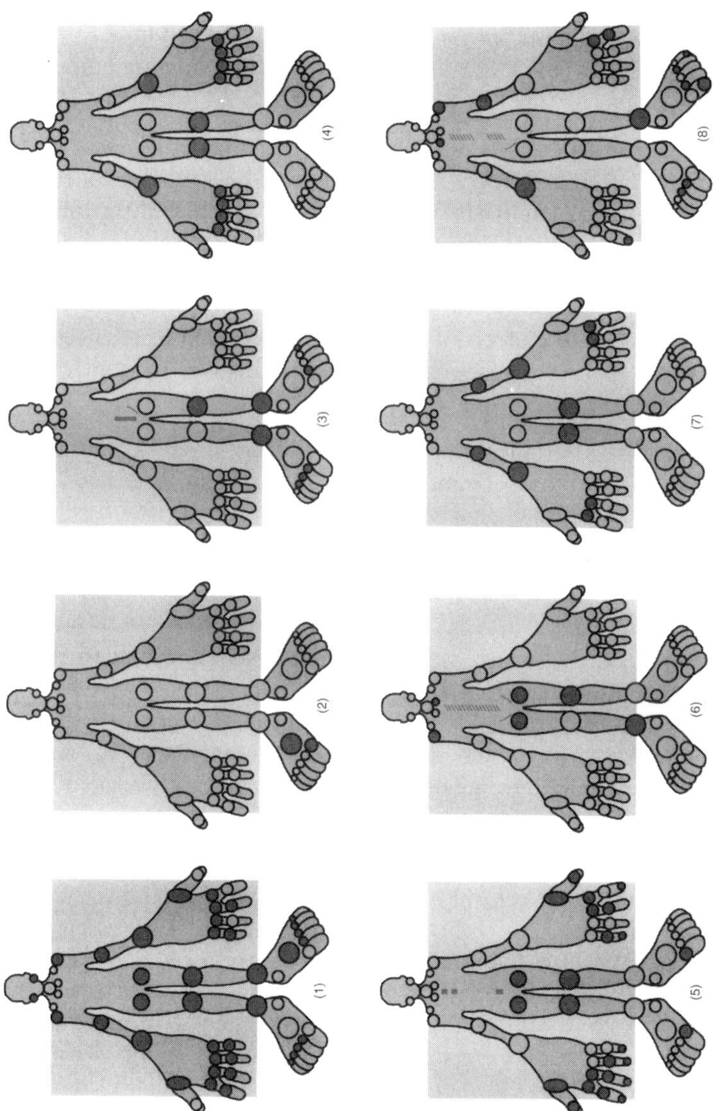

Figure 2.1 Distribution pattern of affected joints in a number of rheumatic diseases.

the past, such as peptic ulcer, nephrolithiasis, menopause, hysterectomy. In addition, relevant information from the family history should be listed.

1.3.3 Differential Diagnosis

On the basis of the synoptic problem list the physician can now formulate the differential diagnosis — a working diagnosis. The following points have been found useful:

> First attempt to identify a diagnosis that suits most of the problems of the list. Often a group of symptoms can be grouped together in clusters, which might already point in a particular direction, e.g., the cluster oligoarthritis, postenteritis, fever, young adulthood, which is suggestive of a post-*Yersinia* reactive arthritis. Experienced physicians look for the diagnosis that gives the best account for the different clusters of problems, whereas unexperienced clinicians try to find a diagnosis and technical investigation for each problem.

One must remember that uncommon presentations of common diseases are more frequently found than common presentation of rare diseases.

> Second, formulate an alternative diagnosis, which also could account for the problem list. If the initial diagnostic consideration is not confirmed, then one is already well advanced for solving the patient's problem.
>
> Elderly people often have multiple diagnoses in addition to the primary diagnosis based on the main complaint.
>
> When a long list of possible diagnoses appears it is good to eliminate the diagnoses for which there are few arguments or for which a number of counterarguments can be formulated. This way of working will save time and cost.

In daily practice, during history taking and physical examination the physician will often think of a central hypothetical diagnosis and direct specific questions accordingly. Although this is good practice, it is dangerous to rely too much on the first hypothesis; biases are introduced and apparently irrelevant or conflicting information may become lost or misinterpreted. Therefore, at this stage it is also desirable to formulate two or more alternative diagnostic hypotheses, except in the most classical patients. For example, gout is a great mimic that should be considered under many guises.

1.3.4 Complementary Investigations

When the list of differential diagnostic possibilities is formulated, the next step is to formulate the least invasive and least expensive investigations that will confirm/establish the proposed working diagnosis. On occasions, the physician may not need any further studies, e.g., polyarticular psoriatic arthritis, scleroderma, longstanding rheumatoid arthritis (RA). Also this clinical thinking will give more intellectual satisfaction than blind demands for a number of tests. In addition to diagnostic investigations, it is of course necessary to delineate the stage or the extent of the disease in order to have a baseline for follow-up.

The above process of clinical thinking is summarized in Table 2.1 and illustrated in two examples.

Example 1. A 28-year-old man comes to the outpatient clinic because of a pain and swelling of the right ankle, nodules on the lower leg, general malaise, shortness of breath on exercise, and fever the last 3 weeks. Physical examination reveals a warm, swollen right ankle and red, hard nodules in the skin, 1–3 cm diameter, on the lower legs. Temperature is 38°C.

SYNOPTIC PROBLEM LIST. Man, 28 years, married, a clerk

Chief problem:

1. Synovitis of the right ankle 3 weeks

Additional findings:

2. Erythema nodosum
3. Dyspnoa
4. Fever

On the basis of this synoptic problem list, the following differential diagnoses can be formulated:

Table 2.1   Differential Diagnosis: Problem Solving Strategy

1. Demographic profile of the patient: age — gender — profession — social status
2. Problem identification: integration history taking and physical examination
   2.1.   Chief problem at presentation
   2.2.   Extraarticular features
   2.3.   Past history: significant events — family history
3. Differential diagnosis list:
   3.1.   Diagnosis that best fits cluster of problems
   3.2.   Alternative diagnosis
   3.3.   Concomitant disease(s)
4. Complementary investigations
   4.1.   To confirm clinical diagnosis
   4.2.   To stage disease

1. Sarcoidosis with arthritis
2. *Yersinia* arthritis
3. Tuberculosis with arthritis

ADDITIONAL INVESTIGATIONS.

1. X-ray chest
2. Antibodies against *Yersinia enterocolitica*
3. Acute phase reactants in blood (erythrocyte sedimentation rate, C-reactive protein)
4. Mantoux test
5. Lung function: bronchoscopy?

DISCUSSION. The most common disease in this context is sarcoidosis. A less probable diagnosis is tuberculosis, but this should not be overlooked.

Example 2. A 42-year-old housewife, mother of three children, returns from summer holidays in the South of Europe with fever, pain in the joints and muscles, shortness of breath, pain in the chest on deep inspiration, and a rash on the face. In the past she often had white-purple-reddish fingers in the cold. On clinical examination there are inflamed follicles at the cheeks, mottling cutaneous vasodilation of the hands, pain on flexion of the wrist and knees, no swelling, precordial friction rub, no murmurs. Temperature is 39°C.

SYNOPTIC PROBLEM LIST. Woman, 42 years old, housewife, three children

Chief problem:

1. Arthralgia myalgia, 3 weeks, UV exposure

Additional findings:

2. Fever 39°C
3. Pericarditis? Pleuritis?
4. Raynaud's phenomenon
5. Erythromelalgia of the hands
6. Folliculitis

DIFFERENTIAL DIAGNOSIS.

1. Systemic lupus erythematosus
2. Systemic sclerosis
3. Mixed connective tissue disease

ADDITIONAL INVESTIGATIONS.

Blood:

ANA (antinuclear antibodies)
White cell count — differential — thrombocytosis
Liver function test
Muscle enzyme test, CK (creatine phosphokinase)

X-ray chest

Electrocardiography; echocardiography

DISCUSSION. The items in the synoptic problem list are very suggestive of the possibility of systemic lupus erythematosus. The patient is a woman; 90% of SLE cases are women. A possible trigger factor for SLE is UV irradiation. Fever, pericarditis and pleuritis are part of a systemic disease. Folliculitis at this age is unusual and is more often seen in a younger age. Folliculitis and/or butterfly rash are the most frequent skin lesions in SLE. Raynaud's is seen in almost all of the inflammatory connective tissue diseases and often as the first manifestation, in particular for systemic sclerosis. Erythromelalgia is a skin disorder with red mottling skin changes of the fingers and palm, accompanied by neuralgia. Also this clinical sign is often seen in SLE.

As an alternative diagnosis, systemic sclerosis and mixed connective tissue disease has been formulated because these diseases have clinical features that are very similar to those of SLE.

2 PATHOGNOMONIC CLINICAL SIGNS

In rheumatology there are a number of findings in the history, physical examination, and laboratory tests that are very suggestive for a particular disease. However, one must be careful; these typical findings must fit with the overall pattern of the patient's problem. So clinical interpretation remains mandatory. These remarks are also valid (even more so) for the laboratory and radiographic findings: the significance of an increased serum uric acid level, positive rheumatoid factor, antinuclear factor, or a positive HLA B27 estimation is very limited.

2.1 Specific Disease Manifestations

When a certain disease has existed for a number of years, the typical clinical features may allow a "spot diagnosis." So it is possible to make a clinical diagnosis from paintings and artworks of the past. These clinical features, however, will not help us to make an early diagnosis in the first stages of the disease.

> *Rheumatoid arthritis.* Ulnar deviation of the fingers, swan neck, and boutonnière deformities of the fingers. These features are in rare cases also seen in systemic lupus erythematosus.
>
> *Gouty arthritis.* Tophi on the ear, the hand, and the big toe.
>
> *Primary osteoarthritis.* Heberden's and Bouchard's nodes, respectively, at the DIP and PIP hand joints, hallux valgus, genu valgum, genu varum, and hip complaints.

Ankylosing spondylitis. Ankylosis of the spine in flexion with or without a hip lesion.

Systemic sclerosis. Ulceration of the fingers, flexion contractures of the fingers (claw hand), vitiligo, small mouth, and pointed nose.

Primary osteoporosis. Old frail woman, dowager's hump, or hip fracture.

2.2 Typical Physical Features

2.2.1 Joints

Heberden's and Bouchard's nodes: primary osteoarthritis

Synovitis, swelling, luxation of the hand and feet joints, swan neck, Boutonnière deformity, ulnar deviation: rheumatoid arthritis

Ankylosis of the spine: ankylosing spondylitis

Palms of the hands on the floor, thumb against lower part of the arm, cubitus valgus, genu recurvatum: hypermobility

2.2.2 Skin

Subcutaneous nodules on pressure points (e.g., elbows): seropositive rheumatoid arthritis

Tophi on the earlobe, fingers, knee (white–yellow subcutaneous nodules): gout

Rash: SLE, Still's disease, viral infections

Butterfly erythema and folliculitis in the face: SLE

Erythema: erythema nodosum, erythema chronica migrans (Lyme disease), erythema marginatum (acute rheumatic fever)

Eczematous violet–purple spots around MCP and PIP joints, muscle weakness: dermatomyositis

Cushions at the PIP joints: knuckle pads

Papyrus-like skin, edema of the fingers, vitiligo, ulcerations of the fingertops, teleangiectasia on the face: systemic sclerosis

Adhesion of tendon and skin in the handpalm: Dupuytren's contracture

Sausage-like fingers: psoriatic arthritis, reactive arthritis

Psoriatic nails, DIP arthritis: psoriatic arthritis

Keratodermia blenorrhagica of palms of hands or of feet: Reiter's disease

Purpura, vasculitis spots: rheumatoid arthritis, connective tissue diseases

Hyperelastic skin, large scars: Ehlers–Danlos syndrome

Xanthoma of the tendons: hyperlipoproteinemia

Scrotal/vaginal ulcers: Bechçet's disease

Balanitis circumscripta: Reiter's disease

2.2.3 Cartilage (of Ear) or Rib

Inflammation: chondritis; (ear–nose–rib): relapsing polychondritis
Pain and swelling at the transition of the rib: Tietze's syndrome

2.2.4 Eyes

Dry eyes, keratoconjunctivitis: Sicca Sjögren's syndrome
Blue sclerae and fractures: osteogenesis imperfecta

2.2.5 Blood Vessels

Inflammation of the temporal arteries: polymyalgia rheumatica arteritis temporalis
Nodular vessel wall thickening: periarteritis nodosa
Absent radial pulse: Takayasu's disease
Triangular pigmentation of the sclera: ochronosis

2.2.6 Joint Fluid

Pus and monoarthritis: septic arthritis
Crystals in polymorphs: needle-like, gout arthritis; bar-like, CPPD arthritis

2.2.7 Blood

Uric acid elevated and monoarthritis: gout
Creatinine phosphokinase content elevated and muscle weakness: myositis
Multisystem disease, positive ANA, anti-ds-DNA positive, young woman: SLE
Systemic disease and positive c-ANCA: Wegener's disease
Antibodies against *Yersinia enterocolitica*: *Yersinia* arthritis
Antibodies against *Borrelia burgdorferi* + knee synovitis: Lyme disease
Granulocytopenia (thrombocytopenia) + hypersplenomegaly and rheumatoid arthritis: Felty's syndrome

2.2.8 Bone

Curving of the femur or tibia ("Sabre Ribia"): Paget's disease
Micrognathia and arthritis: Still's disease

2.2.9 Muscles

Atrophy of thumb muscle: carpal tunnel syndrome, median nerve compression

3 DIFFERENTIAL DIAGNOSIS ARTHRITIS AND TENDONITIS

Arthritis and tendonitis are symptoms and thus not yet a diagnosis. In order to facilitate the differential diagnosis of arthritis and tendonitis, arthritis can be specified as mono-, oligo-, or polyarthritis and as acute or chronic, and tendonitis as local or systemic. For each of these categories a number of diagnostic possibilities can be listed.

3.1 Arthritis

Acute monoarthritis
    Septic arthritis
    Gout
    Pseudogout
    Traumatic (traumatic synovitis, hemarthrosis, internal derangement) hemarthrosis (not traumatic: hemophilia).
    Foreign body
    Reactive arthritis
    Palindromic rheumatism
    Atypical onset of polyarthritis
Chronic monoarthritis
    Monoarthritis is considered to be chronic when lasting for more than 6 weeks
    Septic arthritis (tuberculosis, fungi)
    Rheumatoid arthritis (starting phase)
    Lyme arthritis
    Juvenile chronic arthritis (oligoarticular form)
    Hypermobility syndrome
    Osteoarthritis
    Internal derangement
    Osteonecrosis (SLE, prednisone use)
    Malignancy (synovium, periarticular)
    Pigmented villonodular synovitis, chrondromatosis, hemangioma
    Sarcoidosis
Acute oligoarthritis
    Septic, bacterial, mycobacterial, fungal
    Viral
    Reactive arthritis
    Psoriatic arthritis
    Seronegative spondylarthropathies
    Gout
    Pseudogout
    Sarcoidosis
    Paraneoplastic
    Subacute bacterial endocarditis
    AIDS

Acute polyarthritis >5 joints
    Rheumatoid arthritis
    SLE — other connective tissue diseases
    Serum sickness
    Psoriatic arthritis
    Juvenile chronic arthritis
    Still's disease (systemic form)
Chronic polyarthritis
    Rheumatoid arthritis
    SLE
    Scleroderma
    Seronegative spondylarthropathies
    Hypermobility syndrome
    Gout
    Pseudogout
    Sarcoidosis

3.2 Tendonitis

Overuse injury (especially in local tendonitis)
Systemic diseases ("polytendonitis")
Hyperlaxity
Rheumatoid arthritis
SLE
Scleroderma
Gout
Reactive arthritis
Amyloidosis
Sarcoidosis
Tuberculosis
Fungus infection
Hyperlipidemia
Gonorrhea

3
Infectious and Postinfectious Arthritis

Acute arthritis associated with any suspicion of infection as fever or recent throat, gut, urinary tract, or skin infection has to be explored immediately because there is a possibility to intervene before major damage occurs.

Microorganisms can be involved with rheumatic diseases in several ways. When infectious agents enter the joint they can proliferate and damage the joint directly by stimulating recruitment of polymorphonuclear leukocytes, which produce cytokines and proteases leading to destruction of cartilage and pus formation. This situation is called *septic arthritis*. Infective agents, however, can induce arthritis without proliferation of microorganisms in the joints by inciting at a distance or locally by their antigenic capacity immunologic pathways, some of them by molecular mimicking. This situation is called *reactive arthritis*. Although the microorganisms might not be present in the joint, molecular parts of the microorganisms may play a pathogenic role. This is particularly true for viral and Lyme's arthritis.

In septic arthritis as well as reactive arthritis host factors may play a role and should be taken into account. In septic arthritis the host might have an immune-compromised constitution, lack of defense by poverty, by agammaglobulinemia, by frequent intravenous injections (drug abuse), or by HIV-induced T-cell-mediated immunodeficiency.

Table 3.1   Infectious and Postinfectious Arthritis

Septic arthritis: microorganisms profilerating in the joint
Reactive arthritis: microorganisms stimulate immune-induced arthritis at distance
                or locally
Predisposition: HLA B27 + in urogenital or gastrointestinal microorganism
                Immune-compromised constitution

In reactive arthritis triggered by a urogenital or gastrointestial microorganism, HLA B27 constitution is often found (Table 3.1).

1   SEPTIC ARTHRITIS

1.1   Definition (Table 3.2)

Septic arthritis is an acute bacterial infection in a joint, usually one (monoarthritis) producing severe pain, tenderness, and loss of function. When the infection is in the disc space it is called discitis. When the infection is localized in the bone it is called osteomyelitis. Early diagnosis and antibiotic therapy are urgently required to prevent joint damage.

1.2   Main Clinical Features

1.2.1   Early Manifestations

Any monoarthritis or acute exacerbation of a joint in a patient already suffering from polyarthritis should be suspected of being septic arthritis. Most articular infections involve a single joint but 20% are polyarticular. Joints commonly involved include the knee (50%), hip (13%), shoulder (9%), wrist (8%), ankle (8%), elbow (7%), and small joints of the hands and feet (5%). Vesicopustular and hemorrhagic skin lesions are suspicious for disseminated gonococcal infections (see atypical form). Sometimes the port of entry is obvious, e.g., a wound, pustulotic acne, gastroenteritis, pyelonephritis, a bedsore, or a recent intraarticular injection, or the patient

Table 3.2   Septic Arthritis

Acute bacterial joint infection
Monoarthritis(discitis)–osteomyelitis
Immediate broad-sprectrum antibiotic therapy
Synovial fluid culture — Gram staining
Specific antibiotic therapy

---

belongs to the group of people at risk for infection or is under immunosuppressive therapy. A particular person at risk is the patient who has a joint prosthesis of the hip or knee. When the septic arthritis is in the disc (discitis), the presenting symptom is very severe localized back pain with or without fever. Bacterial infection of the bone—osteomyelitis—affects mostly the metaphyseal part of the tibia or femora. Tuberculous synovitis or discitis should be suspected when there is low-grade monosynovitis or localized chronic backache, particularly of the thoracic spine.

1.2.2 Late Manifestations

In septic arthritis, joint destruction and sometimes ankylosing and, in cases of osteomyelitis, skin ulcerations and fistulae with elimination of bone sequesters are observed if early antibiotic therapy has not been given. In case of tuberculous discitis (Pott's disease), a marked angulation of the spine, kyphosis, is the end stage of the disease (gibbus deformity).

1.3 Confirming the Diagnosis—Investigations

Clinical suspicion and an extraarticular focus of infection should prompt a search for septic arthritis. A positive Gram strain and culture of the synovial fluid are the fundamental criteria for the diagnosis of bacterial arthritis but are diagnostic in only one half to three fourths of patients. Blood tests usually have nonspecific abnormalities. Peripheral white blood cell (WBC) counts are elevated in approximately one half of cases, but the erythrocyte sedimentation rate (ESR) and C-reactive protein (CRP) are usually elevated. Blood cultures are positive in approximately 50% of cases and may be the only method to identify the causative organism.

Synovial fluid analysis is the most important test in acute septic arthritis. The WBC is intensely inflammatory ($> 50,000/\text{mm}^3$) in 50–70% of the cases and moderately inflammatory ($2000–50,000/\text{mm}^3$) in the remainder.

Gram stain of synovial fluid will reveal organisms in 50–70% of infected joints and will distinguish gram-positive from gram-negative organisms but sometimes not staphylococci from streptococci. Fluid should be cultured aerobically and anaerobically. If gonococcal infection is likely, chocolate agar medium should be plated as soon as the specimen is obtained to avoid drying. The use of blood culture bottles for synovial fluid may improve the frequency of bacteria isolation. The operational rule should be to culture all orifices, body fluids, and foci of infection.

Ziehl staining for tuberculosis should be added if the arthritis is low grade or other suspicious symptoms are available. Early in acute bacterial arthritis the only radiographic abnormality evident is soft tissue swelling and signs of synovial effusion. A plain radiograph should be obtained at the time of diagnosis to search for a contiguous focus of osteomyelitis and to provide a baseline to monitor adequacy of treatment. After 10–14 days of bacterial infection, destructive changes of joint space narrowing (reflecting cartilage destruction) and erosions or foci of subchondral osteomyelitis may become evident. Early treatment is designed to prevent this. Gas formation within the joints suggests infection with *E. coli* or anaerobes.

Other studies may be performed but are not required, particularly in the presence of a positive culture.

^{99m}Technetium methylene diphosphonate bone scans demonstrate increased uptake with increased blood flow in the septic synovial membrane and at metabolically active bone. Gallium citrate- or indium-labeled WBC scans may demonstrate enhanced activity in septic joints. Gallium tends to concentrate at sites of increased protein concentration and leukocytes whereas technetium uptake results from increased blood flow.

Bone scans normally may show increased uptake for a year after prosthesis insertion. After a year, increased uptake occurs with septic or aseptic loosening of the prosthesis. Gallium has a low sensitivity for prosthesis infection and the utility of indium-WBC scans has not been established.

1.4 Diagnostic Difficulties

1.4.1 Osteitis

Osteitis, a warm painful bone segment as seen in Paget's disease (osteitis deformans) and in Reiter's and SAPHO (*S*ynovitis, *A*cne, *P*ustulosis, *H*yperostosis, *O*steitis) syndrome, can be confused with chronic septic osteomyelitis. In these cases there is no fever or WBC elevation. In Paget's disease a raised alkaline phosphatase activity will help to differentiate it from Reiter's and SAPHO syndromes. The other characteristic symptoms occurring in other systems—urethritis, conjunctivitis, vasculitis, and arterial occlusion—will be helpful to differentiate it from osteomyelitis.

1.4.2 Fungal Arthritis

In immunocompromised patients such as those on renal dialysis, chronic antibiotic therapy may cause fungal arthritis, which usually presents as an indolent arthritis much like tuberculous arthritis. Synovial biopsy and cultures are generally needed for diagnosis. In regions where leprosy still exists this diagnosis has also to be considered in low-grade symptoms.

1.5 Epidemiology and Historical Data

Joint infection in children is monoarticular in 93% of cases and half of the cases occur in children less than 2 years of age. In adults with septic arthritis approximately 40% are over age 60. In this older age group 75% of the infection occurs in patients with prior arthritis and 75% involves the hip or knee. The majority have significant comorbidity, e.g., diabetes 24%, malignancy 19%, renal failure 14%, and other diseases such as rheumatoid arthritis, SLE, chronic lung disease, or alcoholism. Steroid use is seen in up to one third of cases.

Intravenous drug abuse is increasingly associated with infection of joints. The risk of joint infection following intraarticular corticosteroid injection is well recognized but is probably less than 0.01%. The rate of early prosthetic joint infection ($<$12 months) is 2% or less and the annual rate of late infection ($>$12 months) is 0.6%.

1.6 Pathophysiology

Gram-positive organisms cause 65–85% of nongonococcal bacterial arthritis, gram-negative bacilli cause 10–15%, and less than 5% are caused by mixed aerobic and anaerobic infections. Mycobacteria and fungi cause less than 5% of joint infections.

1.7 Management

Therapeutic decision must be made before and without causative organism identification. Initial therapy selection is based on the clinical picture and on the synovial fluid Gram stain (revealing in 50–60%) and the most likely causative organism given the clinical setting. Ongoing therapy is later modified according to synovial fluid culture results, specific antibiotic sensitivity testing results, and whether clinical response indicates improvement.

Treatment of joint prosthesis infections is arduous and prolonged. Duration of antibiotic therapy must be guided by the clinical response. Parenteral administration should generally be continued for 2 weeks then followed by oral antibiotics for 1–6 weeks given at 2–3 times the usual dose. Staphylococcal infection requires longer treatment, at least 6 weeks of IV treatment. The joint should be aspirated adequately to drain intraarticular pus and should be rested in a splint in order to reduce pain and contractures.

1.8 Atypical Forms

1.8.1 Gonococcal Arthritis

Gonococcal arthritis is discussed as a separate entity from other forms of supperative bacterial arthritis because it is in a number of countries the most common form of acute bacterial arthritis and has a distinctive clinical picture and excellent response to appropriate therapy.

A frequent presentation of gonococcal arthritis is in a sexually active individual with a 5- to 7-day history of fever, shaking chills, multiple skin lesions (petechiae, papules, pustules, hemorrhagic bullae, or necrotic lesions), fleeting migratory polyarthralgias, and tenosynovitis in the fingers, wrists, toes, and ankles that typically evolves into a persistent mono- or oligoarthritis. Skin lesions occur in up to 50%, starting as an erythematous macule that progresses to a papule, then pustule with necrosis or ulceration on the trunk and extremities including palms and soles. The oral mucosa is spared. Lesions of different ages are usually present at the same time. Affected individuals may not have symptoms of genitourinary tract infection: 80% of men and women with disseminated gonococcal infection have asymptomatic local gonococcal infection, urethritis (up to 50% asymptomatic), cervicitis (majority asymptomatic), proctitis (90% asymptomatic), or pharyngitis (most asymptomatic). Women are often menstruating or pregnant. Additional risk factors for disseminated gonococcal infection include inherited deficiencies of the late complement components (C5, C6, C7, C8).

Isolation of the organism can be difficult because it is very sensitive to drying. The operational rule for diagnosis is to culture all orifices and plate at the bedside on chocolate agar or Thayer–Martin medium. Proof of infection by culture of the organism requires 24 hr, but treatment must be initiated according to diagnosis based on the characteristic clinical features described above. Antibiotics should be administered to eradicate all foci of infection and prevent further recurrences of bacteremia. Treatment for disseminated gonococcal infection in the early febrile tenosynovitis phase or the later frank arthritis is the same. Current treatment recommendations are initial ceftriaxone 1 g/day for 7 days; if found to be sensitive, penicillin 10–20 million units/day or ampicillin 4 g/day for 7 days. Daily needle aspiration of synovial fluid should be performed as long as it continues to accumulate. Gonococcal infections most often do not produce permanent joint damage.

1.8.2 Tuberculous Arthritis

Tuberculous arthritis should be considered in the differential diagnosis of monoarticular and pauciarticular arthritis at any age. The arthritis is frequently insidious in onset. It tends to lack some of the usual signs of active inflammation, especially erythema and heat. Pott's disease, tuberculous involvement of the spine, classically involves the thoracolumbar junction. Anterior destruction of vertebral bodies and discs eventually leads to angulation of the spine and kyphosis (gibbus deformity). While constitutional signs of tuberculosis (fever, malaise, or weight loss) may be present, active pulmonary tuberculosis is unusual. A history of infection may be absent. A positive skin test for tuberculosis is helpful, although a negative test in the presence of anergy does not rule out the diagnosis. Diagnosis is based on finding acid-fast bacilli in synovial fluid, but usually a synovial biopsy is needed to document caseating granulomas. Tuberculosis and its complications should be considered in patients with acquired immune deficiency syndrome (AIDS) or a history of immigration from an endemic area. Atypical mycobacterial infections also occur and should particularly be considered in the setting of immune compromise, especially AIDS. Long-term therapy over months with multiple antituberculous drugs is required for eradication of infection.

1.9 Impact of Disease and Prognosis

Mortality rates have decreased from approximately 20% before 1980 to 5% after 1980. Poor joint outcome has decreased from 70% to 33%. Improved outcome is probably due to more effective antibiotics and improved control of underlying medical illness.

Infection is the most devastating complication of prosthetic joint surgery because it leads to prosthesis loosening, failure, and sepsis. There is a high rate of reinfection (38%) in new implants whether replaced immediately or after 2–3 months of antibiotic therapy.

2 VIRAL ARTHRITIS

2.1 Definition (Table 3.3)

Many viral infections are associated with concurrent arthralgias and occasional arthritis, and many forms of viral arthritis occur subsequent to the viral infection. Almost all forms of viral arthritis are self-limited and generally do not cause damage to articular cartilage, in contrast to bacterial or fungal arthritis. Therefore, one of the primary reasons to identify viral arthritis is that most viral anthritides are associated with a very good prognosis. Various forms of viral arthritis will be described below.

Table 3.3 Viral Arthritis

Viral infection or vaccination
1–6 days later arthralgias-arthritis
Oligoarticular to polyarticular
Transient synovitis hip (children)
Self-limited (weeks)

2.2 Main Clinical Features

2.2.1 Rubella Virus

Rubella virus arthritis has become a prominent clinical problem in the use of rubella vaccines. It is generally not seen in childhood but occurs in up to one third of adolescent and adult females. The arthritis usually occurs 1–6 days after the rubella rash, generally symmetric and polyarticular involving the small joints of the hands, as well as knees and wrists, therefore mimicking rheumatoid arthritis. It may be accompanied by inflammatory synovial fluid, with WBC of 10,000 or more, and occasionally rheumatoid factor may be seen. The arthritis generally continues for less than 2 weeks.

Rubella immunization is also associated with two types of neuropathic syndromes. The first mimics carpal tunnel syndrome with numbness and tingling in the hands and shooting pains in the arms. The second involves pain in the back of the legs, particularly in the morning, which leads children to assume a crouching position. These syndromes may persist for many years on the basis of presumed neurologic involvement.

2.2.2 Parvovirus

Parvovirus arthritis was initially described as erythema infectiosum, "Fifth's disease," which was initially thought to be a variant of rubella arthritis. There is a characteristic three-stage rash, characterized by an initial bright so-called slapped-cheek rash of the face, followed by a lace-like eruption of the trunk, and a third stage with recurrence of both lesions. Joint pain is relatively uncommon in infected children but may be seen in up to $>50\%$ infected adults.

2.2.3 Adenovirus

Adenovirus VII, a common upper respiratory infection, is associated with an arthritis that generally develops 1–2 weeks subsequent to a clinical infection manifested by fever and sore throat. Occasionally a nonpruritic macular erythematous rash accompanies the arthritis, which may lead to oligoarticular synovitis.

2.2.4 Herpesvirus

Arthritis has been found in association with several herpes-type viruses, including herpes simplex, cytomegalovirus, varicella, and Epstein–Barr virus. All of these arthritides have been found to be self-limited, as in other viral arthritis arthritides.

2.2.5 Mumps

Arthritis occurs in less than 0.05% of patients infected with mumps, generally in males. The joint symptoms occur 1–2 weeks after salivary gland swelling and generally persist for about 2 weeks.

2.2.6 Arbovirus

The term arbovirus represents a group of viruses transmitted by arthropods, primarily seen in Africa and Asia, including Ross River epidemic polyarthritis in Australia, and Chikungunya in Africa and Southeast Asia, a disease whose meaning is literally "bends up" and was noted in soldiers in Vietnam. O'nyong-nyong, which means "bone breaks," presents a similar picture in regions of Africa. Sindbis is an arbovirus isolated in Egypt associated with joint symptoms. Again, symptoms may persist for about 2 weeks and are self-limited.

2.2.7 Smallpox

Smallpox is no longer a clinical problem because it has been eradicated through public health measures in most parts of the world. A form of smallpox known as osteomyelitis variolosa is of historical interest in that a severe musculoskeletal pain resulted from direct extension of the virus from the metaphysis of the bone to the articular surface. The elbow joint was most commonly involved, followed by the wrist, ankle, and knee joint. This complication fortunately is only of historical interest, but awareness may be helpful for understanding other forms of potential viral infection causing arthritis.

2.2.8 Hepatitis B

Hepatitis B arthritis is a common form of viral arthritis seen in general practice. Initially, it may appear as an early rheumatoid arthritis involving the metacarpophalangeal joints and proximal interphalangeal joints of the hand, and may then settle in a few large joints, such as knees, ankles, shoulders, and wrists. Patients with hepatitis B frequently report fatigue, anorexia, and fever. The arthritis typically occurs prior to development of clinical jaundice, although liver enzymes are generally elevated while the bilirubin is normal. About half of the patients have an urticarial rash and maculopapular or petechiae are seen less frequently. Angioneurotic edema of the soles may be seen as a variant of the urticarial rash.

Curiously, the hepatitis B arthritis improves to remission as the patient becomes jaundiced. Therefore, hepatitis B antigen is recoverable from the blood in most patients at the time of the arthritis, and as the arthritis disappears, hepatitis B antibody is detectable. This arthritis generally persists for less than 3 weeks.

A more severe rheumatic condition associated with hepatitis B is vasculitis, initially reported in 1970. Signs and symptoms of hepatitis B vasculitis are similar to those of other forms of vasculitis, ranging from a mild clinical presentation to a chronic vasculitic process that persists over years.

2.3   Confirming the Diagnosis—Investigations

Apart from the previous vaccination with rubella vaccine and typical clinical signs of specific viral infection, the diagnosis can be established definitely in most cases with a serologic test identifying antibodies against rubella, parvovirus, adenovirus, herpes, arbovirus, and hepatitis B. Because the arthritis is self-limited, the test results generally become available when the arthritis has resolved. Sonography of a hip joint in a child may show fluid and hypertrophic synovitis (Fig. 3.1). Nothing diagnostic is to be expected from radiologic and other imaging techniques.

2.4   Diagnostic Difficulties

The clinical signs of oligoarthritis and polyarthritis of viral arthritis may mimic acute bacterial arthritis, rheumatoid arthritis, or reactive arthritis as in Reiter's syndrome. Indeed, one of the primary rationales to identify a virus in arthritis is to reassure the clinician and patient that the process is not either an acute bacterial or fungal process, or rheumatoid arthritis, Reiter's syndrome, or other potentially persistent rheumatic disease.

2.5   Epidemiology and Historical Data

Arthritis has been found in 15–30% of patients affected by rubella and 12% of hepatitis B during epidemics. Approximately 10% of children with Fifth's disease (parvovirus B19) have arthralgias and 5% have arthritis, and up to 78% of infected symptomatic adults develop joint symptoms.

2.6   Pathophysiology

Rubella virus has been cultured from joint fluid in some patients with rubella vaccine-induced arthritis, suggesting direct involvement of the virus in joint disease. However, the presence of arthritis (and rash) generally is coincident with the appearance of circulating antibodies several days after viremia, more consistent with an immune complex–type mechanism than a direct effect of virus.

Of interest is the identification in the serum and synovial fluid of patients affected by adenovirus arthritis of cryoprecipitates which include intact virus immunoglobulin and complement, suggesting a mechanism involving immune complexes. Circulating immune complexes containing hepatitis B antigen and antibody are thought to be important in the pathogenesis of the arthritis.

A variant of hepatitis B vasculitis is essential mixed cryoglobulinemia in which hepatitis B antigen and antibody are identified in the cryoglobul-

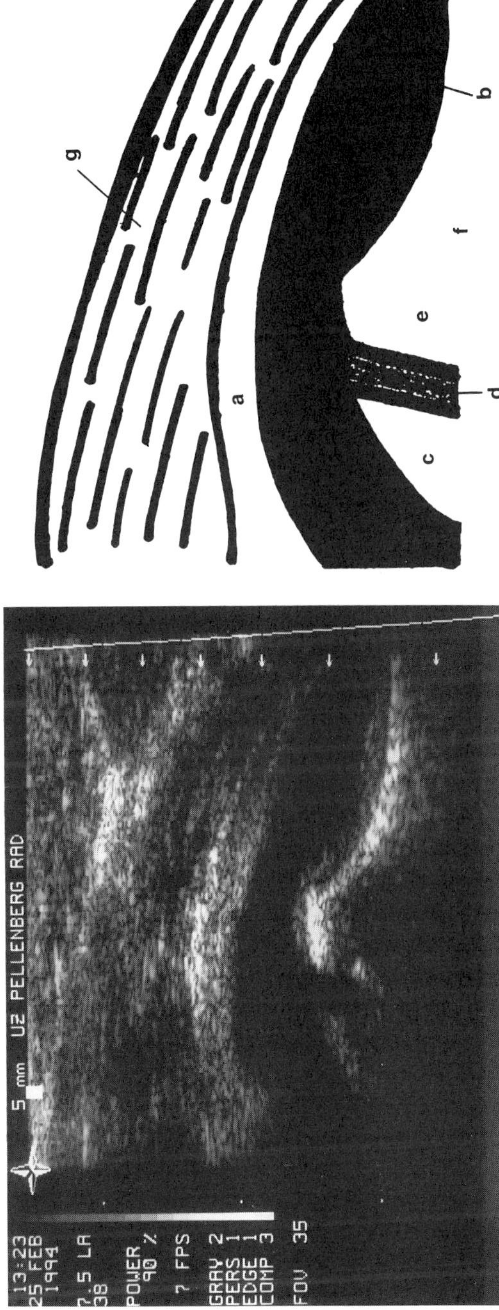

Figure 3.1   Transient synovitis: (a) joint capsule, (b) distended anterior recessus, (c) femoral epiphysis, (d) femoral growth plate, (e) femoral metaphysics, (f) femoral neck, (g) iliopsoas muscle.

ins. These findings suggest the presence of immune complexes of hepatitis B in the etiology of cryoglobulins.

Cryoglobulins are immunoglobulins that precipitate in cold and are isolated by collecting blood from a patient at a warm temperature and then holding the serum in the refrigerator to detect cold-reacting globulins. These globulins often contain immune complexes that can be identified specifically.

2.7 Management

Management of viral arthritis generally is symptomatic as, in almost all cases, the process is self-limited and the patient recovers. Caution must be observed in the use of salicylates and nonsteroidal antiinflammatory drugs for possible hepatic or renal toxicity in individuals who have severe acute illnesses. Nonetheless, these agents are often used quite effectively as is acetaminophen and analgesic drugs. Corticosteroids may be used with caution but may be very helpful in ameliorating symptoms and any possible long-term damage resulting from inflammation.

2.8 Impact of Disease and Prognosis

Most viral arthritides are associated with a very good prognosis. Symptoms persist for about 2–4 weeks, are self-limited, and do not lead to long-term joint damage. Occasionally patients experience recurrent attacks of rubella arthritis, most prominently affecting the knee, which may last as long as 5 years. It is possible that rare cases of "chronic" rubella arthritis may involve individuals who have rheumatoid arthritis, which develops coincident with a rubella vaccine. This type of coincidence may be expected in as many as 100,000 cases because of the common use of rubella vaccine and common presentation of rheumatoid arthritis.

Parvovirus arthritis is generally self-limited. A few isolated reports suggesting a possible role of parvovirus in the etiology of rheumatoid arthritis may represent coincident isolation of parvovirus in an individual who had rheumatoid arthritis, as in the case of rubella virus.

3 REACTIVE ARTHRITIS

3.1 Definition (Table 3.4)

Reactive arthritis is a sterile joint inflammation that develops after a distant infection. The disease is systemic and not limited to the joints. Triggering infections most commonly originate in the throat, urogenital organs, or

Table 3.4 Reactive Arthritis

Postinfectious sterile joint inflammation
Oligoarthritis lower limbs
HLA B27–associated posturogenital-postenteric
Extraarticular manifestations skin, mucous membranes
Good prognosis: 1/3 self-limiting, 1/3 intermittent, 1/3 chronic

gastrointestinal tract. The disease also occurs without obvious preceding infection, e.g., in association with inflammatory bowel disease.

Within the broad group of reactive arthritis a wide range of syndromes and disease entities have been distinguished based on symptom clusters, e.g., Reiter's syndrome, triggering infection, e.g., *Yersinia* arthritis, port of entry, e.g., postdysenteric arthritis or genetic susceptibility as HLA B27+ (HLA B27–associated arthritis) (Table 3.5).

Table 3.5 Classification of Reactive Arthritis

(a) HLA B27–associated
    1. Urogenital infection
       Neisseria gonorrhoeae
       Chlamydia trachomatis
       Ureaplasma urealyticum

    2. Gut infection (enterocolitis)
       Salmonella
       Shigella flexneri
       Yersinia enterocolitica
       Campylobacter jejuni

    3. Undifferentiated reactive arthritis
       No infectious agent demonstrable

(b) Not HLA B27–associated
    Acute rheumatic fever
    Sarcoidosis
    Virus-associated reactive arthritis (hepatitis B, rubella)
    Neisseria gonorrhoeae
    Mycoplasma
    Herpes genitalis
    Lyme arthritis

3.2 Main Clinical Features

3.2.1 Early Manifestations

The patient is most often a young adult who comes to consult for tendonitis and arthritis in a few joints, in particular at the lower limbs. Careful history indicates a "flu"-like syndrome, an enteric or urogenital infection a few days or a couple of weeks ago. The triggering infection is often mild and in about 10% of cases the infection has passed unnoticed. The joints most often affected are the weight-bearing joints—knees, ankles, and hip—but quite commonly other large joints such as the shoulders, elbows, and wrists are also involved. Occasionally, small joints of hands and feet and a sacroiliac joint are affected. Plantar fasciitis and tendovaginitis of the ankle region often results in difficulties in walking. Reactive arthritis is associated with general symptoms as fever, malaise, and a number of inflammatory skin, gastrointestinal, and ocular manifestations. Based on the presence or absence of these associated symptoms a number of syndromes and disease entities have been described.

The most common skin and mucous membrane symptoms are keratoderma blenorrhagica, also called pustulosis palmoplantaris, onicholysis, erythema nodosum, urethritis, circinate balanitis, cystitis, prostatitis, cervicitis, salpingitis, and oral and genital aphtosis. Enteritis, ocular symptoms such as conjunctivitis, episcleritis, acute uveitis, carditis, valvular disease, conduction disturbance, and mild renal manifestations as proteinuria and microhematuria may occur.

3.2.2 Late Manifestations

In some cases of chronic arthritis bilateral sacroiliitis and spondylitis, recurrent iridocyclitis, and cardiac conduction disturbance may become prominent.

3.3 Confirming the Diagnosis—Investigations

ESR and CRP are elevated in many cases of acute reactive arthritis. The blood cell count will reveal moderate leukocytosis and mild anemia. Urine analysis should be carried out to detect possible aseptic pyuria and urethritis. The best simple diagnostic test for urethritis is a so-called two-glass urine test (cell count in first and second urinary void). In urethritis the first urine void will contain the washed out inflammation cells of the urethra and look cloudy whereas the second void contains clear urine (Fig. 3.2).

Microscopic cell count will confirm it. Tests for rheumatoid factor are usually negative and should not be done if the clinical picture suggests Reiter's syndrome. Joint fluid should always be aspirated when possible. Gram stain and bacterial culture should be performed for a differential

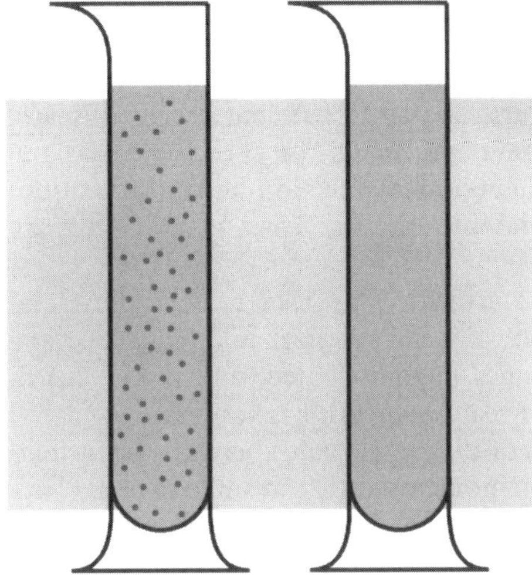

Figure 3.2 Two-glass urine test.

diagnosis. In reactive arthritis bacteria are not demonstrable either by staining or even extensive culturing. Microbiological and serologic studies form a cornerstone of diagnosis. Every effort should be taken to isolate the causative microorganism from the throat, feces, or urogenital tract. Isolation of *Yersinia* requires special methods, and it is easily missed in routine fecal culture. In most cases, however, results are negative, which emphasizes the role of serology. The serologic tests to be considered include antibodies against *Salmonella*, *Borrelia burgdorferi*, and β-hemolytic streptococci.

Depending on the infection history of the patient, antibodies against various viruses may yield a specific diagnosis. It should be stressed that not all microorganisms triggering reactive arthritis have been identified, but the list is rising steadily. Thus, negative serology does not rule out a diagnosis of reactive arthritis; furthermore, in some patients the antibodies rise slowly and yield a positive result only a few weeks after the onset of disease and sometimes are negative as one does not test for the organism (some are unknown).

Detection of the HLA B27 antigen may be helpful in the diagnosis and in considering the treatment and follow-up of the patient. As noted before, however, the disease may occur also in HLA B27–negative individuals.

Radiographic studies of symptomatic joints normally are helpful as the findings in reactive arthritis are somewhat scanty, such as periarticular osteoporosis and soft tissue swelling. They might be done not so much to confirm the diagnosis of reactive arthritis as to rule out erosive disease, e.g., rheumatoid arthritis. In recurrent and chronic cases they increase and may include erosions. More often, periosteal reaction and proliferation, especially at the insertion sites of tendons, are seen. Thus, plantar spurs are a common sign in chronic cases.

Chronic or recurring reactive arthritis may lead to sacroiliitis and spondylitis that may be radiographically indistinguishable from ankylosing spondylitis. However, the changes remain limited, and severe ankylosing spondylitis as a late sequela of reactive arthritis is very rare.

Biopsy of the synovium is not of diagnostic value because the inflammation is nonspecific. It has been demonstrated that in some patients with reactive arthritis inflammatory bowel disease (ulcerative colitis or Crohn's disease) may be a background factor.

Ileocolonoscopy has revealed that inflammatory conditions are present in the absence of subjective symptoms. However, endoscopy or radiographic investigation of the colon is not recommended routinely.

3.4 Diagnostic Difficulties

The most important question at admission is whether the patient has reactive arthritis or true septic infection of the joint. Especially in children, a purulent arthritis may rapidly lead to destruction of the joint. As discussed above, the question may be difficult to solve rapidly. Therefore it is advisable to proceed with therapy on the assumption of purulent arthritis in uncertain cases. In case of intensive inflammation, the redness may lead to a suspicion of erysipelas.

Gout or pseudogout may present with similar symptoms and findings to reactive or infectious arthritis, but careful history taking and identification of crystals in the joint fluid clarify the situation in most instances.

Patients express much concern on the question of whether the disease is rheumatoid arthritis or ankylosing spondylitis. Demonstration of rheumatoid factor and radiographic observations may be helpful, but if negative does not exclude it. Sometimes the diagnosis can be established only after follow-up. Especially in chronic cases, it is of great value for the patient if rheumatoid arthritis or ankylosing spondylitis can be excluded. Chronic reactive arthritis can be like rheumatoid arthritis.

Psoriatic arthropathy may resemble reactive arthritis, but collectively radiography, history, and observation over a period of time yields the correct diagnosis.

3.5 Epidemiology and Historical Data

Because the clinical severity varies greatly and milder cases apparently go unnoticed, the true incidence of reactive arthritis is hard to assess. Certainly, increasing awareness of reactive arthritis as a diagnostic possibility will increase the number of cases recognized. According to a Finnish estimation, the incidence of seronegative oligoarthritis (probably often reactive arthritis) is 40 per 100,000. Reactive arthritis has been described from several countries and can be assumed to affect people all around the world. Rheumatic fever, also a type of reactive arthritis, occurs often in developing countries but has practically disappeared elsewhere.

Reactive arthritis affects males and females with the same frequency. Typically it is a disorder of young adults, rare in small children and in old people. Most of the patients are aged between 20 and 40 years. Genetic factors play a role in susceptibility to the disease. Most patients report relatives who have had a similar disease. Patients with reactive arthritis are positive for HLA B27 in 65–96% of cases. Conversely, persons with the HLA B27 antigen have a strongly increased risk of developing reactive arthritis. The association is not absolute: HLA B27–positive individuals do not always get reactive arthritis even after a suitable triggering infection, and it can occur even in HLA B27–negative individuals.

The frequency of reactive arthritis following enteric infections due to *Salmonella*, *Shigella*, and *Campylobacter* has been reported to be 1–4% in unselected populations. In some yersiniosis outbreaks the frequency of this complication has been quite high and in others negligible.

3.6 Pathophysiology

There is no disagreement regarding the etiology of reactive arthritis: it is a response to infection. With increasing awareness of this condition, the list of causative agents is still growing. Although effort has been made to characterize the microorganisms linked to reactive arthritis, no common or definite feature has so far emerged. Many of the bacteria implicated are gram-negative, have cell membranes that contain lipopolysaccharide and peptidoglycan, and are intracellularly invasive, i.e., able to enter cells and to survive (and even multiple) intracellularly. Many are quite common in the environment, and infection does not necessarily lead to reactive arthritis. In most instances, the triggering infection affects the throat, the intestine, or the urogenital tract. Therefore it appears that mucosal immune defense mechanisms must be of importance, but how and why are not known. The frequency of reactive arthritis in connection with outbreaks of *Yersinia*, *Salmonella*, and *Shigella* varies quite considerably. The evidence implies that some features of a microbe are important for its arthritogenicity.

The term reactive arthritis acknowledges the facts that the joint inflammation develops some time after the actual triggering infection and that the causative agent cannot be isolated from the site of inflammation. This strongly suggests that a breakdown of immunologic defense mechanisms plays a central role.

The role of HLA B27 is of interest. Although not all HLA B27–positive individuals develop reactive arthritis after a suitable triggering infection whereas some negative individuals may do so, this tissue antigen undisputably is associated with reactive arthritis. It has been suggested that the granulocytes of HLA B27–positive individuals would be especially active metabolically, perhaps thus enhancing an inflammatory response. Another very plausible possibility is that HLA B27 would lead to an aberrant immune response by presenting the HLA B27–specific (microbe-derived?) peptides to helper T cells, leading to recognition of autoantigens by cytotoxic T cells.

A hypothesis much studied and discussed has been that HLA B27 could act as a receptor for a microbial antigen, which would modify the HLA B27 antigen to be a target for harmful immune response.

Another theory that has gained wide attention is that of molecular mimicry, i.e., that the microorganisms share a structure with the HLA B27 molecule. The role of HLA B27 remains unclear. Recent studies on the immune response suggest that in patients with reactive arthritis the microorganism may persist somewhere in the body, e.g., in the intestinal mucosa or in the mesenteric lymph nodes. Furthermore, microbial components might actually enter the site of inflammation itself, i.e., the synovium or the synovial fluid.

Currently it seems, therefore, that reactive arthritis involves persistence of the triggering microorganisms in the host and the spread of its components either as parts of immune complexes or within phagocytosing cells into the joints, where they activate the inflammatory cascade. This would explain the inflammation of many different sites. However, many questions remain unanswered. The relation of infection microbial and antigen persistence and the development of autoimmunity is illustrated in Fig. 3.3.

3.7 Management

3.7.1 Articular Disease

Nonsteroidal antiinflammatory drugs (NSAIDs) form the basis of therapy. They should be used regularly over some time in order to achieve maximum antiinflammatory effect, and patients should be informed of this; otherwise

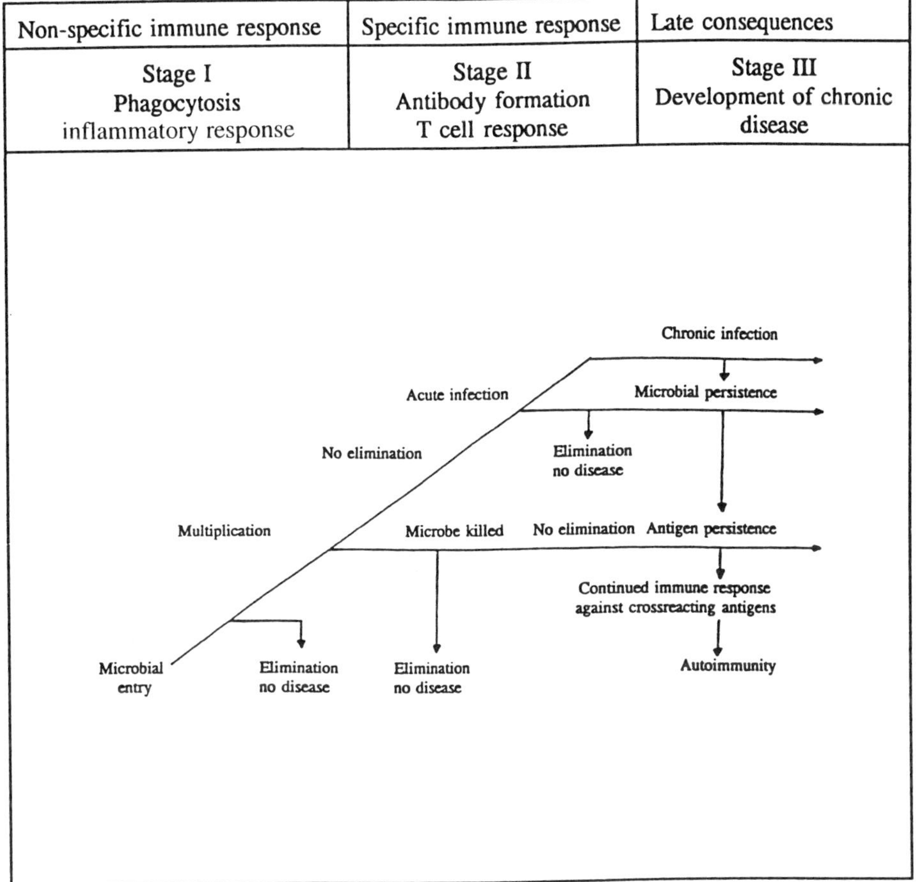

Figure 3.3 Relationship of infection, microbial and antigen persistence, and autoimmunity.

they consider the drug as an analgesic. There is no definite drug of choice because patients' responses differ.

Corticosteroids may be a valuable asset in the treatment of reactive arthritis. In many cases, intraarticular administration gives prompt relief. However, purulent arthritis must be excluded before the injection. Systemic treatment with low-dose corticosteroids may be of benefit. They should be used in cases in which NSAIDs have not had a sufficient effect and when many joints are affected. Oral corticosteroids should be withdrawn slowly while continuing NSAIDs. Corticosteroids should not be used more than for 2–4 months. Antibiotic treatment should be given if a microbe is isolated. However, this is more to diminish spread of the infection than to influence the ongoing course of the disease. All of the available information indicates that at the time of the first joint symptoms—when the patient usually comes to the physician—the pathogenic process cannot be reversed. The new quinolones offer a good alternative to the trimethoprim-sulfamethoxazole or tetracyclines often used. For streptococcal throat infection, penicillin or erythromycin are the drugs of choice. Recently lymecycline, administered for 3 months, has been studied and found to have some beneficial effect in patients with *Chlamydia*-triggered disease. Currently, further studies on the value of long-term antibiotic therapy in reactive arthritis are underway.

Physical therapy using cold pads may alleviate the pain and edema of an inflamed joint. Rest is advisable, and splinting may be used to alleviate pain at night. However, immobilization should not be complete, with some periods of gentle exercises daily. In severe cases, muscle wasting may be a problem and systematic rehabilitation may be required. During convalescence many patients tend to stop the analgesics too early; it is better to use them until pain no longer inhibits full use of muscles and joints, in order to ensure a good end result.

Sulfasalazine is of interest because of the observations that patients with reactive arthritis often have more or less asymptomatic inflammation of the bowel. In some instances, it may give good results. The drug should be started at low dose, increasing to 2 g or even 3 g if tolerated by the patient. Unfortunately, some patients cannot continue with the drug because of gastrointestinal intolerance.

The possibility of microbial persistence has opened the question of whether long-term antibiotic treatment should be used in chronic reactive arthritis. For rheumatic fever, permanent penicillin prophylaxis is commonly used to prevent relapses.

3.7.2 Extraarticular Disease

Ocular inflammations must be diagnosed and treated promptly to prevent irreversible damage to the eyesight. If possible, the patient should be referred to an ophthalmologist because the diagnosis of uveitis requires use of a slit lamp. Therapy consists of corticosteroids in the form of eye drops or even systemically, and of mydriatics. The patient should be informed about the strong possibility of recurrence.

Including the carditis of rheumatic fever, the most common cardiac complications are conduction disturbance. In these instances a cardiac pacemaker is often required when indicated.

The nephritis that can be associated with reactive arthritis is usually mild, subsides spontaneously, and does not require any treatment. The skin lesions, which by many dermatologists are considered identical to psoriasis, are treated accordingly. In mild cases keratinolytic agents, such as salicylic acid ointment or topical corticosteroid, may be used. In more severe cases, the patient is best referred to a dermatologist; retinoids or methotrexate are most commonly used (Table 3.6).

Impact of Disease and Prognosis. The prognosis of reactive arthritis is generally good. The duration of the disease varies from a few days to several weeks. Even patients who are severely incapacitated and bedridden can look forward to full recovery. However, recurrences are frequent, and they can be triggered not only by new infections but also by nonspecific stress factors. Urogenital and eye inflammations particularly have a tendency to recur. Many patients complain of abdominal discomfort and occasional diarrhea for months and even years after the initial attack of the disease. Back pain and arthralgia are common; also frank synovitis may be seen. Tendonitis and enthesopathy may lead to erosion or proliferation of bone at the tendon insertions. These joint symptoms may be precipitated by rather nonspecific factors, such as changes in the weather, and many patients report discomfort during the fall and winter seasons. Conversely, a new infection by bacteria known to trigger the disease may pass without any sequelae. The nonsymptomatic period between recurrences may last for several years.

Follow-up studies of reactive arthritis suggest that 20–70% of patients later suffer some joint discomfort or other symptoms. For the individual patient it is important to know that, in spite of unpleasant symptoms, severe destructive disease as a sequel of reactive arthritis is extremely rare. Observations of sacroiliitis and radiologic findings suggest that ankylosing spondylitis can occur, but even in these cases the disease usually remains mild.

Table 3.6 Treatment of Reactive Arthritis

Antibiotics if infection is still present
Rest
Nonsteroidal antiinflammatory drugs
Intraarticular corticosteroids
Rarely: systemic steroids
In chronic cases: sulfasalazine

3.8 Atypical Forms

3.8.1 Acute Rheumatic Fever

Definition (Table 3.7). An acute systemic inflammatory condition that follows a group A β-hemolytic streptococcal infection and may involve joints, heart, skin, central nervous system, and subcutaneous tissue. The most relevant clinical manifestations are polyarthritis, carditis, subcutaneous nodules, Sydenham's chorea, and erythema marginatum.

Main Clinical Features. Acute rheumatic fever occurs most frequently in children age 5–20 years and is characterized by fever, migratory arthritis for 4–6 weeks, erythema marginatum, and, in some, destructive inflammatory lesions within the myocardium, endocardium, pericardium, heart valves, joint, periarticular regions, lungs, subcutaneous tissues, and, rarely, chorea.

Confirming the Diagnosis—Investigations. Laboratory studies used to confirm the diagnosis of rheumatic fever are serologic studies confirming recent A group of streptococcal infection—residual elevation of antistreptococcal antibodies such as ASO or anti-DNA-ase β levels. However, it is important to recognize that high titers of these antibodies may be seen in the absence of acute rheumatic fever.

Leukocytosis, ESR, and CRP often remain elevated long after clinical signs have returned to normal. An ECG will frequently show conduction disturbance, with slight or moderate lengthening of the P-R interval. Chest X ray and echocardiography will demonstrate heart involvement and active carditis.

Establishing an accurate diagnosis of acute rheumatic fever is often difficult but has been aided considerably by application of the revised Jones criteria (Table 3.8).

Diagnostic Difficulties. The differential diagnosis of acute rheumatic fever has been expanding. Particularly when polyarthritis is the main presenting problem, other possibilities to be considered include reactive arthritis, ankylosing spondylitis, gonococcal arthritis, subacute bacterial

Table 3.7 Acute Rheumatic Fever

Acute migrating reactive arthritis in children
Now rare in developed countries
Post–group A streptococcal infection: angina
Carditis, heart valve involvement, and chorea may be associated
Prognosis determined by cardiac sequellae/lesions
Prophylaxis for recurrence is important

Table 3.8 Jones Criteria (Revised) for Guidance in the Diagnosis of Rheumatic Fever

Major manifestations	Minor manifestations
Carditis	Clinical
Polyarthritis	Fever
Chorea	Arthralgia
Erthyem marginatum	Previous rheumatic fever
Subcutaneous nodules	or rheumatic heart disease

Plus:

Supporting evidence of preceding streptococcal infection:
    Increased ASO or other streptococcal antibodies
    Positive throat culture for group A streptococcus
    Recent scarlet fever

The presence of two major criteria, or of one major and two minor criteria, indicates a high probability of the presence of rheumatic fever if supported by evidence of a preceding streptococcal infection. The absence of the latter should make the diagnosis suspect, except in situations in which rheumatic fever is first discovered after a long latent period after the antecedent infection (e.g., Sydenham's chorea or low-grade carditis).

endocarditis, Lyme disease, viral infections, acute leukemia, Still's disease, and serum sickness. When carditis is the outstanding feature, additional diagnostic considerations include congenital lesions, mitral valve prolapse, infection with *Yersinia enterocolitica*, viral myocarditis, Lyme disease, and SLE with valvular disease. In all of these situations, evidence of a prior streptococcal infection strongly suggests a diagnosis of acute rheumatic fever, particularly if there is a curve with rising titer of antibodies. The possibility of a coincidental streptococcal infection with another disease must always be considered.

Epidemiology and Historical Data. The incidence of rheumatic fever has declined steadily in the last decades, leading to the near disappearance of the disease in developed countries. In the poorer areas of the world and in (certain) developed countries, incidence has been substantially reduced, although in some of them its frequency is still high.

A steep descent in mortality began before the introduction of antibiotics and was attributed to general improvement in health conditions, less crowding, and better access to medical care. Additional elements could be related to changes in host susceptibility and modifications in the virulence of streptococci. With the advent of penicillin and clear treatment guidelines for streptococcal pharyngitis, the number of cases diminished even further.

Recently, several outbreaks have occurred in the United States. The cause of this resurgence is not clear, but the reappearance of heavily encapsulated, highly virulent rheumatogenic streptococcal strains may be important. Also, a decrease in the general awareness of the disease and the relaxation of some epidemiologic control measures, particularly related to prophylaxis in large groups, may have contributed to a resurgence of acute rheumatic fever.

Pathophysiology. A link between streptococci and acute rheumatic fever has been clearly established both clinically and epidemiologically. The incidence of an acute rheumatic episode after a streptococcal pharyngitis is in the range of 0.5–3%. Although the pharyngeal infection may be clinically inapparent, it can be documented by culture or increasing antibody titers to diverse streptococcal antigens in 95% of patients. Furthermore, appropriate treatment clearly prevents the disease as well as its recurrences. Interestingly, skin or other types of streptococcal infections usually do not cause the disease.

Acute rheumatic fever represents one of the most well-documented instances of molecular mimicry between a foreign agent and autologous host tissue. A large number of antigens or components of group A streptococci have been shown to cross-react directly with various human tissues. The mechanism whereby this molecular mimicry induces acute rheumatic fever remains incompletely understood. The most straightforward explanation would be that components of the streptococcus, such as the streptococcal membrane, the group-specific glycoprotein, or carbohydrate components, induce both a humoral and a cell-mediated immune response which may cross react directly with vulnerable autologous host tissues. For example, this may involve sarcoplasmic membranes within myocardial cells and valvular connective tissues, inducing a pancarditis, or even neurons within the caudate nucleus of the brain, inducing chorea.

Management. Eradication of the β-hemolytic streptococci, symptomatic treatment of acute disease manifestations, and medicosurgical treatment of cardiac sequelae are the main goals in the management of patients with rheumatic fever. The standard form of therapy involves suppression of inflammation with antiinflammatory drugs and simultaneous elimination of any concomitant or residual β-hemolytic streptococcal pharyngeal infection. Salicylates given in adequate doses are effective at suppressing signs of inflammatory reactions in many patients, and a dramatic positive response is usually observed 12–24 hr after therapeutic blood levels (20–30 mg/dl) have been attained. Initial dosages are usually 80–100 mg/kg/day in children and 4–8 g/day in adults. Other nonsteroidal antiinflammatory agents may be equally effective. The use of corticosteroids is generally unnecessary for arthritis alone, and their overall long-term benefit in the treatment of carditis is not established. Bedrest or diminished physical activity may be required until virtually all signs of active carditis subside.

After the diagnosis is firmly established, eradication of infection is achieved by a single dose of intramuscular benzathine penicillin (600,000 units in children or 1.2 million in adults). An alternative is oral phenoxymethyl penicillin (250,000 units 4 times daily for 10 days) if appropriate compliance is assured. Erythromycin is a choice in those allergic to penicillin. Sulfa derivatives do not eradicate the streptococcus from the pharynx and are not recommended.

Secondary prophylaxis, a major breakthrough in the control of the disease, is extremely important. It should be carefully planned, once the acute stage has been adequately controlled, to avoid recurrences or further cardiac damage by repeated infections. Prophylaxis is achieved with monthly benzathine penicillin (1.2 million units by intramuscular injection). In highly endemic areas or in patients with severe cardiac sequelae, it has been suggested that prophylaxis should be repeated every 3 weeks. Oral phenoxymethyl penicillin (250,000 units daily) can also be used in compliant patients.

Depending on the weight of the patient, sulfadiazine (500–1000 mg/day orally) is the treatment of choice in individuals who are allergic to penicillin. Duration of secondary prophylaxis is a crucial question. Although there is no absolute consensus, some guidelines are firmly established and should be followed.

It is well known that the risk of a new episode of rheumatic fever is higher within the first 5 years following an acute attack, and all patients should have prophylaxis at least during this period of time or until they reach 18 years of age. In those patients who have had carditis, but without residual valvular damage, prophylaxis may be prolonged particularly if they live in poor or crowded areas and are at high risk of repeated streptococcal infections. When chronic valvular sequelae are present, prophylaxis should be indefinite or until the chances of recurrence are definitely reduced. Prophylaxis is also indicated in patients with chorea, in whom the same principles can be applied. In addition, it should be maintained after cardiac surgery. Secondary prophylaxis requires special follow-up, and attention has to be given to patients at high risk to maximize adherence.

Impact of Disease and Prognosis. The course followed by a patient after a first attack of rheumatic fever is highly variable and unpredictable. Ninety percent of the episodes last less than 3 months, and only a minority persist longer in the form of unremittent rheumatic carditis or prolonged chorea. Established mitral regurgitation, aortic insufficiency, or mitral stenosis are the most important chronic consequences of acute rheumatic fever. Their frequency is higher in patients who have more than one episode of the disease, so that 50–100% have valvular damage after two or more recurrences. A minority of patients following an acute bout present with an unremitting course leading to multiple valvular disease and cardiac failure. Permanent cardiac sequelae frequently require both medical and surgical procedures, such as mitral valve replacement.

Sydenham's chorea is usually a late neurologic event of an acute rheumatic episode, appearing weeks or months after a streptococcal infection when other symptoms have abated. Its frequency has declined in recent years affecting 5–10% of all patients.

3.8.2 Reiter's Syndrome

Definition (Table 3.9).   Historically a reactive arthritis characterized by the triad urethritis, conjunctivitis, and arthritis has been called Reiter's syndrome. In French-speaking countries it is also called Fiessinger–Le Roy syndrome. It has become clear that Reiter's syndrome develops in genetically susceptible host (HLA B27 +) following an infection by bacteria such as *Chlamydia trachomatis* in the genitourinary tract or by *Salmonella, Shigella, Yersinia*, or *Campylobacter* in the gastrointestinal tract.

Main Clinical Features.   Arthritis and local inflammation of insertion of a tendon, ligament, or articular capsule into bone (enthesopathy) typically appear within 1–3 weeks of the inciting urethritis or diarrhea. Constitutional symptoms are usually mild. Joint stiffness of the lower limbs, myalgia, and low back pain are prominent symptoms.

UROGENITAL TRACT.   Men experience increased frequency of a burning during urination. Examination of the penis revels meatal erythema and edema, and a clear mucoid discharge can be expressed. Pyuria is best detected in a first-void urine. Prostatitis is common and has been reported in up to 80% of patients. Hemorrhagic cystitis may develop and may clear spontaneously. Silent cystitis or cervicitis without urethritis may be the only urogenital involvement in women; salpingitis and vulvovaginitis have also been reported.

Urogenital symptoms do not necessarily indicate infection at that site. Patients who develop postdysenteric Reiter's syndrome may experience a sterile urethritis within 1–2 weeks of the initial bout of diarrhea. It is therefore difficult at times to determine whether the arthritis is postdysenteric or postvenereal.

Table 3.9   Reiter's Syndrome

Reactive arthritis with triad: urethritis (cervicitis), conjunctivitis, arthritis
More often in males than in females
Oligoarthritis lower limbs
Osteitis may occur
Strongly associated with HLA B27

MUCOUS MEMBRANES AND THE SKIN. Two characteristic sites of lesions, on the penis and on the skin, are diagnostic of Reiter's syndrome. Small shallow painless ulcers of the glans penis and urethral meatus, termed balanitis circinata, have been described in 25% of post-*Chlamydia* and post-*Shigella* Reiter's syndrome.

Keratodermia blenorrhagica is a hyperkeratotic skin lesion that is seen in 12–14% of patients. It begins as clear vesicles on erythematous bases and progresses to macules, papules, and then to small keratotic nodules (Fig. 3.4). The lesions are frequently found on the soles of the feet but may involve the toes, scrotum, palms, penis, trunk, and scalp. They cannot be distinguished either clinically or microscopically from pustular psoriasis, and their presence or course does not predict or correlate with the course of the disease. The keratotic material also accumulates under the nail and lifts it from the nailbed (onycholysis).

EYE. In 40% of patients there is unilateral or bilateral apparently noninfectious conjunctivitis. This most often occurs early in the disease and is usually mild as well as transient. A more significant involvement is uveitis that is acute and unilateral; however, subsequent attacks may also affect the other eye.

Confirming the Diagnosis—Investigations. The first group of *laboratory tests* to be considered consists of those that attempt to document the

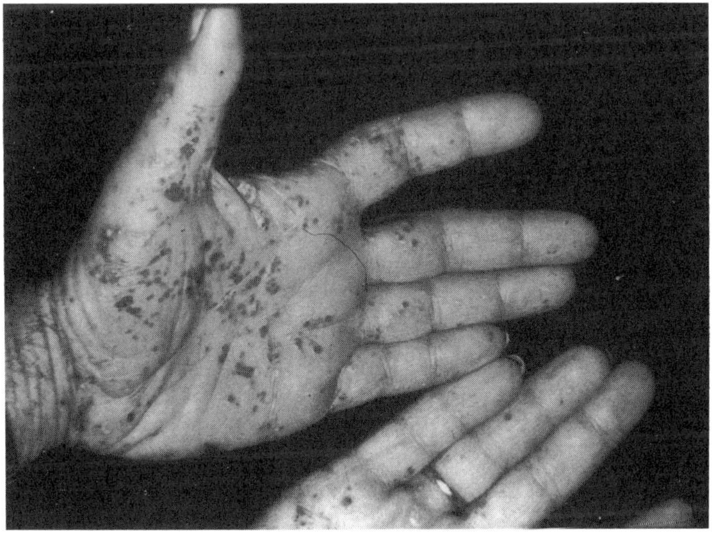

Figure 3.4 Keratodermia blenorrhagica.

urethritis (cell count in first and second urinary void) and the presence of a specific bacterial infection. Since chronic antimicrobial therapy is possibly beneficial in *Chlamydia*-induced Reiter's syndrome, it is now important to look for *Chlamydia* in every case of Reiter's syndrome or to treat empirically as culture techniques are unreliable. *Chlamydia trachomatis* is an obligate intracellular parasite that cannot be grown on artificial media. It is better to submit urethral swabs and cervical cytobrushings for either direct fluorescent antibody and enzyme immunoassay tests or preferably DNA probe for chlamydial ribosomal RNA. Stool cultures are useful for confirming the diagnosis of infection by an appropriate triggering microbe even when bowel symptoms are unapparent or mild, and these can support the diagnosis of reactive arthritis in an otherwise undefined case.

The second group of laboratory tests reflects the presence of inflammation. A moderate neutrophilic leukocytosis, elevated ESR, and CRP are common during the acute illness.

Synovial biopsies show nonspecific inflammatory changes. HLA B27 typing is helpful when characteristic extraarticular features are absent. HLA B27 is positive in 80% of Reiter's syndrome cases. There is increasing evidence that the possession of the HLA B27 antigen correlates with axial disease, carditis, and uveitis.

Radiologic findings can be found only in the late stage. Soft tissue swelling is prominent around affected joints. Sacroiliitis occurs in 10% of patients with early disease. Its presence can confirm the diagnosis of Reiter's syndrome in a patient with a suggestive asymmetric oligoarthritis. Eventually up to 70% of patients with chronic Reiter's syndrome show either unilateral (early) or bilateral (late) sacroiliac abnormalities. Asymmetric paravertebral comma-shaped ossification is a distinctive finding in Reiter's syndrome and psoriatic arthritis, typically involving the lower three thoracic and upper three lumbar vertebrae. Squaring of vertebrae is uncommon, but bone density is surprisingly well preserved even in chronic disease. Joint space narrowing is often restricted to the small joints of the hands and feet where erosions with indistinct margins and fluffy periostitis can be seen. Linear periostitis occurs along metacarpal, metatarsal, and phalangeal shafts, and exuberant periosteal spurs can be seen at the calcaneus, ischial tuberosity, and trochanter.

Diagnostic Difficulties.   Because of the skin and nail lesions as keratodermia and onycholysis, Reiter's syndrome in particular in cases with incomplete triad with asymptomatic urethritis can be confused with psoriatic arthritis or with enteropathic arthritis.

Reiter's syndrome can be associated with human immunodeficiency virus (HIV) infection and symptoms of arthritis may precede any overt sign of acquired immune deficiency syndrome (AIDS).

Epidemiology and Historical Data. Reiter's syndrome was reported initially during the First World War (1914–1918). Reiter's and Fiessinger–Leroy were military doctors. The incidence of Reiter's syndrome has not been well documented because of the variable nature of its presentation. In Rochester, during epidemics of enteric infections with *Shigella* and *Salmonella*, 1–4% of unselected populations subsequently develop arthritis. Reiter's syndrome has been reported worldwide, but it is rare in blacks.

Reiter's syndrome is rarely seen in children; most reported cases are postenteric rather than postvenereal. Traditionally it has been claimed that Reiter's syndrome is 20 times more common in men than in women. With the recognition that the initiating infectious episode might be silent cystitis or cervicitis, the male-to-female ratio is more likely 5 : 1. Postdysenteric reactive arthritis shows an equal sex distribution.

Pathophysiology. Reiter's syndrome is considered to be one of the typical examples of reactive arthritis to an infection associated with a genetic host susceptibility, in particular HLA B27 antigen (see Section 3).

Impact of Disease and Prognosis. The natural history of Reiter's syndrome is highly variable and probably related to the particular infective organism and host factors, including the presence or absence of HLA B27. Most patients experience recurrent symptomatic episodes of arthritis lasting for several weeks to 6 months. A few patients have only a single self-limiting period of arthritis, but 15–50% have recurrent bouts. Recent evidence suggests that recurrent arthritis may be caused by unapparent chlamydial infection of the synovium. The presence of heel pain has been reported to correlate with a poorer prognosis. A few patients (3%) may develop axial disease indistinguishable from ankylosing spondylitis. About 20% develop chronic peripheral or axial arthritis and may become unemployed or be forced to change their occupations. The presence of HLA B27 correlates with persistent low back pain and sacroiliitis but not residual symptoms in peripheral joints.

3.8.3 Whipple's Disease

Definition (Table 3.10). Whipple's disease is characterized by polyarthritis, steatorrhea, and weight loss and is probably a form of enterogenic arthritis caused by an infection of the intestine.

Main Clinical Features. The arthritis is polyarticular, symmetrical, and usually transient, but it may become chronic. The joint symptoms may antedate the intestinal complaints by more than 5 years. Arthritis flares are not related temporally to exacerbation of intestinal symptoms. The main intestinal symptoms are diarrhea with steatorrhea and weight loss.

Confirming the Diagnosis – Investigations. Acute phase reactants are elevated. Rheumatoid factor is negative. The diagnosis is based on

Table 3.10 Whipple's Disease

Polyarthritis associated with steatorrhea and weight loss
Nonerosive polyarthritis antedating gastrointestinal symptoms by years
PAS+ staining in macrophages of small intestine
Cured with antibiotics

microscopic examination of small intestine. Characteristic periodic acid–
Schiff (PAS) staining deposits are found in the macrophages of the small
intestine and in the mesenteric nodes. These cells also contain rod-shaped
free bacilli best seen by electron microscopy.

Diagnostic Difficulties. When no gastrointestinal symptoms are
present, the polyarthritis is usually diagnosed as seronegative rheumatoid
arthritis, rarely erosive. Later in the course of the disease—sometimes years
later when steatorrhea occurs—the diagnosis of Whipple's disease should
be considered and intestinal biopsy studies performed.

Epidemiology and Historical Data. Whipple's disease is rare and
was first described by G. H. Whipple in 1907.

Pathophysiology. The rod-shaped fine bacilli in the macrophage of
the small intestine are considered to be the etiologic agent because they
disappear when the patients are successfully treated with antibiotics. Phylo-
genetic analysis showed the bacteria to be a gram-positive actinomycete
that is being designated *Tropheryma whippelii*. Some synovial morphologic
studies suggest that joint can also be directly invaded by the causative agent.

Management. A correct diagnosis is important, as the condition responds well to appropriate antibiotic therapy, usually tetracycline 1 g/day,
which must be continued for more than a year.

3.8.4 Erythema Nodosum and Arthritis

Definition (Table 3.11). Arthritis associated with an acute tender
and nodular skin eruption with marked erythema and bruising as a consequence of inflammation of subcutaneous fat. Erythema nodosum and ar-

Table 3.11 Erythema Nodosum and Arthritis

Acute arthritis lower limbs associated with erythema nodosum
Triggered by multiple hypersensitivity factors
Often seen in association with sarcoidosis
Self-limited course

thritis can be triggered by infection, drugs, sarcoidosis, and rarely, neoplasia (Table 3.12).

Main Clinical Features. Cutaneous nodules 1–10 cm in diameter occur on extensor aspects of the legs (Fig. 3.5). The eruption lasts for 6–8 weeks. Fever, polyarthralgia, ankle synovitis, and hilar adenopathy are often associated. The synovitis usually resolves with the skin lesions; joint pain and stiffness may persist for up to 6 months but resolves eventually. The acute arthropathy of erythema nodosum is readily distinguishable from the persistent anthropathy of chronic sarcoidosis.

Confirming the Diagnosis—Investigations. In 75% of patients with erythema nodosum, the ESR is raised to 50 mm/hr or more and will fall to normal once the rash has resolved. Further investigations are required to establish the cause, as the diagnosis of the skin lesions is usually apparent. Virologic and *Yersinia* titers may be helpful. The chest radiograph may be abnormal, with bilateral hilar lymphadenopathy found in 20–50%. The combination of erythema nodosum and bilateral hilar lymphadenopathy is a form of acute sarcoidosis that has an excellent prognosis, as there is usually a complete resolution of the adenopathy within 12 months in 90% of cases and only a few will progress to a more chronic sarcoidosis. Histologic examination of palpable lymph nodes, when present, will often confirm the diagnosis. Measurement of serum angiotensin converting enzyme is not discriminatory in establishing the diagnosis of sacroidosis in the presence of erythema nodosum and hilar lymphadenopathy.

In erythema nodosum triggered by streptococcal infection, there is usually a history of sore throat preceding the eruption, and significant

Table 3.12   Associations with Erythema Nodosum

Medications
    Sulfonamides, estrogen, oral contraceptives
Infections
    Bacterial: *Streptococcus*, tuberculosis, *Yersinia*, leprosy, *Leptospirosis*, tularemia, cat scratch disease
    Fungal: Coccidioidomycosis, blastomycosis, histoplasmosis, dermatophytes
    Viral: Paravaccinia, infectious mononucleosis
Sarcoidosis
Inflammatory bowel disease
Malignancy
    Lymphoma and leukemia, postirradiation therapy
Behçet's syndrome
Pregnancy

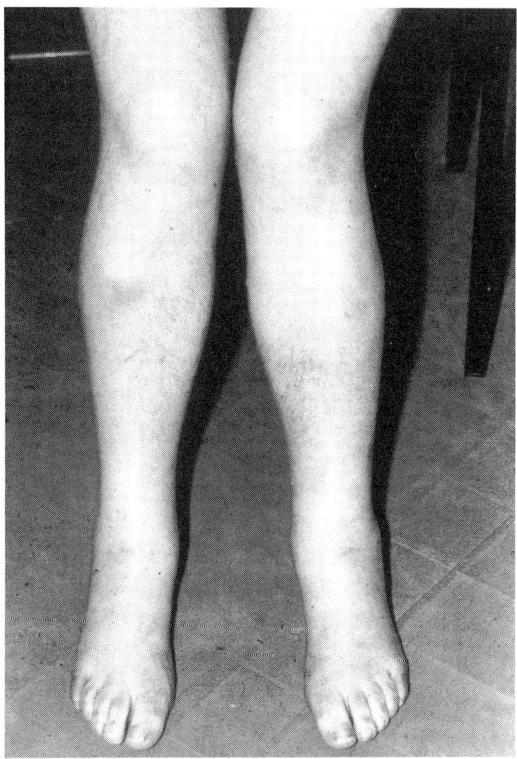

Figure 3.5   Erythema nodosum on lower limbs.

infection is confirmed by a rise in antistreptolysin O titer. Although uncommon in industrialized societies, active tuberculosis should be considered, especially in children under 5 years old. In children and adults with active tuberculosis, the Mantoux test will be strongly positive. In contrast, the Mantoux is usually negative when erythema nodosum and hilar lymphadenopathy are the manifestations of acute sarcoidosis.

In those with hilar lymphadenopathy, follow-up chest radiography should be performed to monitor status and document resolution. If the lymph nodes fail to diminish in size or enlarge, a lymphoproliferative disorder should be considered, although, fortunately, erythema nodosum as a manifestation of neoplasia is unusual.

Diagnostic Difficulties.   The early lesion of erythema nodosum is commonly mistaken for insect bites by those who have not seen the skin disorder before. Otherwise, erythema nodosum is distinct and normally is easily distinguished from other causes of subcutaneous fat inflammation. Erythema nodosum does not ulcerate and heals without a scar, and these properties should distinguish the lesion clinically from vasculitic lesions such as nodular vasculitis and polyarteritis nodosa. *Weber–Christian disease*, a widespread vasculitic disease of subcutaneous fat, differs from erythema nodosum in that punched-out lesions of fat necrosis, situated predominantly over the buttocks, occur with scarring. Widespread fat necrosis of skin is occasionally seen in acute pancreatitis, in which case the symptoms of pancreatitis itself should provide the diagnosis. A biopsy of the lesion should be diagnostic.

Epidemiology.　The annual incidence per 100.000 is 2–3. The rash is more common in women (F/M ratio 4 : 1) and occurs in young people 25–40 years old.

Pathophysiology.　Erythema nodosum is a form of cell-mediated hypersensitivity initiated by circulating immune complexes. Cellular hypersensitivity results from an exaggerated interreaction between antigen and cell-mediated immune mechanisms, exemplified by the formation of granulomata.

Management and Prognosis.　Erythema nodosum is generally an acute, self-limiting disease. Treatment of any underlying condition is appropriate. NSAIDs and, occasionally, oral glucocorticosteroids can be helpful. The prognosis is usually good but will be determined by the underlying condition.

3.8.5 Lyme Arthritis

Definition (Table 3.13).　Lyme arthritis is a disease named for a small town in the state of Connecticut in the United States, in which the disease was initially recognized. Lyme disease results from infection with a spirochete, *Borrelia burgdorferi*, which is transmitted through a tick vector.

Table 3.13　Lyme Arthritis

Borrelia burgdorferi infection
Transmitted by tick bite — forest area
Erythema chronicum migrans
Arthralgia — oligoarthritis
Chronic synovitis knee
Carditis
Meningitis — encephalitis
Cure by antibiotic therapy

Main Clinical Features.

EARLY MANIFESTATIONS.   The early manifestation of Lyme disease is
a characteristic skin rash known as erythema chronicum migrans, generally
seen in a proximal extremity or the trunk, especially in the thigh, buttocks,
or axilla. This lesion begins in a red macule or papule that extends to form
an annular lesion, as large as 5 cm in diameter.

The annular lesion has an intensely red outer border that is usually
flat, a middle area showing partial clearing, and a center that is sometimes
indurated in a deeper red. Occasionally, the lesion remains intensely reddish
showing secondary rings within the initial one. Nearly half the patients who
develop the initial lesion develop smaller additional lesions that lack an
indurated center. During resolution, evanescent lesions may occur.

There is no mucosal involvement. Lesions may produce a burning
sensation and be hot to the touch. They usually last for a few weeks and
then regress. Skin lesions are seen in about three quarters of patients who
ultimately develop arthritis, generally preceding the arthritis by at least a
few weeks to several months, although the interval may be as long as 2
years. About one patient in five remembers a tick bite, generally a week to
1 month prior to the appearance of erythema chronicum migrans.

If musculoskeletal symptoms occur early in the illness, the typical
pattern is one of migratory pain in joints, tendons, bursae, muscles, or
bones. The pain is usually without joint swelling and lasts for hours or
several days in one or two occasions at a time. Three stages of Lyme disease
are described. In the first stage the symptoms are mainly skin lesions and
arthralgia (Table 3.14).

LATE MANIFESTATIONS.   Late manifestations of Lyme disease include
stage II arthritis and cardiac lesions, and stage III neurologic problems.

Months later, about 60% of untreated patients in the United States
develop frank arthritis. The typical pattern is brief, intermittent attacks of
monoarticular or oligoarticular arthritis in a few large joints, especially
knees. Although the pattern varies, episodes of arthritis often become

Table 3.14 Stages of Lyme Disease

Stage	Organ involved	Clinical findings
I	Skin	Erythema chronicum migrans arthralgia
II	Joints	Oligoarthritis
	Heart	Carditis
III	Nervous system	Neurologic

longer during the second or third years of illness, lasting for months rather than weeks. In about 10% of these patients, chronic arthritis — defined as 1 year or more of continual joint inflammation — begins during this period. Chronic Lyme arthritis, which usually affects only one or both knees, may lead to erosion of cartilage and bone. Even among patients with chronic arthritis, objective joint swelling lasting longer than 5 or 6 years is rare, although brief episodes of joint pain may still occur after the period of frank arthritis. A few patients have been reported with osteomyelitis, panniculitis, or myositis.

Cardiac abnormalities are also seen, primarily in young males. Two thirds of patients who develop heart disease Lyme carditis also have joint involvement, equally divided between polyarthritis and oligoarthritis. Cardiac involvement generally occurs about 3 weeks after the skin rash, presenting with either a rapid or slow heart rate. On electrocardiogram, 18 of 20 patients had atrioventricular (AV) block.

Neurologic sequelae of Lyme disease are seen generally 2–8 months after the initial erythema chronicum migrans. The most common neurologic finding was meningismus, manifested by headache, stiff neck, nausea, vomiting, photophobia, developing over several weeks. Cerebrospinal fluid may contain up to 450 leukocytes, most of which are lymphocytes. Encephalitis was the next most common symptom, manifested by somnolence, emotional lability, depression, poor memory, behavioral changes, and chorea. These patients had an abnormal electroencephalogram (EEG). Cranial neuritis, including multiple cranial neuropathies, was seen in about half of patients.

Confirming the Diagnosis — Investigations.

EARLY PHASE.   The diagnosis of early Lyme disease is based primarily on the rash of erythema chronicum migrans. It cannot be based on a serologic tests for *Borrelia* because 5% of the normal population has a positive test for Lyme disease, indicating that most people who have positive serology do not have the disease. If erythema chronicum migrans is seen, a positive IgM antibody for *Borrelia burgdorferi* will confirm the diagnosis. However, patients with other spirochetal diseases, including syphilis, relapsing fever, leptospirosis, infectious mononucleosis, as well as many normal individuals, may cross-react and have false-positive serologic results.

LATE PHASE.   All patients with stage II or III disease have IgG antibodies to *B. burgdorferi*. However, again 5% of the general population, including people with rheumatoid arthritis (RA), have antibodies that are reactive with the *Borrelia* and do not have Lyme disease. Therefore, the diagnosis of Lyme disease must be established on the basis of clinical criteria and the laboratory tests must be consistent with the diagnosis.

Diagnostic Difficulties.

DIFFERENTIAL DIAGNOSIS. The differential diagnosis of Lyme disease includes any type of inflammatory arthritis, including RA, although Lyme arthritis generally is an oligoarthritis. Reiter's syndrome, or other forms of oligoarthritis, villonodular synovitis, and chronic meniscus lesions, must be included in the differential diagnosis.

Epidemiology and Historical Data. Lyme disease occurs primarily in endemic areas which, in the United States, include Connecticut, Massachusetts, Rhode Island, New Jersey, Delaware, Wisconsin, and Minnesota. All of these areas have a population of ticks known as *Ixodes dammini* in Eastern states and *Ixodes pacificus* in Western states. The discovery of Lyme disease is of great interest in that a woman in Lyme had telephoned the State Health Department of Connecticut to report that her daughter had been diagnosed as having juvenile RA, but several other children in the area had a similar type of arthritic complaint. A second lady from Lyme had called Yale University School of Medicine with the observation that two of her children were diagnosed as having juvenile RA, which would be most unusual in itself, but particularly so as she and her husband had similar symptoms as well. Further investigation led to recognition that the disease occurred in geographic clusters leading to the name of Lyme disease. Discovery of the tick vector and the spirochete *B. burgdorferi* represents one of the most exciting developments in rheumatology during the 1980s.

Lyme borreliosis is widely disseminated throughout Europe, where *Ixodes Ricinus* is the vector. Cases have also been noted in China, Japan, and Australia. Because the tick vector becomes infectious by contact with deer that are the reservoir for the spirochete *B. burgdorferi*, its endemic areas are forest areas.

Pathophysiology. The pathophysiology of Lyme disease is now well understood. The tick vector *Ixodes dammini* becomes infected by contact with deer. Spirochetes were found in 61% of ticks collected from a focus of disease in Long Island. The ticks then bite humans who become infected with the spirochete and develop the lesions of erythema chronicum migrans.

The spirochete has been cultured from blood, skin, cerebrospinal fluid and joint fluid, and has been seen in skin, mycocardial, retinal, and synovial lesions. These findings and the usual response of all stages of the disease to antibiotic therapy suggest that the organism invades and persists in affected tissues throughout the illness even a period of months to years. The specific cellular and humoral immune responses develop to an increasing array of spirochetal antigens.

As the specific immune response develops, the disease often seems to localize to a few joints that become markedly inflamed. At that time, antigen-reactive mononuclear cells are concentrated in the joint fluid.

Management. Lyme disease is well cured with antibiotics. Initial studies involved the use of penicillin or tetracyclines. Because occasional patients have resistant neurologic symptoms, use of ceftriaxone (Rocephin) to cross the blood–brain barrier has been advocated as treatment for Lyme disease, certainly for resistant patients. Concomitant use of corticosteroids for severe inflammatory problems, as well as nonsteroidal antiinflammatory drugs, is advocated for symptomatic relief in certain patients.

In general, Lyme disease is curable with antibiotic therapy, and if after 10 days of treatment the patient is not better, strong consideration must be given to alternative diagnoses.

Atypical Forms. The most difficult problem involves a patient who has Lyme disease without the typical rash of erythema chronicum migrans in whom the diagnosis may be difficult. A common clinical problem is the patient who may have a tick bite and musculoskeletal problems, both of which are very common; 5% of such individuals will have a positive serologic test for *Borrelia*, but 99% will not have Lyme disease.

Impact of Disease and Prognosis. Lyme disease became a subject of popular media attention in the United States and Western Europe in the early 1990s, in general, is over-diagnosed. During the height of the interest in Lyme disease, many patients with longstanding RA suggested that they might have Lyme disease, which was not the case. The costs of inappropriate therapy of Lyme disease are considerable, and the medical community should strive to reduce these costs.

On the other hand, the discovery of Lyme arthritis has advanced our knowledge of chronic inflammatory rheumatic diseases and brought back the attention of the medical world to the role of infection even in the chronic phase of the disease. It also has given new hope that so-called incurable diseases eventually may be cured if we know the etiopathogenesis.

4

Polyarthritis: Rheumatoid Arthritis and Related Conditions

1 RHEUMATOID ARTHRITIS

1.1 Definition (Table 4.1)

Rheumatoid arthritis (RA) is a systemic autoimmune disease, affecting all age groups but occurring three times more often in women than in men. Rheumatoid arthritis is characterized by polyarthritis of the small and large peripheral joints; it becomes progressive and erosive over time. The majority of the patients have elevated titers of serum rheumatoid factors. Nonarticular manifestations include subcutaneous nodules, dry eyes, vasculitis, pleuritis, pericarditis, pulmonary fibrosis, and episcleritis. The severity of the joint disease may fluctuate over time and the final outcome is joint destruction, deformity, and disability.

In a number of countries, the term progressive chronic polyarthritis is used instead of rheumatoid arthritis. This term is confusing, on the one hand because other arthritides can be chronic and progressive, and on the other hand because rheumatoid arthritis is not always progressive and chronic. Also for patients it is not pleasant to be confronted with a diagnostic term that includes a bad prognosis.

Table 4.1 Rheumatoid Arthritis

Most common systemic autoimmune disease
Polyarthritis or peripheral joints for months
Female/male ratio 3:1; prevalence 0.8% of adults
Majority rheumatoid factor (RF)–positive
Progressive and erosive
Extraarticular manifestations: subcutaneous nodules, vasculitis, pericarditis,
   pleuritis, dry eyes
Fluctuating course: severity related to extraarticular manifestations
Possible final outcome: joint destruction — deformation — disability
Early disease-modifying therapy might change outcome

1.2 Main Clinical Features

1.2.1 Early Manifestations

The disease usually begins acutely or insidiously with symmetric swelling of
the small hand and/or feet joints, in particular the second and third metacarpal phalangeal, proximal phalangeal, and wrist joints. Patients complain
for weeks of pain in the fingers and experience stiffness and difficulty
closing fingers in the morning. The pain may resemble that of carpal tunnel
syndrome, being worse at night. The initial presentation of RA often lacks
the characteristic symmetry seen as the disease progresses. In early rheumatoid arthritis, patients may note fatigue and general malaise with prominent
joint swelling and pain. In the elderly, the first manifestations may be
stiffness in the shoulders at night and in the morning.

On clinical examination, symmetric synovitis, firm pasty-like, spindle-
shaped swellings of the small hand and/or feet joints and eventually the
knee, and tenderness on squeezing metacarpal (tarsal) joints is found. Distal interphalangeal joints (DIPs) are usually spared. Tenosynositis of the
extensor digitorum at the dorsum of the hand is frequently seen and nodular thickening of the flexor tendons can be palpated in the palm of the hand
and give rise to locking and snapping of the fingers (Fig. 4.1).

In about one third of the cases, subcutaneous nodules are felt at the
elbow (Fig. 4.2) or other pressure points and palpation of the radial head
may disclose tenderness and crepitus on pronation-supination.

1.2.2 Late Manifestations

After many months to years, typical joint deformities can be seen. Ulnar
deviation (coup de vent deformity) at the metacarpal phalangeal joints is
often associated with radial deviation at the wrist. Swan neck deformities
with hyperextension of proximal interplalaneal (PIP) joints plus fixed

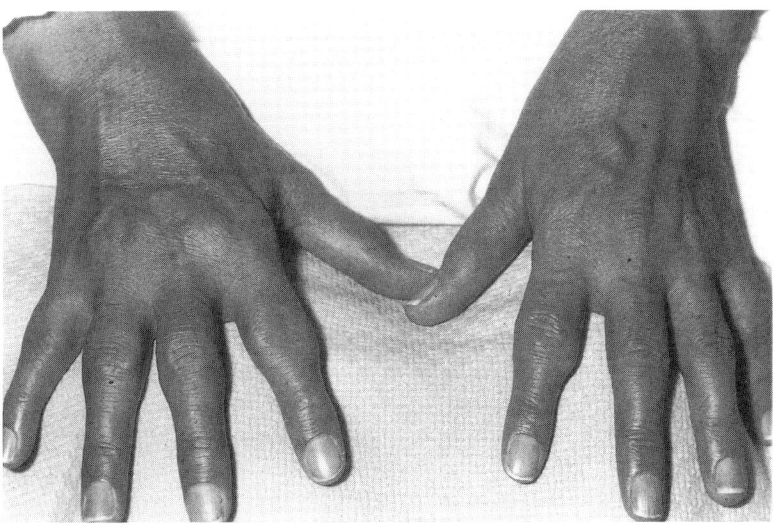

Figure 4.1 Synovitis PIP joints in rheumatoid arthritis.

flexion of DIP joints may develop, as may boutonnière deformities with flexion at the PIP joints and hyperextension at the DIP joints (Fig. 4.3).

Tendon rupture may occur at any site of inflammation, most commonly in the extensor pollicis longus that extends the DIP joint of the thumb and in the extensor tendons of the third, fourth, and fifth fingers. Tendon ruptures usually present with a history of abrupt and usually painless loss of function. The characteristic discrepancy between active and passive motion is seen on physical examination.

Vasculitis may be observed in the early and chronic phase, manifested by peripheral neuropathy, weight loss, splinter hemorrhage under the nail or nailfold infarcts (Fig. 4.4), and purpura hyperglobulinemia (Fig. 4.5). Fortunately, vasculitis is unusual.

Sometimes middle sized arteries are involved and give necrotic skin ulcers usually at the legs. Peripheral neuropathy and adenopathy may be part of severe disease. Episcleritis and scleritis occur but more frequently patients complain of dry eyes (Sjögren's syndrome). When splenomegaly is present in RA, then a subdiagnosis of Felty's syndrome and when hepatomegaly is diagnosed, amyloidosis associated with RA has to be envisaged. The figure illustrates the location of the extraarticular manifestations of RA (Fig. 4.6).

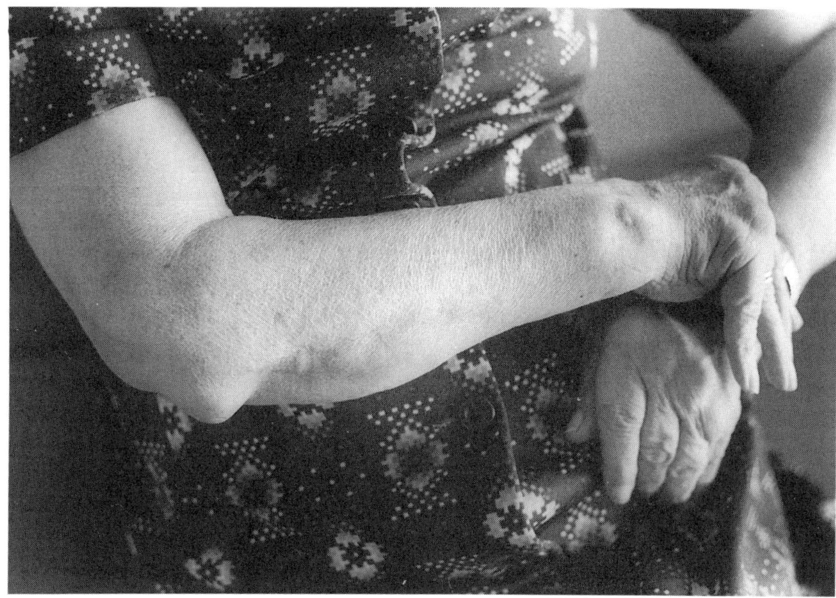

Figure 4.2 Subcutaneous nodule elbow, ulnar deviation metacarpophalangeal joints.

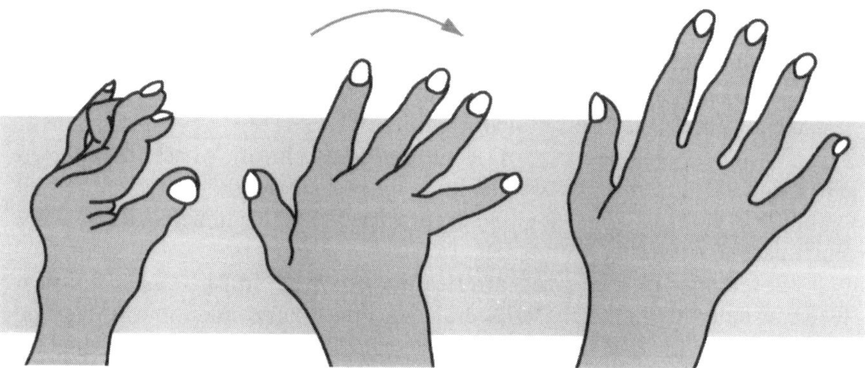

Figure 4.3 Typical finger deformities in rheumatoid arthritis.

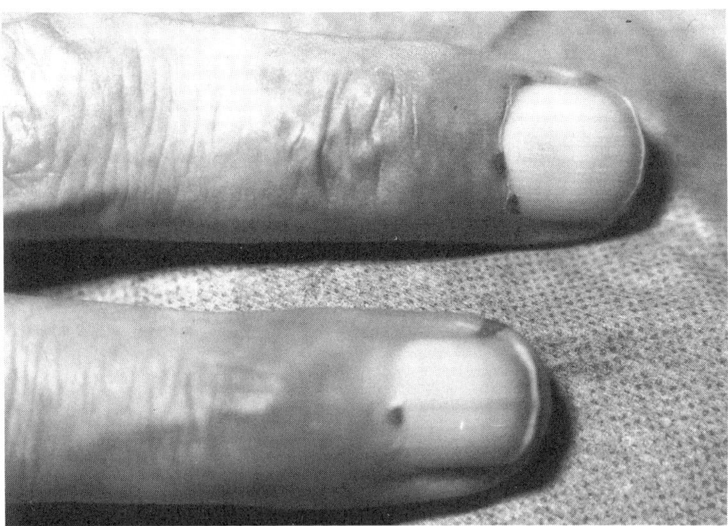

Figure 4.4 Nailfold vasculitis.

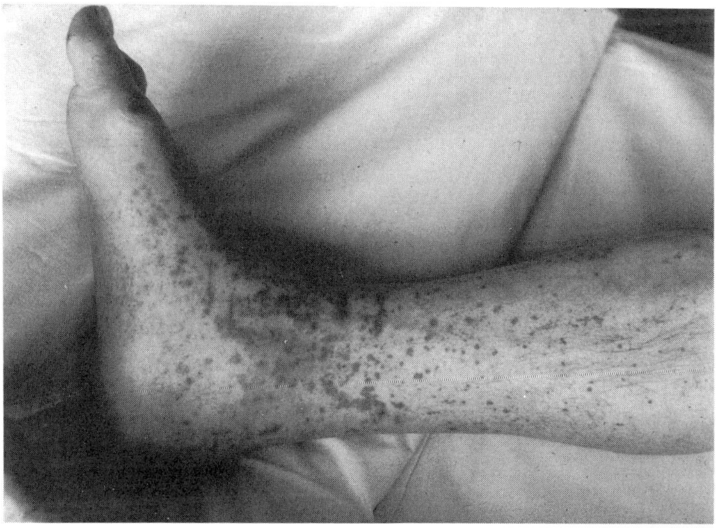

Figure 4.5 Purpura hyperglobulinemia.

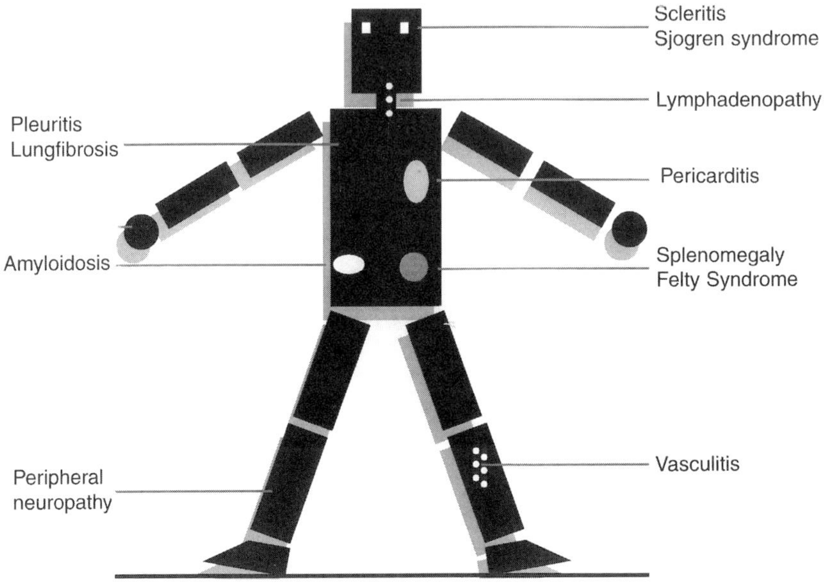

Figure 4.6   Extraarticular manifestations of RA.

1.3   Confirming the Diagnosis—Investigations

1.3.1   Early Phase

The diagnosis of RA is in the first phase clinical. No laboratory test, histo-logic or radiographic finding conclusively indicates a definite diagnosis of RA. The most important finding essential for the diagnosis of RA is identi-fying the presence of an inflammatory polyarticular synovitis, although extraarticular manifestations may be found in some patients. Another diag-nostic feature is the evolution of the disease process in a pattern consistent with RA. By definition RA cannot be diagnosed until the condition has been present for at least 6 weeks.

Other conditions causing synovitis must be excluded. Although this can often be done on initial evaluation, certain conditions such as systemic lupus erythematosus (SLE) or psoriatic arthritis may initially be indistin-guishable from RA.

Rheumatoid factor is found in the serum of 75–90% of patients with RA. The detection of the factor in patients with RA is of clinical value because its presence and, in particular, the titer tend to correlate with severe and unremitting disease, nodules and extraarticular lesions of RA. How-ever, rheumatoid factor is detectable in fewer than 50% of patients who ultimately develop rheumatoid arthritis during the first 6 months of disease. Rheumatoid factor can occur also in the normal population (5–10%) depending on age and other diseases, including several inflammatory disorders associated with synovitis.

In RA, the acute phase reactants, erythrocyte sedimentation rate (ESR), and the C-reactive protein (CRP) vary according to the degree of inflammation. CRP is less influenced by anemia and other serum factors than ESR. ESR and CRP are useful to monitor the level of inflammation. Other laboratory abnormalities may include anemia of chronic disease, hypergammaglobulinemia, thrombocytosis, and a positive antinuclear factor. Rarely, hypocomplementemia may be seen associated with vasculitis. All of these findings are more common in patients with more severe disease.

Synovial fluid analysis and synovium biopsy will document inflammation. These data, however, are nonspecific as inflammatory synovial tissue indistinguishable from RA may be seen in other inflammatory diseases of the joints.

Sonography is useful, if available, for documenting and quantitating soft tissue swelling, synovitis, and hydrops in the joint (Fig. 4.7). The demonstration by sonography of a Baker's cyst or Baker's cyst rupture (pseudophlebitis) (Fig. 4.8) is particularly helpful for differential diagnosis.

1.3.2 Late Phase

After months, characteristic radiologic features of arthritis can be documented (Fig. 4.9). In RA the following features are seen: soft tissue swelling, periarticular osteoporosis, global joint narrowing, marginal erosions, subluxation, and in the later stage complete joint destruction or ankylosis (Fig. 4.10). However, it should be remembered that erosions are seen in more than 50% of patients within the first 2 years of disease.

RA may affect the cervical spine and in particular the C1–C2 region, without much pain. Tenosynovitis of the transverse ligament of C1, which stabilizes the odontoid process (dens) of C2 may produce significant C1–C2 instability allowing myelopathy due to pressure on the cord. Careful neurologic examination is mandatory for, e.g. positive Hoffman–Trömer sign of the fingers, sensation of electricity in the fingers and general power loss in the limbs are alarming signs of myelopathy. A spinal lateral X ray of the cervical spine in flexion will show the subluxation of the C1–C2 region (Fig. 4.11) and a through-the-mouth picture will show the erosions of the odontoid and eventually instability of the apophyseal joint (Fig. 4.12).

Preoperatively, a more accurate evaluation to stage a neurologic compression using magnetic resonance imaging (MRI) is indicated. MRI is for this situation a better imaging procedure than computed tomography (CT) (Fig. 4.13).

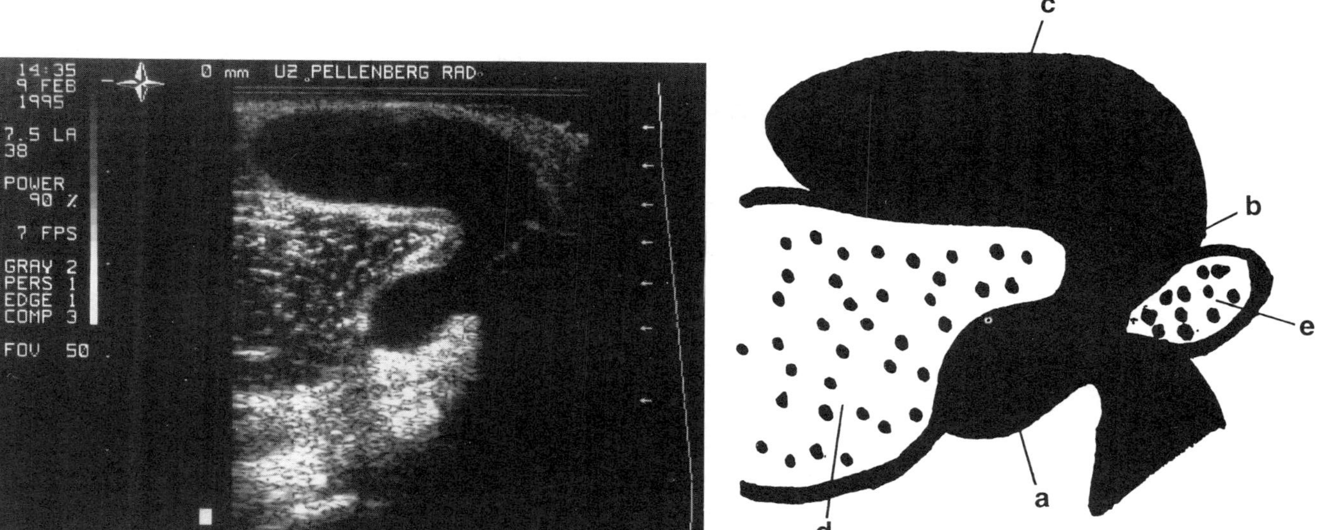

Figure 4.7   Sonography of Baker's cyst: (a) base, (b) neck, (c) superficial part, (d) medical gastrocnemius, (e) semimembranosus tendon.

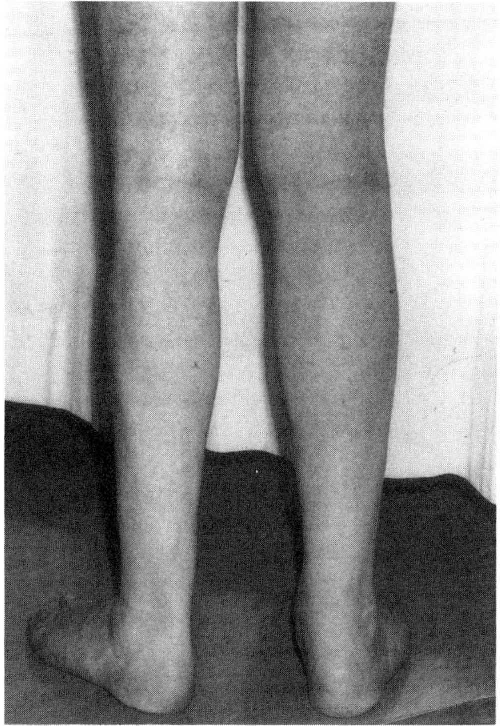

Figure 4.8 Clinical picture of ruptured Baker's cyst presenting as pseudophlebitis.

1.3.3 RA ACR Criteria

The American College of Rheumatology established criteria for classification of RA in 1958, which were revised in 1987 (Table 4.2a) and for clinical remission (Table 4.2b). These criteria were established to assure uniformity for clinical trials and epidemiologic studies of the disease. They are not intended to be used in clinical practice to establish a diagnosis in a specific patient but are often so used.

1.4 Diagnostic Difficulties

In the early phase of RA, the diagnosis may be confounded with fibromyalgia, SLE, reactive arthritis, psoriatic arthritis, knuckle pad disease, generalized osteoarthrosis, and calcium pyrophosphate dihydrate (CPPD) disease, and also with polymyalgia rheumatica in the elderly and hypertrophic osteoarthropathy.

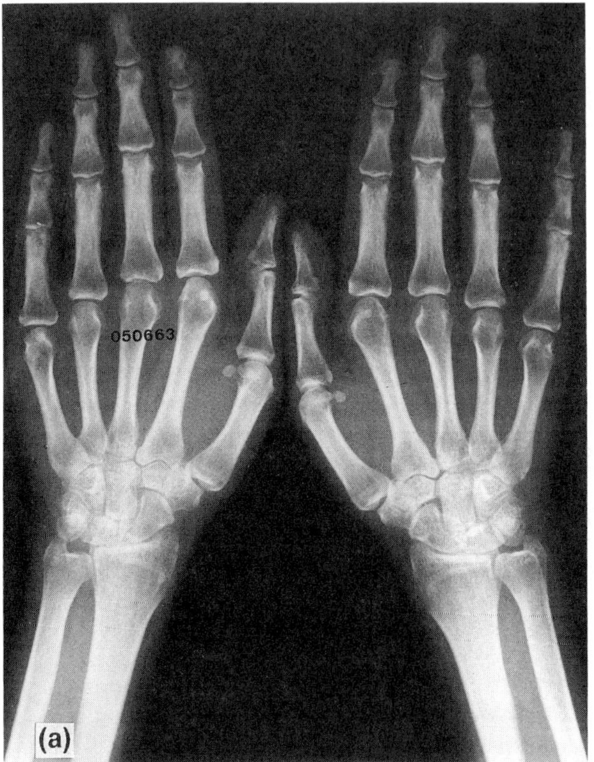

Figure 4.9   X-ray findings at the hand and wrist in RA in three patients.

1.4.1 Systemic Lupus Erythematosus

SLE has to be considered in the differential diagnosis, particularly in young women, because of a number of common clinical features: symmetric polyarthritis, pleuritis-pericarditis, and vasculitis. The joint involvement tends to be nondestructive in SLE. The most important discriminative features in favor of SLE are ultraviolet (UV) exposure, skin rash, hypocomplementemia, leukopenia, and a normal CRP.

Joint luxations, typical for Jaccoud's syndrome, can be seen in long-standing SLE. Erosions, however, are rare (Fig. 4.14).

1.4.2 Reactive Arthritis: Spondylarthropathies

Reactive arthritis and spondylarthropathies may mimic rheumatoid arthritis. Helpful differential diagnostic features in favor of reactive arthritis or spondylarthropathy are prearthritic illness (flu-like symptoms, enteritis,

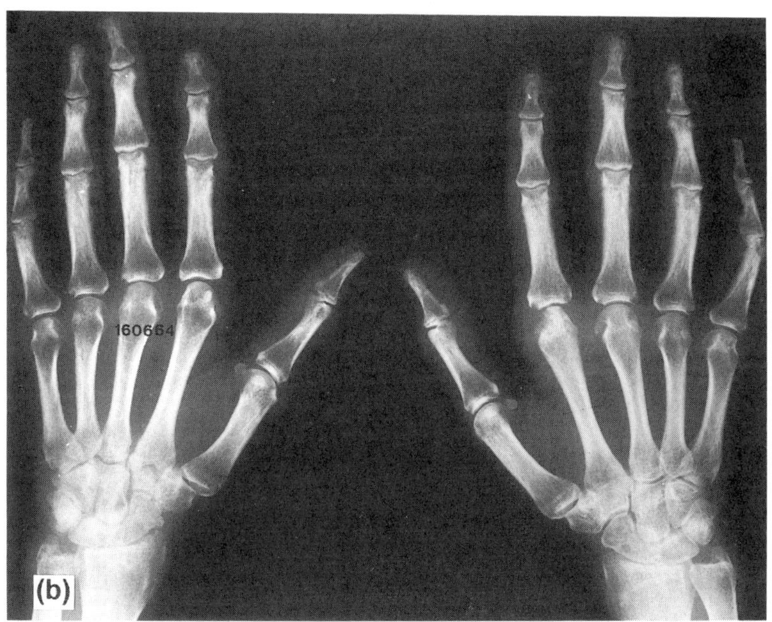

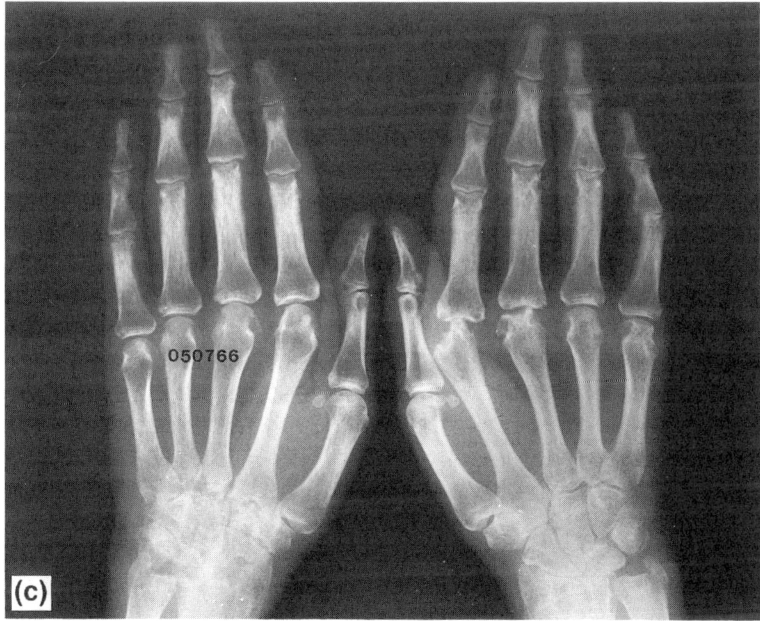

Figure 4.9 Continued.

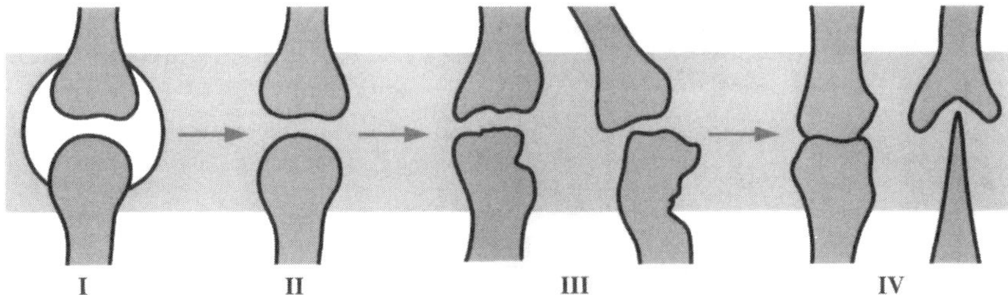

Figure 4.10 Different radiologic stages or joint alterations in RA. Stage I: normal bone, periarticular osteopenia, soft tissue swelling. Stage II: slight global joint narrowing. Stage III: cartilage and bone destruction with subluxation. Stage IV: fibrous or bony ankylosis.

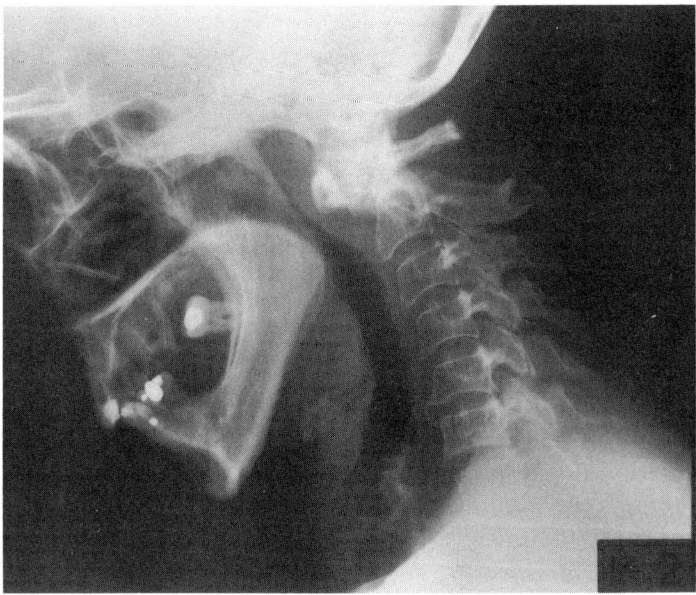

Figure 4.11 Lateral X-ray cervical spine in flexion.

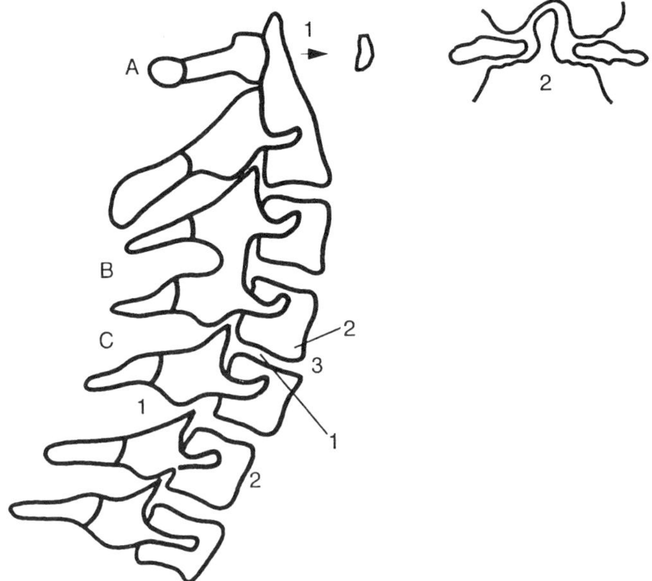

Figure 4.12 Graph showing X-ray alterations in the cervical spine in RA. (A) Subluxation C1–C2 (1). The atlas (C2) is more than 3 mm separated from the anterior face of the odontoid (C1) on a lateral X-ray of the cervical spine in flexion. Erosion of the odontoid (2). (B) Fusion apophyseal joint C3–C4. (C) Rheumatoid spondylodiscitis: disc narrowing (1), erosion of the vertebral deckplates (2), moderate osteophyte formation (3). (D) Destruction apophyseal joint C5–C6 (1) with anterolisthesis of C5–C6 (2).

urethritis, uveitis, cervicitis), oligoarthritis of the lower limbs, skin eruption (e.g., erythema nodosum, psoriasis), sacroiliitis, and spondylitis.

1.4.3 Knuckle Pad Disease (Maladie des Coussinets)

Fatty pads over the proximal interphalangel joints of the hands and prepatella at the knee should not be confused with synovial swelling. These pads are subcutaneous fibrofatty depositions and are of no clinical significance.

1.4.4 Polymyalgia Rheumatica

In the elderly may be difficult in the early phase to differentiate RA from polymyalgia rheumatica (PMR) because RA can start with shoulder and hand pain, and in polymyalgia synovitis of one or more joints, e.g., the knee and wrist without hand involvement are not unusual. If the pain dominates in the shoulder girdle and hip girdle and is associated with a very

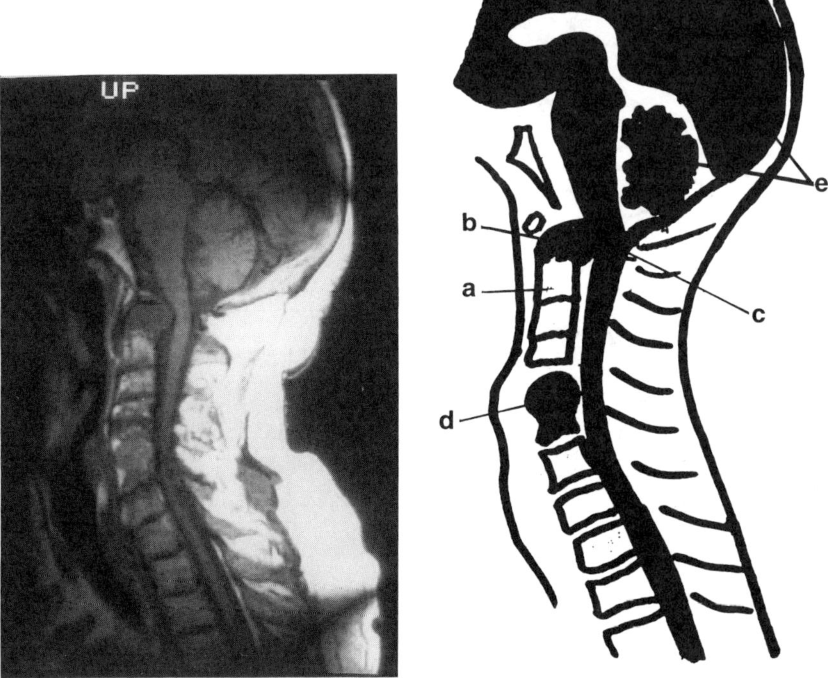

Figure 4.13 MRI sagittal T1-weighted SE image of the cervical spine: (a) corpus of C_2, (b) pannus tissue, (c) replaced upper cervical, (d) cerebellum, (e) rheumatoid discitis C5–C6.

high ESR, polymyalgia is more likely to be diagnosed. Temporal arteria biopsy may be positive for giant cell arteritis but may be negative in PMR.

1.4.5 Hypertrophic (Pulmonary) Osteoarthropathy

Occasionally rheumatoid arthritis can be confounded with the hypertrophic osteoarthropathy or achropachy syndrome, often associated with a thoracic disorder, in particular lung cancer. This syndrome is characterized by excessive proliferation of skin and bone at the distal parts of the extremities associated with deep-seated symmetric pain, more prominent in the lower extremities. Physical examination is the key to the diagnosis: clubbing of the fingers and soft tissue swelling of the ankles and wrist accompanied by tenderness of the affected area will be seen. There is no detectable hypertrophy of the synovial capsule; correction of a heart malformation, removal of a lung tumor, and successful treatment of endocarditis can produce rapid progression of all symptoms.

Table 4.2a American Rheumatism Association 1987 Revised Criteria for the Classification of Rheumatoid Arthritis

Criterion	Definition
1. Morning stiffness	Morning stiffness in and around the joints, lasting at least 1 h before maximal improvement.
2. Arthritis of 3 or more joint areas	At least 3 joint areas simultaneously have had soft tissue swelling or fluid (not bony overgrowth alone) observed by a physician. The 14 possible areas are right or left PIP, MCP, wrist, elbow, knee, ankle, and MTP joints.
3. Arthritis of hand joints	At least 1 area swollen (as defined above) in a wrist, MCP, or PIP joint.
4. Symmetric arthritis	Simultaneous involvement of the same joint areas (as defined in 2) on both sides of the body (bilateral involvement of PIPs, MCPs, or MTPs is acceptable without absolute symmetry).
5. Rheumatoid nodules	Subcutaneous nodules, over bony prominences, or extensor surfaces, or in juxtaarticular region observed by a physician.
6. Serum rheumatoid factor	Demonstration of abnormal amounts of serum rheumatoid factor by any method for which the result has been positive in $<5\%$ of normal controls.
7. Radiographic changes	Radiographic changes typical of rheumatoid arthritis on posteroanterior hand and wrist radiographs, which must include erosions or unequivocal bone decalcification localized in or most marked adjacent to the involved joints (osteoarthritis changes alone do not qualify).

For classification purposes, a patient shall be said to have rheumatoid arthritis if he or she has satisfied at least 4 of these 7 criteria. Criteria 1–4 must have been present for at least 6 weeks. Patients with 2 clinical diagnoses are not excluded. Designation as classic, definite, or probable rheumatoid arthritis is *not* to be made.

1.5 Epidemiology and Historical Data

The prevalence, representing all known cases of RA, is about 0.8% of adults in the USA and Europe, and increases with age for both males and females. The prevalence is clearly higher in females than in males with a ratio of 3 : 1. The prevalence is lower in African and Asian rural areas but not in urban areas. In all populations there is a female excess. The inci-

Table 4.2b ACR Criteria for Clinical Remission of Rheumatoid Arthritis

A minimum of five of the following for at least two consecutive months:

1. Morning stiffness not to exceed 15 min
2. No fatigue
3. No joint pain
4. No joint tenderness or pain on motion
5. No soft tissue swelling in joints or tendon sheets
6. ESR (Westergren's method) less than 30 mm/hr (females) or 20 mm/hr (males)

Exclusions prohibiting a designation of complete clinical emission:

Clinical manifestations of active vasculitis
Pericarditis
Pleuritis or myositis
Unexplained recent weight loss or fever secondary to RA

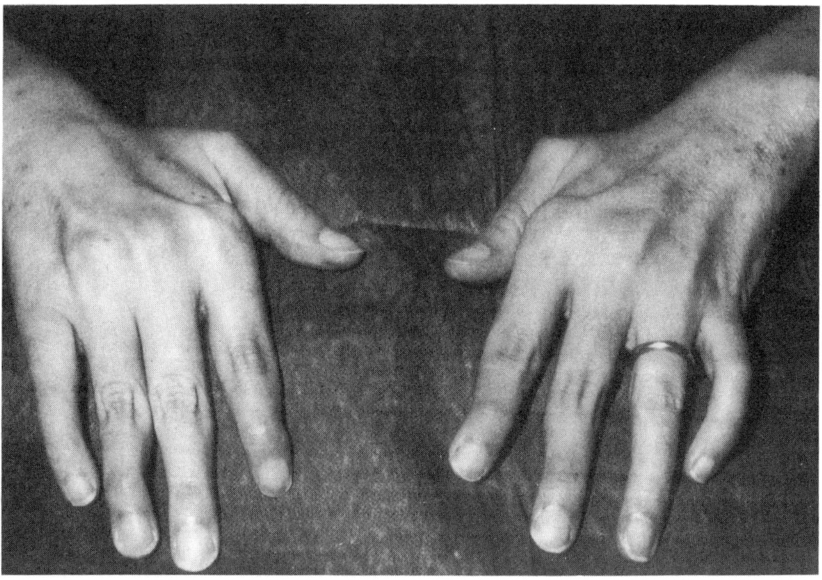

Figure 4.14 Joint luxation seen in Jaccoud's syndrome.

dence, defined as the rate of new cases arising in the population at risk over a given time period, is 0.15 per 1000 for males and 0.36 per 1000 for females per year in the UK (1992).

The disease may begin at any age, but most frequently it appears between 40 and 60 years.

Rheumatoid arthritis was not seen in antiquity, but is not a new disease and has been described in historical writings and portrayed in paintings for at least 300–400 years. The first entirely convincing description of RA was published in 1800 by Landré Beauvais. He named the disease "la goutte asthénique primitive."

1.6 Pathophysiology

The etiology of rheumatoid arthritis is unknown (Table 4.3). RA is found in all races and in all countries where it has been looked for. It is believed that there is only one naturally animal disease that resembles it pathologically — a retroviral arthritis found in goats or sheep. This finding has raised the possibility that the human disease may have a viral etiology. However, no virus has been definitively established as being its cause. Another possibility is that it may be an autoimmune disease. Although a number of autoantigens have been postulated, such as collagen, there is no unanimity as to a single antigen seen consistently in all patients. More recently, evidence has been produced that the disease, at least in its chronic form, may be maintained by immune reactivity, both by antibody and by T lymphocytes, to chondrocyte autoantigens.

Family studies have shown that the disease is dependent on at least two genetic factors. One of these is the DR4 antigen on the major histocompatibility human leukocyte antigen (HLA). HLA DR4 has been found linked to rheumatoid arthritis in most populations studied but to a variable degree. In patients of northern European origin HLA DR4 and its molecular variants are found in up to 80% of patients. By contrast, in southern

Table 4.3 Etiologic Factors in Rheumatoid Arthritis

Virus	No definitive proof
HLA DR4	Necessary for antigen presentation to CD4 and T cells
Autoantigens	
Type II collagen	Only a minority of patients exhibit autoimmunity to them
	Autoimmune response not linked to HLA DR4
Chondrocyte antigens	More patients exhibit autoimmunity to them

European populations such as the Greeks and Israeli Jews, the prevalence may vary from about 40% to 60%. Nevertheless, the association of the disease with HLA DR4 provides an important clue as to the etiopathogenesis of the disease.

HLA-DR molecules are found on the surface of antigen presenting cells such as macrophages and dendritic cells. These cells phagocytose antigen and process it into small antigenic peptides, of some 18 amino acids in length, which are then transported in the groove of the HLA DR molecule on to the surface of the antigen presenting cell. CD4+ T cells, equipped with the appropriate T-cell receptor, are then able to recognize this complex of antigenic peptide and the HLA DR molecule. They are stimulated to release lymphokines, such as interleukin-2 and interferon-γ, which then initiate the inflammatory events described above. Thus, the association of rheumatoid arthritis with HLA DR4 implies that unknown antigen(s) may be involved in the initiation and the maintenance of the disease.

The pathogenesis of rheumatoid arthritis (RA) may be understood from the histology of the synovial membrane itself and secondly by the histology of the rheumatoid nodules.

1.6.1 Synovial Membrane

The rheumatoid synovial membrane is characterized by hypertrophy and hyperplasia of the synovial lining cell layer, which can be thickened to 10 layers deep. The subsynovial lining layer is characterized by exuberant new blood vessel formation, increased numbers of specialized synovial fibroblasts or synoviocytes, and the entry of large numbers of lymphocytes and monocytes from the circulation (Figs. 4.15 and 4.16). The lining cell layer itself consists of the type A cells, which are bone marrow–derived cells that have arrived from the blood and are macrophage in nature, and the type B cells, which are synoviocytes that have arisen locally. The lymphocytes which are found within the subsynovial lining layer consist of T lymphocytes and B lymphocytes. The T lymphocytes are usually found as perivascular aggregates at whose periphery there may be large collections of B lymphocytes and plasma cells. T lymphocytes are also found scattered diffusely within the subsynovial tissue. The T lymphocytes belong predominately to the CD4 helper variety. T lymphocytes are activated and are participating in the inflammatory response by cell-to-cell interactions and the release of lymphokines. The B lymphocytes and particularly the plasma cells are secreting immunoglobulins but only a proportion of them are secreting rheumatoid factors. The specificity of the nonrheumatoid factor antibodies produced is not known, nor is their relationship to a possible etiologic agent.

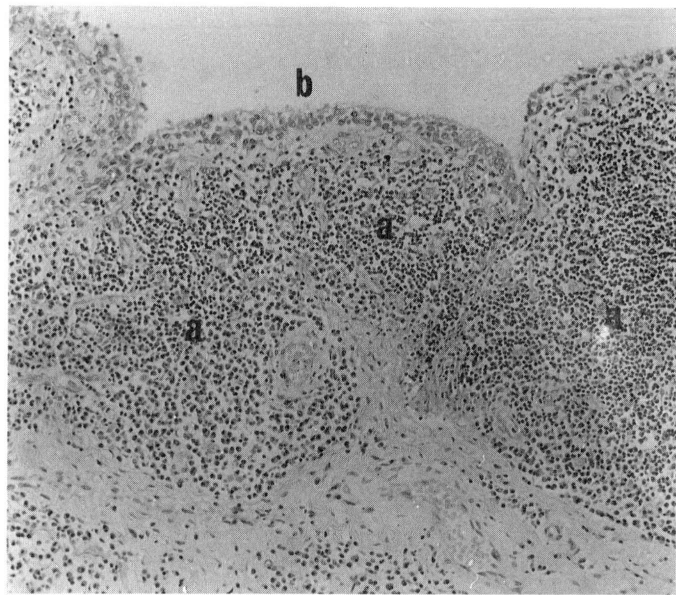

Figure 4.15 Anatomopathology of synovial membrane in RA. Synovial membrane of a case of rheumatoid arthritis showing (a) dense perivascular mononuclear cell infiltrates that consist of T lymphocytes and macrophages, (b) hypertrophic lining cell layer. Hematoxylin and eosin, ×40.

1.6.2 Rheumatoid Nodules

Rheumatoid nodules are characterized by a central necrotic but noncaseating center surrounded by palisaded tissue macrophages intermingled with CD4+ T cells (Fig. 4.17). As with the rheumatoid synovial membrane, neutrophils are sparse or absent. Both in the synovial membrane and the rheumatoid nodule the macrophages and the fibroblasts are secreting inflammatory cytokines of various types including interleukin-1, tumor necrosis factor–α, interleukin-6, and interleukin-8 (Table 4.4). These cytokines not only are involved in the local inflammatory response but also provide help for the activation and differentiation of the B cells into immunoglobulin-secreting plasma cells within the lesion and, when released systematically, will stimulate the liver to secrete acute phase proteins. This is particularly true for interleukin-1, tumor necrosis factor–α, and interleukin-6. The stimulation of the liver leads to the increased synthesis and secretion of fibrinogen, which is responsible in part for the elevated ESR

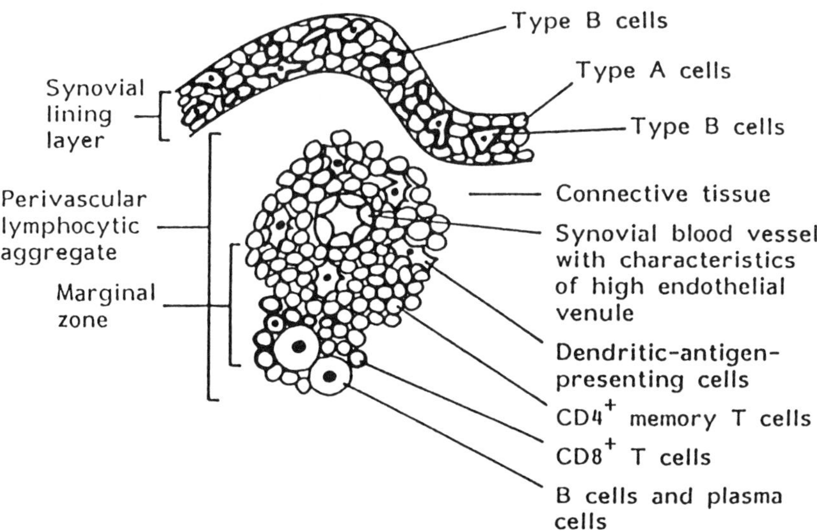

Figure 4.16 Schematic diagram illustrating the main features of rheumatoid synovitis. (Reproduced with permission from Kluwer Academic Publishers, Ref. 1.)

and for increased serum CRP, providing laboratory markers of clinical activity. In addition to these factors already mentioned, synoviocytes and macrophages release enzymes, such as collagenase and other neutral proteases, which are responsible for tissue destruction. The actual erosion of bone and articular cartilage is carried out by the inflammatory tissue called the pannus, which consists primarily of macrophages and synoviocytes (Fig. 4.18).

1.6.3 Angiogenesis in the Synovial Membrane

One of the striking features of the rheumatoid synovial membrane is that of new blood vessel formation or angiogenesis. The marked increase in the amount of synovial tissue requires new blood vessel formation for its continued nutrition, analogous to malignant tissue. The mechanisms of angiogenesis are not completely understood but one of the main mediators may very well be interleukin-8, a cytokine involved not only in angiogenesis but in the chemotaxis of neutrophils from the blood into the tissue as well as the entry of the CD4+ T cells into the synovium. Neutrophils are not found in the synovial tissue or synovial fluid because they lack receptors that allow them to anchor themselves in the synovium.

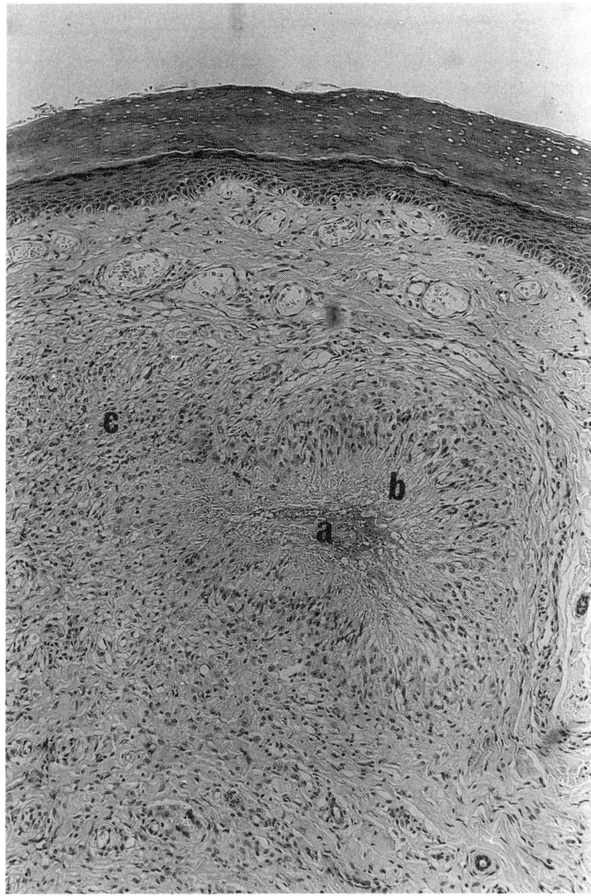

Figure 4.17 Anatomopathology of rheumatoid nodules. Skin showing a rheumatoid nodule in the dermis. Notice the necrotic center (a) surrounded by a palisaded layer of macrophages (b). There is also an increase of lymphocytes in the surrounding dermis (c).

1.6.4 Pathogenesis of Extraarticular Features

Rheumatoid arthritis is characterized by extraarticular manifestations, including nodules, vasculitis, which can involve peripheral nerves to cause a peripheral neuropathy, and involvement of lungs, pericardium, and heart, and other organs. The vasculitis is thought to be dependent on the deposition of immune complexes, which then activate complement. These immune complexes contain rheumatoid factor. Rheumatoid factors are autoanti-

Table 4.4 Some Lymphokines and Cytokines Found in the Rheumatoid Synovial Membrane

	Function
Lymphokines	
Interleukin-2	Activate T cells
Interferon-γ	Activate macrophages
Interleukin-10	Activate B lymphocyes
Cytokines	
Interleukin-1	Proinflammatory; stimulate acute phase response
Tumor necrosis factor-α	Proinflammatory; stimulate acute phase response
Interleukin-6	Stimulate acute phase response; activate B lymphocytes
Interleukin-8	Attract and activate neutrophils; stimulate angiogenesis recruitment CD4 and T cells

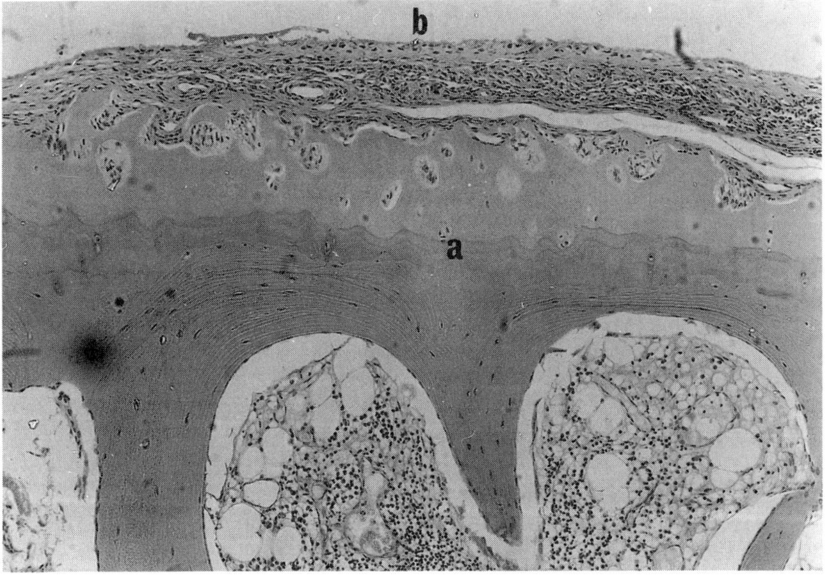

Figure 4.18 Anatomopathology of pannus and erosion in RA. Articular cartilage (a) from a case of rheumatoid arthritis showing erosion by the pannus (b).

bodies whose antigen is a region of the Fc fragment of normal IgG immunoglobulin. There are two main isotypes of rheumatoid factor, namely, IgM and IgG. An IgG molecule, which also has rheumatoid factor activity, can self-associate to form immune complexes that can directly activate complement. IgM rheumatoid factors can form the immune complexes either with normal IgG or with IgG with rheumatoid factor activity and then activate complement.

The anemia of active rheumatoid disease, which can be considered an extraarticular feature of the disease, is due to two main mechanisms, namely, the sequestration of iron within macrophages in the bone marrow and in the synovial membrane as well as the suppression of erythropoiesis within the bone marrow by circulating inflammatory cytokines.

1.7 Management

1.6.5 Treatment of RA

Nondrug Therapy in RA. The foundation of therapy for RA does not involve drugs but rather building a foundation of patient education, including establishment of the therapeutic relationship with a caring and knowledgeable health professional. It is most important to overcome some serious traditional misconceptions concerning RA including beliefs that "there is nothing one can do about arthritis" or that "crippling is an inevitable consequence of aging." It is also important to establish efforts that delve into such areas as joint preservation through occupational therapists, exercise programs through physical therapists, impact of arthritis on work and family through social workers, an understanding of drugs through nurses, and occasionally intervention regarding vocational matters through rehabilitation counselors. These matters have been approached in certain centers traditionally through a "team" of health professionals who interact with patients with RA. However, a team is not always available for every patient. Therefore, it would appear appropriate to recommend that any type of health professional who has interactions with a person with RA become somewhat familiar with principles of the various disciplines involved in RA, recognizing that in an optimal situation, a specialist within a certain field would provide optimal care for an individual patient. In a sense, a health professional who interacts with a person with RA or other rheumatic disease assumes a role of an "AT" (arthritis therapist) in providing knowledge and information that is needed for the patient.

Drug Therapy in RA. Notwithstanding the above, drugs are an important component of RA management (Table 4.5). Four types of drugs are important in patient management: analgesics, nonsteroidal antiinflammatory drugs (NSAIDs), corticosteroids that act quickly and are therefore

Table 4.5 Role of Therapeutic Regimens in the Management of Rheumatoid Arthritis: Early and Late Stage of Diseases

Therapeutic regimen	Early and established disease	End-stage disease
Nondrug therapy		
Patient education	+ + +	+
Rest		
Systemic/therapeutic	+ +	+
Local/protective	+ +	+ +
Physiotherapy		
Maintenance range of motion	+ +	+
Prevention of disuse atrophy of		
muscle, support of condition	+	+ +
Occupational therapy		
Joint protection	+ +	+
Adaption	+	+ +
Drug therapy		
NSAIDs	+ +	+ +
Second-line drugs	+ +	+
Steroids (systemic)	+	±
Intraarticular therapy	+ +	+
Surgical intervention		
Therapeutic (synovectomy)	+	−
Reconstructive	+	+ +
Joint replacement	−	+ + +

used as first-line agents, and second-line agents that have been developed for treatment of RA and of which the effects come on more slowly and are more profound. Therefore they have also been called slow-acting antirheumatic drugs (SAARDs) or disease-modifying antirheumatic drugs (DM-ARDs).

ANALGESIC DRUGS. Analgesic drugs are often ignored in treatment of patients because it is certainly optimal if control of inflammation results in lessening of pain. Nonetheless, it is often appropriate that patients be directly treated for pain with such drugs as paracetamol, acetaminophen, propoxyphene, and small amounts of narcotics when necessary as an adjuvant. It should be emphasized that there is very little value in a patient experiencing chronic pain and considerable evidence that the capacity to control pain is important in enhancing self-efficacy and development of positive reinforcement for therapeutic intervention. An analgesic therapy alone for chronic rheumatic pain may induce addiction and harm the patient.

NONSTEROIDAL ANTI-INFLAMMATORY DRUGS (NSAIDS). The prototype nonsteroidal antiinflammatory drug (NSAID) is aspirin, which was regarded traditionally as the mainstay of management of RA. However, aspirin is found to have limited usefulness, primarily because doses in the antiinflammatory range required for optimal control frequently result in gastrointestinal distress and bleeding. Consequently, long-term use of high doses of aspirin is really not possible for most patients. Newer forms of aspirin have been developed, e.g., aspirin with an antacid, enteric-coated aspirin, and long-acting preparations that release active ingredients slowly. All of these preparations are more likely to have lower toxicity than plain aspirin and are likely to be continued by patients longer than plain aspirin. A class of drugs known as propionic acids includes ibuprofen, naproxen, and ketoprofen, and a group of nonacetylated salicylates show reduced gastrointestinal toxicity but may not have as high an efficacy as acetylated salicylates. Other nonsteroidal antiinflammatory drugs include indomethacin, diclofenac, meclofenamate, piroxicam, meloxicam, and sulindac.

All NSAIDs have activity against prostaglandin synthetase (cyclooxygenase), so that other nondesirable effects of this mechanism of action, including gastrointestinal irritation, interference with kidney function, and headaches and other unpleasant central nervous system effects, may emerge as side effects in some patients.

Inhibition of cyclooxygenase (Cox) by NSAIDs can result in two pathways (isoforms): Cox 1 and Cox 2. The Cox 1 pathway is mainly present in normal physiologic processes and is responsible for production of cytoprotective prostaglandin (TXA_2, PGI_2, PGE_2). Cox 2 is induced in inflammation or during mitosis, and is not detectable in normal tissue. Some NSAIDs (aspirin, indomethacin) inhibit Cox 1 in a potent way, ibuprofen in an equipotent way. Cox 1 and Cox 2 nonacidic naphthylkanones inhibit mainly Cox 2 pathway. Selective inhibition of Cox 2 seems superior for limiting side effects of NSAIDs. The future will determine which of these pathways is the most important for reducing inflammation and limiting these side effects.

CORTICOSTEROIDS. Corticosteroids have a long history in the treatment of RA. They were initially a "wonder drug" used in doses of 20–60 mg of prednisone daily. Use of these daily doses over longer than 6 months led to considerable toxicity and came to be regarded as so toxic as to not be advised for patients with this disease. In recent years the use of low-dose corticosteroid such as prednisone or prednisolone in doses of 7.5 mg or less has become widespread. Patients who take these doses over periods of 10 years or longer have no higher prevalence of diabetes, hypertension, obesity, or other recognized complications of long-term corticosteroid therapy, except osteopenia and fractures. It should be noted that a small dose of corticosteroid steroid may be very helpful to patients, in contrast to a large dose of steroids which will invariably produce toxicity and be deleterious to patients. The most important determinants of bone loss in RA are disability and cumulative corticosteroid dose. Therefore low-dose steroids in postmenopausal women and children should not be used with complacency. Parenteral corticosteroids may be given periodically as an intramuscular injection of 40–80 mg of a long-acting preparation, or as an intraarticular injection into a joint that appears disproportionately involved compared to other joints.

SECOND-LINE DRUGS FOR TREATMENT OF RA. A number of second-line drugs have been documented to be of value for treatment of patients with rheumatoid arthritis. Second-line drugs are also referred to as disease-modifying antirheumatic drugs (DMARDs), slow-acting antirheumatic drugs (SAARDs), and as remission-inducing drugs. However, the term "remission inducing" should not be used as several studies indicate that remission occurs in only a very small percentage of patients, and sustained remission is seen in fewer than 2% of patients over 3 years or more.

Specific second-line drugs used in RA include the following:

(1) *Methotrexate* is at present the most widely used second-line drug, primarily because its use is generally continued considerably longer than other second-line drugs. Furthermore, the toxicity of methotrexate is now documented to be in the range of many NSAIDs. Methotrexate was used initially on the basis of its cytotoxic activity as an antifolic acid agent to destroy activated lymphocytes. However, further research has documented that it has antiinflammatory properties as well, which probably represents the primary mode of action in the doses used to treat RA.

The initial dosage is 7.5 mg/week, in one or three divided doses, which may be increased to 25 mg/week. Patients who take methotrexate should also take folic acid at a dose of 1 mg/day. Potential toxicities of methotrexate include GI distress and less commonly hair loss, which usually can be minimized through dosage reduction, hepatotoxicity — which is common but not serious as long as the liver tests remain within 2–3 times the normal values — and a liver biopsy is rarely indicated in usual practice. The occurrence of methotrexate-induced intracutaneous nodules may necessitate interruption of the therapy. "Methotrexate lung," which may mimic a pulmonary infection, is the most serious clinical toxicity associated with the use of methotrexate in RA. Methotrexate may rarely induce bone marrow suppression in a patient. Hematologic and liver test monitoring is indicated every 6–12 weeks. Methotrexate has the hypothetical potential to promote malignancy, although this has been found to be minimal in careful studies.

Methotrexate is cleared by the kidney and therefore renal function should be good and taken into account. In the elderly, in particular with serum creatinine > 1.2 mg %, MTX should not be given unless careful monitoring is carried out.

(2) The antimalarial drugs *chloroquine and hydroxychloroquine* were discovered to be effective for patients with RA who were taking them for malaria prophylaxis in areas in which malaria was endemic. Chloroquine appears more powerful than hydroxychloroquine, but also is associated with a higher level of ocular toxicity, with loss of visual fields and retinopathy after long-term use at high dosage. Hydroxychloroquine is rarely associated with ocular toxicity, although some gastrointestinal toxicity is seen. The dosage is 200 mg twice a day. Patients should have visual fields checked periodically and see an ophthalmologist annually to monitor ocular status.

(3) Injectable *gold salts* have been a traditional mainstay in treatment of RA. Gold was used initially on the basis of its being bacteriostatic for mycobacteria and RA was thought to represent a chronic mycobacterial infection. Gold salts are given weekly at dosages of 10, 25, and 50 mg/week. After a response occurs they may be given less frequently, e.g., every 2 weeks or even monthly. The important toxicities resulting from gold salts include a rare immediate flushing "nitritoid" reaction seen primarily in water- rather than in oil-soluble preparations, hematologic cytopenia, glomerulitis with proteinuria, pulmonary toxicity, and rash. Blood counts should be monitored at least monthly in the beginning as well as urinalysis before each injection.

(4) In recent years, an oral form of gold therapy, auranofin, has been developed. Although in clinical trials it is documented to be effective, in clinical practice it is generally effective only in patients with relatively mild or early disease. The primary toxicity involves diarrhea, although it may be that there is also potential hematologic toxicity and nephritis, as seen with injectable gold at lower levels. Auranofin is rarely continued over 5 years in patients with RA.

(5) *Sulfasalazine* was developed as a drug to combat rheumatoid arthritis with an active salicylate and sulfonamide moiety. It is the most widely used second-line drug in Europe at this time. The dosage is generally 1000–2000 mg twice a day. Toxicities include GI distress, rash, salicylism, and induction of antinuclear factor (ANF) and lupus.

(6) D-Penicillamine is a drug that interferes with the binding of sulfhydril groups and is thought to possibly interfere with the binding of rheumatoid factor. It generally has been used in a "go-low, go-slow" approach, beginning with 125 mg daily increasing to 200, 500, or even 1000 mg/day. Toxicities of D-penicillamine include rash, nephritis, hematologic toxicities,

so that monthly monitoring of blood counts and urine is appropriate. Although occasional patients have excellent responses to D-penicillamine, its use has been largely supplanted in most settings by methotrexate and sulfasalazine.

(7) *Azathioprine* is an immunosuppressive drug thought to benefit patients with rheumatoid arthritis through destruction of activated lymphocytes. Azathioprine is given in dosages of 50–200 mg daily. At least monthly hematologic monitoring is indicated, which can be reduced to every 2 months after the patient has been stable over a year. There is also some concern that azathioprine may contribute to increased susceptibility to malignancy, but this is not likely to be seen in the doses used to treat rheumatoid arthritis (in contrast to doses used to treat patients who have transplants for immunosuppression with azathioprine).

(8) *Cyclophosphamide* is used primarily for rheumatoid vasculitis. It is an effective drug for joint symptoms in dosage of 50–200 mg/day in some patients, but it is not used in most patients because of the risks of severe toxicities associated with long-term use, including malignancies (in contrast to other cytotoxic agents such as methotrexate and azathioprine, which have little if any oncogenic potential). These toxicities include leukemia and hemorrhagic cystitis leading to neoplasia of the bladder endothelium. Hematologic monitoring including white blood cell counts and platelet counts is indicated at least monthly.

Principles concerning clinical use of drugs in RA include the following:

(1) Inflammatory *activity* is reversible, whereas resulting *damage* is irreversible. Therefore, the traditional teaching that use of second-line drugs should be reserved until there is evidence of severe disease, such as radiographic erosions, has now been revised to recognize that a patient is a candidate for second-line drugs once the diagnosis of rheumatoid arthritis is established, at a relatively early stage.

(2) The doses required for drugs such as methotrexate or azathioprine to be effective in treatment of RA are considerably lower than those used in treatment of cancer or to suppress rejection in transplant patients. Patients with RA can experience substantial clinical improvement even if only 50% of activated lymphocytes are killed. In contrast, patients with neoplasia or transplantation a much higher proportion must be killed, including more than 99.9% of cells in patients with cancer. Therefore, the margin of benefit to toxicity is considerably better in patients with RA treated with cytotoxic or immunosuppressive drugs than in other types of patients treated with these drugs.

(3) Individual patients respond differently to different second line drugs, so that there is no single drug which is optimal for all patients. Figure

4.19 shows the survival curve of second-line therapies over 60 months in a rheumatology practice.

Recognition of severe long-term outcomes in RA and limited long-term effectiveness of current therapies suggests that an optimal treatment strategy in RA is needed to control inflammation as aggressively as possible with as many drugs, including combinations of several drugs, as appropriate (Table 4.6). Considerations of aggressive treatment of RA may leave the health professional with a serious conundrum: the care of a patient with RA may be optimal only when both the professional and patient are concerned that treatment may be too aggressive or involve too many drugs. When it is obvious to the health care team and the patient that aggressive treatment is needed, some irreversible progressive damage has likely already occurred and it is probably too late to gain optimal benefit of treatment. The validity of an aggressive approach may be documented only through long-term studies, which should include a patient self-report questionnaire completed by each patient at each visit. The reassessment of approaches of rheumatology to RA does appear to be leading to improved results to the benefit of people with RA.

(4) Several new approaches to treat RA are currently under investigation, such as anti-TNF-α drugs, anti-CD4 agents, etc. Cyclosporin A, a drug that revolutionized transplantation, has also been tested in RA. The

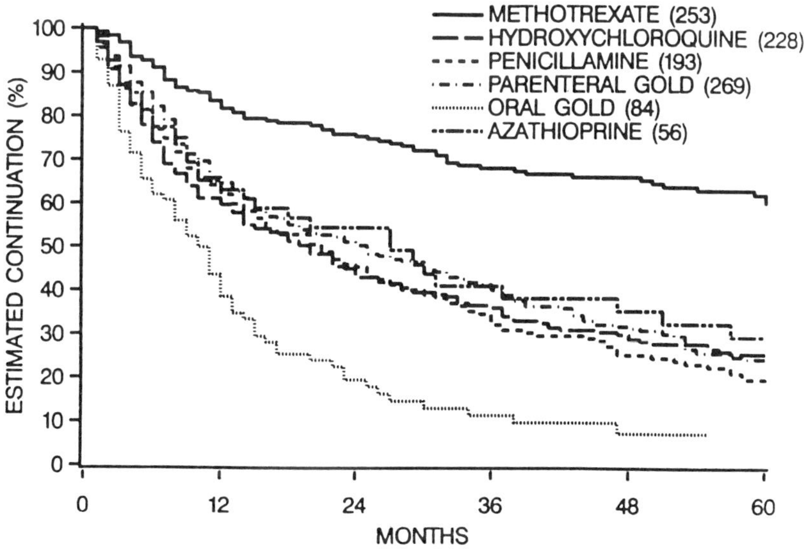

Figure 4.19 Survival curve of second-line drugs.

Table 4.6 Drug Therapy in RA

	First choice NSAID	Adjuvant Analgesics (intermittent)
Early RA NSAID failing to suppress disease (weeks)	Second-line DMARD according to age, stage, contraindications: —Sulfasalazine —Gold —Hydroxychloroquine —Methotrexate —D-penicillamine —Azathioprine	Low-dose corticosteroids (<7.5 mg) IM depo-corticosteroids intermittently

Established disease not controlled by DMARD	—Change DMARD
	—Combination therapy
	    MTX +
	      sulfasalazine
	    MTX +
	      hydroxychloroquine
		Low-dose corticosteroids

Flares + fever + vasculitis	—Methylprednisolone bolus —Cyclophosphamide	
Single-joint inflammation	IA corticosteroids Chemical synovectomy —Osmium —Yttrium	

benefit/side effect ratio, however, is insufficient to recommend cyclosporin A for routine use in RA.

Management of Complications.

VASCULITIS. Pulse corticosteroids (1 g IV) and cyclophosphamide (0.5 g/m^2 IV) are often beneficial in the treatment of severe diseases associated with vasculitis.

ATLANTOAXIAL SUBLUXATION. Conservative treatment with cervical collars is indicated for patients with nonprogressive and mild neurologic symptoms, but surgical intervention is necessary for intractable pain or progressive neurologic disease.

SYNOVIAL CYSTS. The most common synovial cyst is a popliteal cyst (Baker's cyst), resulting from chronic knee effusions. A ruptured popliteal cyst gives a clinical picture similar to that for deep venous thrombosis.

Intraarticular steroids and rest are often effective, but synovectomy may be required.

RHEUMATOID NODULES. There is no effective treatment for subcutaneous nodules, nor is any required because they are usually asymptomatic. Intralesional injections may provide temporary benefit. Surgical removal may help temporarily, but the nodules may recur. Surgery is generally indicated for infected nodules or nodules that mechanically interfere with usual activities, e.g., in pressure points of feet.

Management.

TEAM APPROACH. A number of patients with rheumatoid arthritis will have a chronic course of disease and will develop joint deformities and the consequent social isolation that arises from being house-bound (Fig. 4.20).

As there are at present no reliable indicators of progressive disease, prevention of disability has to start early, before irreversible damage occurs. Therefore education, prevention of contracture, muscle atrophy, support for social and psychological coping problems, and sustained therapeutic control of the inflammatory process are essential for a good outcome of rheumatoid arthritis.

The control of outcome of rheumatoid arthritis is not the sole expertise of the doctor or specialist in rheumatology but rather is the work of a collaborative group, including allied health professionals. This gives the best assurance for success due to presence on the team of rheumatology nurses, physiotherapists, occupational therapists, psychologists, social workers, orthopedic surgeons, and orthesists.

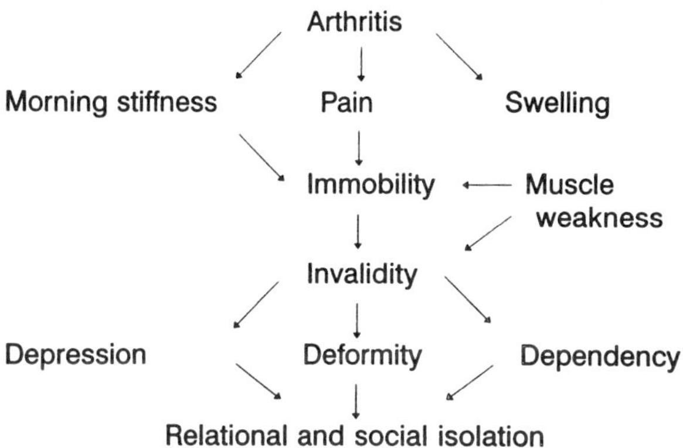

Figure 4.20 Psychosocial consequences of rheumatoid arthritis.

Table 4.7 Essential Elements of
Physiotherapy

Isometric exercises
Relaxation exercises
Preservation of range of joint motion
Physical conditioning exercises
Maintaining good posture

In order to bring the multidisciplinary expertise to the profit of the patient, a patient-centered team conference is essential and the basis of modern therapy of the patient with RA. Each member of the team, according to the plan and the consensus on the goals to be achieved, has to fulfill his role in a concerted action.

The essential elements of physiotherapy and occupational therapy are summarized in Tables 4.7 and 4.8.

SURGICAL THERAPY.   Surgical therapy has an important place in the treatment of RA. Joint replacement can now be done for almost all destroyed joints, but total hip and knee replacements are the most successful. For severe hand deformities, transpositions of tendons and arthrodesis can be necessary to improve function. Replacement of small hand joints can also be done in carefully selected patients. Carpal tunnel release and fixation of cervical spine subluxations for myelopathy are important indications for surgery in RA.

Despite serious deformities of the hands, most patients with rheumatic diseases surprisingly can perform daily activities without too much trouble. Surgery to improve hand function is rarely necessary. For esthetic reasons, however, arthroplasty of metacarpophalangeal joints can be done for a young female patient if she explicitly requests it. The patients, however, should know in advance that hand function probably will not be improved. Repair by grafting or tendon transfer of ruptured tendons have to be done preferably soon after rupture. The tendons likely to rupture are

Table 4.8 Essential Elements of
Occupational Therapy

Advise joint sparing techniques
ADL training (make up, ironing, cooking)
Functional training (games, creative activities)
Testing of aids

---

those with inflamed synovial tendon sheets on the dorsal side of the hand, at the extensor pollices longus, at the extensior digitis minimi, and at the flexor side flexor pollicis longus. Longstanding synovitis should be treated, surgically if necessary, to avoid rupturing.

When the patient's thumb and index finger no longer can be brought together ("the pinch" movement) because of subluxation of the thumb joints, an arthrodesis of the subluxated joints can be considered in order to restore this function. Another simple procedure that can improve hand function, in particular pronation and supination, is the resection of the distal end of the ulna at the wrist and the radial head of the elbow (Fig. 4.21).

The pronation and supination at the wrist becomes difficult because of destruction of the distal end of the ulna or of the radial head. Pronation and supination are necessary when bringing up a spoon to the mouth or to fill a glass. The above-mentioned operation will improve these functions. When the wrist joints are destroyed and despite medical treatment remain painful, an arthrodesis of the wrist is indicated. A bilateral wrist arthrodesis, however, has to be discouraged because the patient might experience difficulties in cleaning himself after defecation.

Surgical resection of hypertrophic synovia (synovectomy) has its place in selected cases, usually when only one or two joints remain involved after good medical treatment. At present, arthroscopic resection of synovial tissue is more often done, with less inconvenience for the patient. Chemical synovectomy (synoviorthesis) with radioactive yttrium or with osmium is

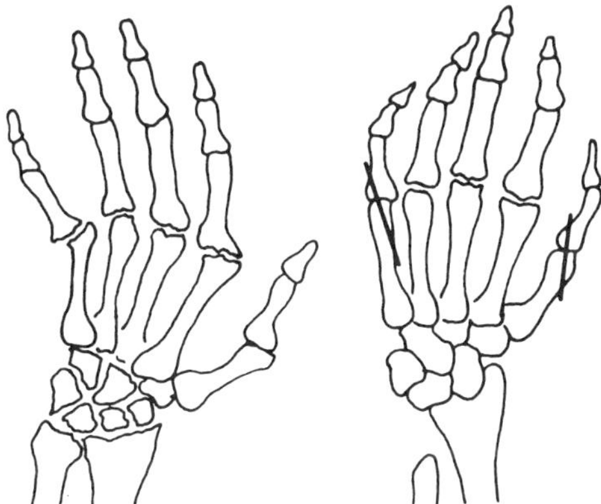

Figure 4.21 Interventions to improve hand function: arthrodesis metacarpal joint I-V; arthrodesis wrist joint; resection ulna, distal end.

also a useful procedure, with almost no side effects. Radioisotopic synovectomy is, however, reserved for older patients because it may cause chromosomal damage.

Reconstructive surgery at the knees, hips, and feet gives good results in selected cases, when there is serious joint destruction, laxity, and important functional deterioration. Before the decision for surgery is made, one has to investigate whether adaptation of the shoes, metatarsal pad for relief of involved metatarsal joints, strengthening of the muscles, in particular the quadriceps, and correction of flexion contractures have been tried out and yielded insufficient results. Often surgery can be prevented or postponed using appropriate physiotherapy.

Because of destruction of toe joints, partial or complete luxation, and bunions, a number of patients, despite good medical treatment and shoe adaptation, experience important functional problems when walking. For them surgical procedures, e.g., resection of destructed metatarsal joints and reconstruction of the foot arch, are very helpful (Fig. 4.22). It is better to have no metatarsal joints than to have anatomic mechanically unfit joints. Mobility and independency will be considerably improved.

Shoulder and elbow prostheses are also indicated when these joints are destroyed and very painful. Mainly the pain component will be improved. Improvement of mobility at the shoulder after prosthesis is rather small.

At the knees, pain is constant and invalidity may result because of laxity due to loss of cartilage, joint capsule destruction, and depression of the loading area of the tibia. Surgery is the preferred treatment. The anatomic disintegration cannot be improved with local injections of corticosteroids or with analgesic drugs. An anatomic reconstruction by either osteot-

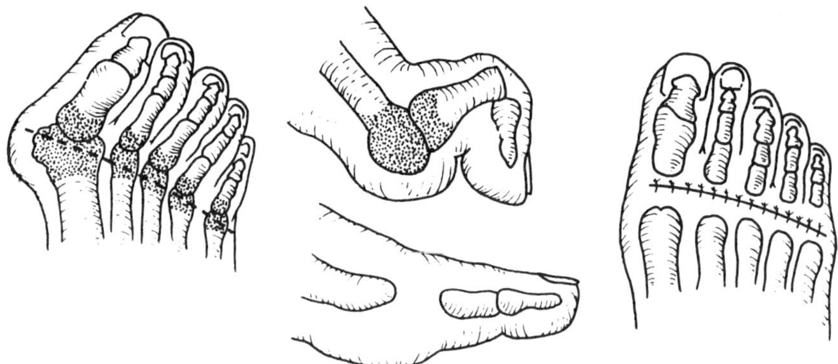

Figure 4.22 Intervention to improve feet function.

omy or total knee prosthesis is strongly indicated in these cases (Fig. 4.23). Due to the improved outcome of total knee arthroplasty, a total knee prosthesis is now often preferred above osteotomy.

The most important progress of the last 20 years in reconstructive surgery lies in the treatment of hip lesions. By introducing total hip replacement with this technique, the destroyed hip as well as the femoral head and the acetabulum are removed and replaced by a polyethylene joint cup and a metallic (Vitalium) femoral head (Fig. 4.24). The two parts of the total hip prosthesis are made from different materials in order to reduce friction.

The postoperative rehabilitation is short because the patient has a pain-free hip and is allowed full weight bearing almost immediately after surgery. The procedure is very well tolerated, even by very elderly and frail patients. When both knee and hip replacement are indicated in general the hip has to be operated first. Because the artificial hip can wear out and loosening can occur, total hip replacement in young persons has to be postponed as long as possible. However, the improvement in quality of life is so important that a correct cost/benefit balance has to be estimated, particularly in juvenile rheumatoid arthritis and ankylosing spondylitis cases with bilateral coxitis. Complications of surgery including infection, fracture of the prosthesis or of the bone beneath the prosthesis, and loosening may occur in 5% of the cases. When infection occurs, the prosthesis might have to be taken out, leaving the patient with an unstable hip (girdlestone hip). New interventions and reconstruction after a failure of hip prosthesis are now done with success, but a longer immobilization postsurgery is usually indicated.

Before modern reconstructive surgery was available, arthrodesis of

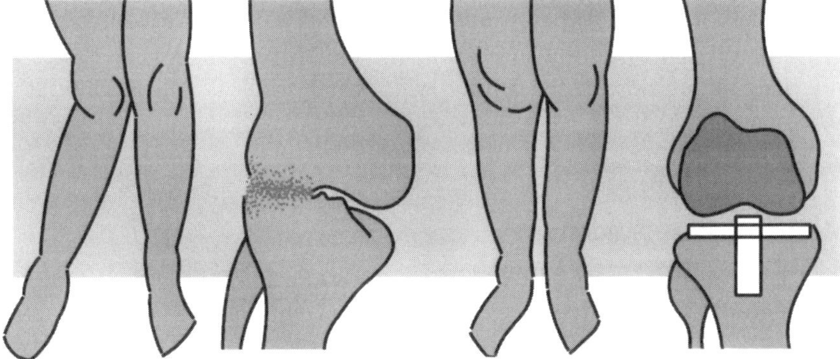

Figure 4.23 Knee prosthesis to correct valgus deformity.

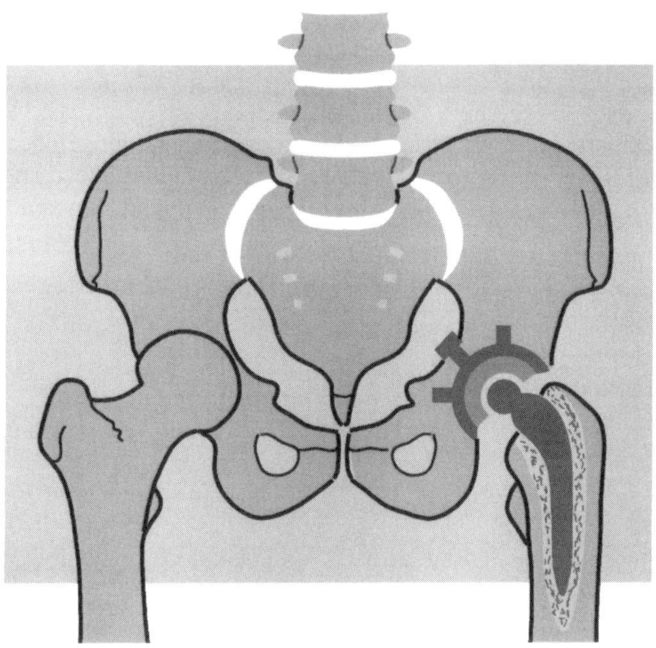

Figure 4.24 Total hip prosthesis.

the hip or knee was often performed. In order to compensate for a stiff hip or knee, the lower back mobility is used, which might increase the possibility of overuse and low back pain. However, arthrodesis of the knee or hip is rarely done, and only after previous failed procedures. The progress of surgical reconstruction now makes it possible to give back an independent life to very incapacitated and elderly patients.

In order to be fully successful, the reconstructive surgery has to be carried out in close collaboration with good medical and rehabilitative treatment.

1.8 Atypical Forms

1.8.1 Sjögren's Syndrome

RA is frequently associated with Sjögren's syndrome. Sjögren's syndrome is a chronic, slowly progressive inflammatory autoimmune exocrinopathy of unknown etiology. The typical clinical presentation of Sjögren's syndrome includes keratoconjunctivitis sicca and xerostomia due to diminished lacrimal and salivary gland secretion. This autoimmune disease may evolve from an organ-specific (exocrine glands) to a systemic (extraglandular) disorder affecting lungs, kidneys, blood vessels, and muscles, as well as a B-cell lymphoproliferative disorder. These features are believed to be the consequence of overt immune system activation, manifested by various autoantibodies and lymphocytic invasion of the exocrine glands and other affected organs. When not associated with other connective tissue diseases, the syndrome is designated primary Sjögren's syndrome. Most of these cases have the characteristic antibodies SSA and SSB.

Secondary Sjögren's syndrome defines the disease complex in the presence of other autoimmune disorders, including rheumatoid arthritis, systemic lupus erythematosus, systemic sclerosis, myositis, biliary cirrhosis, chronic hepatitis, cryoglobulinemia, vasculitis, and thyroiditis (Fig. 4.25).

Sjögren's syndrome is the second most common autoimmune rheumatic disorder, following RA. It progresses very slowly, with 8–10 years elapsing from the initial symptoms to the full-blown development of the syndrome. Although Sjögren's syndrome typically occurs in middle-aged women, the disease is known to appear in all ages and in men.

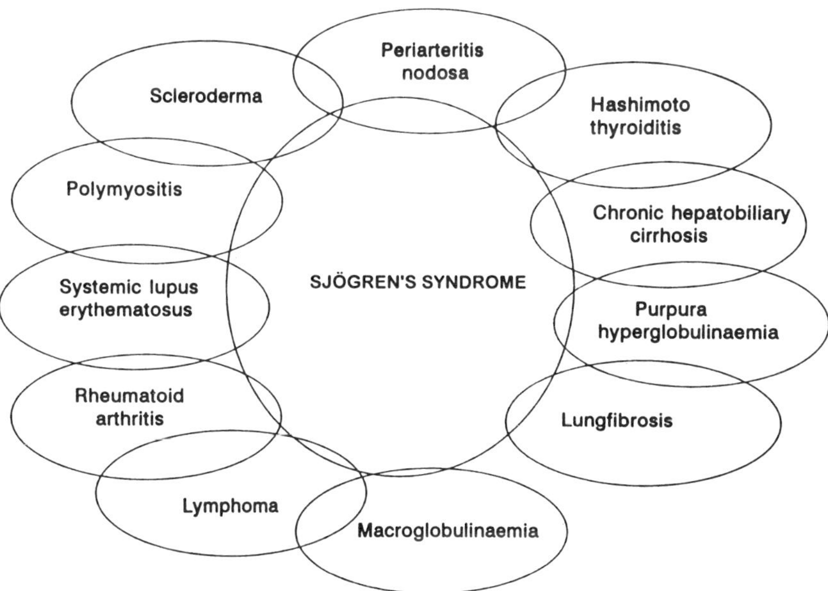

Figure 4.25 Disorders associated with Sjögren's syndrome.

1.8.2 Felty's Syndrome

This unusual complication of severe seropositive RA consists of splenomegaly, granulocytopenia, leg ulcers, and recurrent infections. Splenectomy has only a variable effect on leukopenia. There have been reports of improvement from SAARD therapy, particularly gold, methotrexate, and penicillamine. High-dose corticosteroid or lithium carbonate may provide short-term benefit with increases in neutrophil counts.

1.8.3 Palindromic Rheumatism

Palindromic rheumatism is a recurring acute arthritis and periarthritis with symptom-free intervals of days to months between attacks. Each attack begins suddenly in one or two joints, often in the late afternoon or evening, with pain that may be intense, reaching a peak within a few hours. Swelling, warmth, and redness over or near the affected joints are noted shortly after the onset of pain. These signs usually disappear in 1–3 days but may remain for as long as a week.

Fewer than 10% of patients experience a spontaneous remission but may continue to have attacks without developing persistent synovitis or permanent joint damage. In 30–40% of patients the disorder evolves into typical rheumatoid arthritis. These patients often have rheumatoid factor during the palindromic phase. The treatment is the same as for rheumatoid arthritis. Periarticular swelling can be symptomatically successfully treated with sublesional infiltration of xylocaine.

1.8.4 Intermittent Hydrarthrosis

The term intermittent hydrarthrosis has been used to describe recurrent effusions of unknown cause that occur with equal frequency in both sexes starting in the third to fifth decade. In contrast with palindromic rheumatism, the attacks come at regular intervals, usually with involvement of one knee or occasionally another large joint. Both knees are usually affected, but accompanied by minimal discomfort or signs of inflammation. The effusion resolves within an additional 2–4 days. Between attacks the joints appear entirely normal.

Pathologic changes of mild inflammation in the synovium have been reported, but clinical evolution into RA is rare. No treatment has been shown to abort or prevent attacks.

1.8.5 Rheumatoid Disease

Constitutional features of RA such as fatigue, weight loss, and systemic involvement as pleuritis, vasculitis, and the presence of rheumatoid factor may occur early in the course of the disease and may dominate, overshadowing the joint manifestations. This condition is often called rheumatoid disease (Fig. 4.26).

1.8.6 Adult Onset Still's Disease

Adult onset Still's disease is a form of polyarthritis associated with systemic manifestations identical to those described in children with systemic onset juvenile chronic arthritis or Still's disease. Common clinical features include sudden high spiking fever, sore throat, and an evanescent erythematosus salmon-colored rash. Fever and rash are often the only initial manifestations. The musculoskeletal manifestations consist of myalgias and arthralgias, and oligoarticular or polyarticular arthritis. Peripheral lymphadenopathy may be seen as well as hepatosplenomegaly, pleural pericarditis, and even peritonitis. Laboratory studies reveal high ESR and WBC count.

1.9 Impact of Disease and Prognosis

The course of rheumatoid arthritis tends to be uncertain for at least two reasons. (1) The natural history of groups of patients includes at least three types—I, II, and III (Table 4.9)—which cannot be distinguished definitively by laboratory tests or other studies, although patients with types II and III RA are more likely to have rheumatoid factor and be HLA DR4. Careful

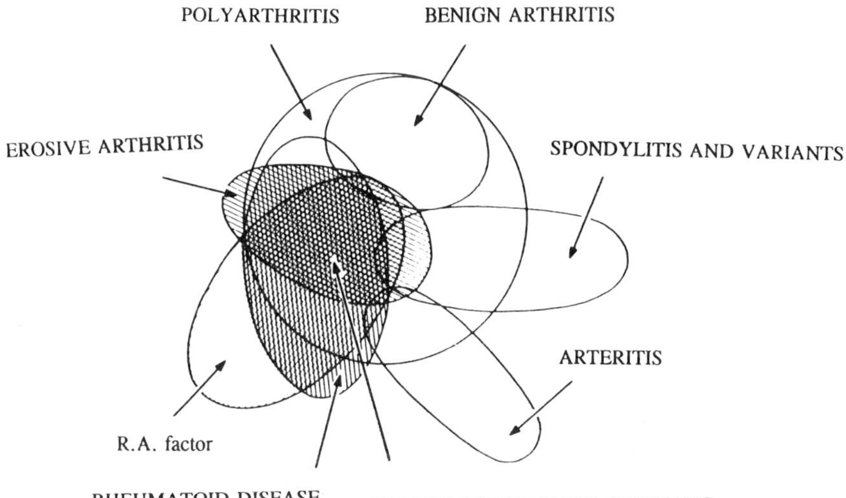

Figure 4.26 Venn diagram illustrating the different expressions of rheumatoid arthritis and their interrelationships.

Table 4.9 Subtypes of Clinical Course of Patients Who May Meet Classification Criteria for Rheumatoid Arthritis

Factor	Type I	Type II	Type III
Type of polyarthritis	Self-limited process	Minimally progressive disease	Progressive disease
Predominant site of identification	Population studies; occasionally in clinic	Clinical settings (unusual)	Clinical settings (unusual)
Estimated proportion of the next 100 patients with RA to be seen by a rheumatologist	5–20%	5–20%	60–90%
% rheumatoid factor–positive	<5%	60–90%	60–90%
Odds of HLA DR4	1:1	3–5:1	3–5:1
% who meet criteria for RA 3–10 years later	0% (by definition)	90–100% (a few may have a different diagnosis)	90–100% (a few may have a different diagnosis)
Response to tradional treatment approach	Long-term treatment not needed	Good, although some progression usually seen	Disease progression continues despite treatment
Markers to distinguish from other types	Rheumatoid factor HLA DR4	Course over 30–80 days ? Baseline clinical markers	Course over 30–180 days ? Baseline clinical markers

Source: Ref. 2.

monitoring over 30–90 days is often the most helpful method to predict the course of disease, if evidence of progressive disease is not apparent at presentation. Clearly, a patient who has 10 swollen joints at presentation but had 30 swollen joints 2 weeks earlier is in a different situation than a patient who has 10 swollen joints and had 3 swollen joints 2 weeks earlier, but the *rate* of change in patient measures the time of the first visit generally has been neglected in development of criteria. (2) The courses of individual patients with types II and III RA may vary considerably, from those who have a rapidly severe course to those with a relatively undulating course, both from patient to patient and within the same patient at different periods (Fig. 4.27).

RA was regarded traditionally in the 1970s and 1980s as, in the majority of instances, a disease with a good prognosis, in part based on the assumption that data from population-based studies in which the majority of patients had type I RA with a self-limited process, applied to most patients monitored in clinical settings. However, most patients with clinical RA have a type III progressive course. It is important to distinguish between measures of inflammatory activity and end-organ long-term damage in assessment of outcomes of RA. Measures of inflammatory activity, including ESR, number of tender joints, and patient global status, may improve over 5 years, even in the face of progressive functional disability. These data indicate that assessment of improvement in RA without a measure of functional disability and radiographic progression may lead to inappropriate optimism concerning the outcomes of therapy, as most patients with type III RA show radiographic damage, severe functional decline, work disability, and premature mortality in long-term clinical studies.

Radiographic damage in RA is often seen within the first 2 years of disease. Increases in radiographic scores according to various quantitative methods, including Larsen and Sharp scores, appear more rapid during

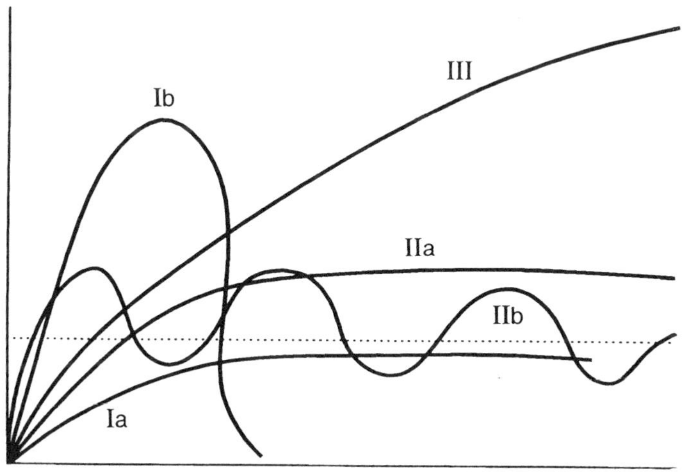

Figure 4.27 Course of RA. Type Ia: low grade not clinically manifest; seen in epidemiologic studies. Type Ib: important system features in the early phase—good recovery. Type IIa: slow progression, stable course. Type IIb: undulating course; drug-induced clinical or spontaneous (not necessarily radiologically) remission. Type III: malignant RA—progressive joint destruction—nonresponse to drugs.

early, rather than late, disease. Radiographic progression has been found in all longitudinal studies of patients with RA.

Most patients show severe declines in functional status over long periods, not explained by age. For example, in analyses over 9 years in 75 patients with RA, most declined in the capacity to perform physical tests of function, grip strength, and the button test, as well as in functional status according to questions concerning activities of daily living (Fig. 4.28). Many patients showed improvement in morning stiffness over 9 years, suggesting that the disease process may "burn out" over time but leave an individual patient with significant losses in functional capacity.

Work disability has been reported after 5 years in 60–70% of patients with RA younger than 65 years who had been working at onset of disease. A high rate of work disability has been recognized not only in patients seen in rheumatology settings, who may have more severe clinical status among all patients with RA, but also in individuals in the general population identified to have symmetric polyarthritis. Among men age 18–64 in the 1978 U.S. population, 87% were working, including 89% of those with no arthritis, versus only 56% of those with symmetric polyarthritis. Similar findings were seen for women.

Patients with RA appear to die from immediate causes substantially similar to those in the general population (Table 4.10). However, patients

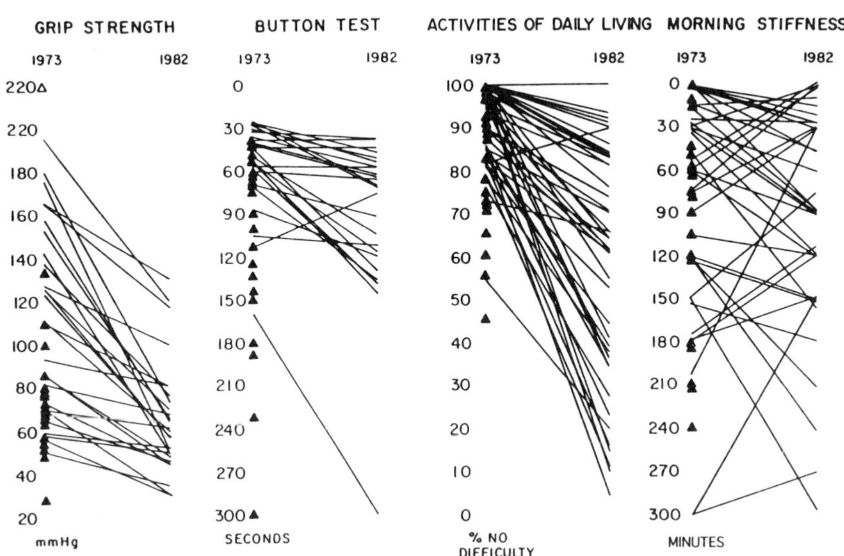

Figure 4.28 Long-term evaluation of function state in RA. (From Ref. 3.)

Table 4.10 Attributed Causes of Death (%) in 2269 Patients with
Rheumatoid Arthritis in 13 Series

Attributed cause of death	Patients with rheumatoid arthritis	1977 U.S. population
Cardiovascular disease	42.1	41.0
Cancer	14.1	20.4
Infection	9.4	1.0
Renal disease	7.8	1.1
Respiratory disease	7.2	3.9
Rheumatoid arthritis	5.3	Not listed
Gastrointestinal disease	4.2	2.4
Central nervous system disease	4.2	9.6
Accidents	1.0	5.4
Miscellaneous	6.4	15.2
Unknown	0.6	Not listed

Source: Ref. 4.

with RA die at an earlier age than would be expected for persons of similar age and sex in the general population. Ten studies from such diverse locations as Massachusetts, Canada, Sweden, England, the Netherlands, Finland, Minnesota, and Tennessee include actuarial life table analyses to examine survival and mortality. All of these studies indicate premature mortality in patients with RA (one study incorporates comparisons with osteoarthritis patients rather than with the general population) (Fig. 4.29).

Mortality in patients with RA, whether attributed to RA or other causes, is associated with more severe disease rather than simply a random event in persons with RA. In analyses over 15 years, significant high subsequent mortality was seen according to the baseline number of involved joints, with similar results in counts which included 50, 36, 28, 12, or even 6 joints. Mortality was also predicted by poorer functional status, documented according to four measures, questionnaire responses regarding activities of daily living, grip strength, walking time, and button test, as well as high age, low socioeconomic status, and comorbid cardiovascular disease. Five-year survivals were in the range of 85–95% in individuals with favorable values, versus 45–55% in patients with unfavorable baseline values for most of these measures. These findings are not explained by age, duration of disease, race or clinical setting, although age, educational level, and cardiovascular comorbidity were also significant predictive markers for mortality in RA.

Patients with poor clinical status according to measures of functional

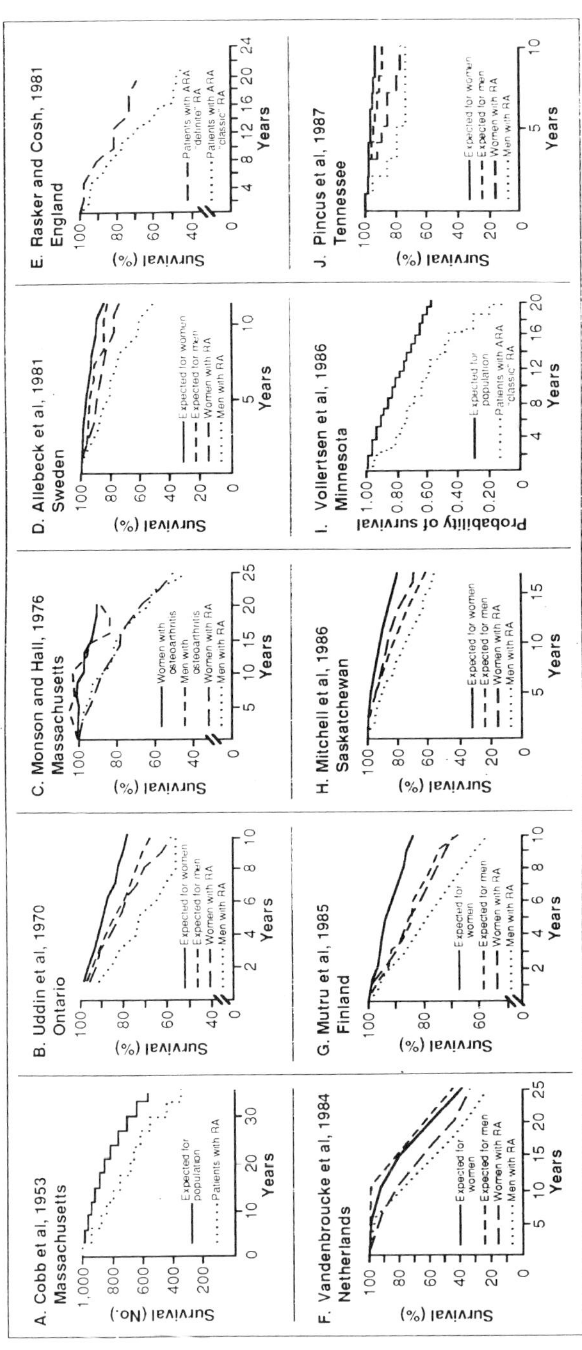

Figure 4.29 Survival and mortality. (From Ref. 5.)

status or the number of involved joints, cardiovascular comorbidities, older age, and low socioeconomic status are 4.4–7.5 times more likely to die over the next 5 years than patients with favorable status according to these measures.

Mortality rates in certain patients with severe RA over long periods may be in the ranges seen in cardiovascular and neoplastic diseases (Fig. 4.30). Patients with more than 20 involved joints or who could perform less

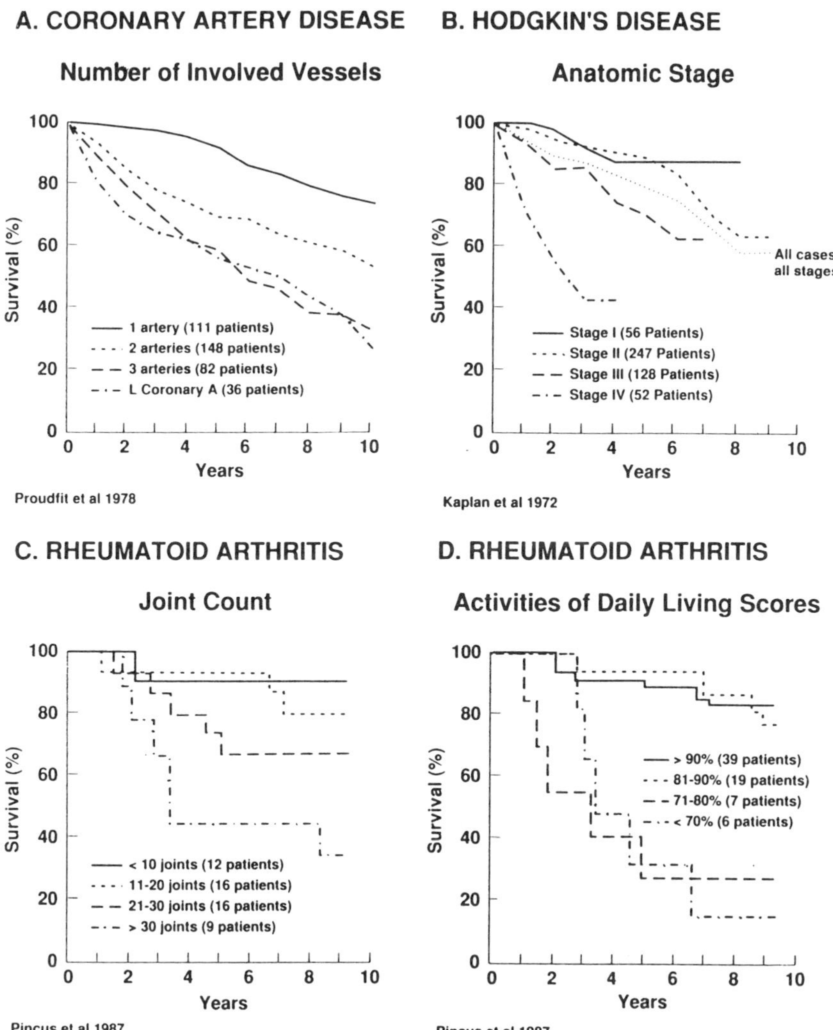

Figure 4.30 Mortality in severe RA. (From Ref. 6.)

than 80% of activities of daily living without difficulty according to a questionnaire were found to experience 5-year survival patterns of about 50%, in the range of patients with three-vessel coronary artery disease or stage IV Hodgkin's disease. A smaller proportion of RA patients appear in the poorest prognostic category compared to patients with cardiovascular or neoplastic diseases, and many patients with coronary artery disease and Hodgkin's disease were studied earlier in the disease course than the RA patients. Nonetheless, certain patients with RA have a poor prognosis for survival comparable with those seen for certain patients with cardiovascular and neoplastic diseases.

2 JUVENILE CHRONIC ARTHRITIS

2.1 Definition (Table 4.11)

Juvenile chronic arthritis (JCA), known as juvenile rheumatoid arthritis (JRA) in the USA, is the most commonly diagnosed rheumatic disease in children and is often an important cause of disability and blindness. However, JCA is not a single disease but rather a heterogeneous group of diseases. The criteria for diagnosis include age of onset under 16 years and the exclusion of other forms of juvenile arthritis. After 6 months three major onset subtypes can be identified that help in clarifying the prognosis:

> Pauciarticular onset (four or fewer joints involved) is the most common form, with 55–75% of cases presenting in this manner.
> Polyarticular onset (five or more joints affected) composes 15–25% of the whole group.

Table 4.11 Juvenile Chronic Arthritis

Chronic arthritis onset before 16 years of age
Heterogeneous group diseases
Three major subtypes according to onset pattern:
    —Pauciarticular: less than 2 years old
                older than 9 years
    —Polyarticular: RAF-negative or positive
    —Systemic
Management has to be multidisciplinary
Prognosis and course of disease differ according to subtype
Prognosis is favorable in 75% of patients
Pauciarticular + ANA — asymptomatic chronic uveitis and blindness
Children with arthritis ankylose earlier than adults

Systemic onset JCA composes 10–20% of the whole group and is defined as arthritis associated with daily temperature spikes to 39.5°C for at least 2 weeks with or without typical rash.

2.2 Main Clinical Features

2.2.1 Early Manifestations

Pauciarticular Onset JCA. By definition these patients have an involvement (synovial swelling and tenderness) of four or fewer joints. One third go on to a polyarticular course and these may very well be different diseases. Two subtypes of pauciarticular onset JCA can be identified: those presenting with lower extremity arthritis before the age of 5 years; those presenting over the age of 9 years with or without sacroiliitis.

PAUCIARTICULAR JCA BEFORE THE AGE OF 5 YEARS. This subgroup occurs more frequently in females with a ratio of 4 : 1. Few children complain of pain; commonly such children are brought to the physician because of a limp. The knee is the most commonly affected joint (47%) followed by the ankle and then either the small joints of the hand or the elbow.

Antinuclear antibodies (ANAs) are present in 40–75% of children with pauciarticular onset JCA with onset before the age of 5 years and are largely associated with chronic anterior uveitis. The child with uveitis is asymptomatic 90% of the time, thus making routine eye examination essential. The course of the eye disease is unrelated to the course of the arthritis and often persists after the arthritis has remitted.

PAUCIARTICULAR JCA AFTER THE AGE OF 9 YEARS. This subgroup affects boys more than girls. The lower extremity tends to be involved (especially the knee and ankle) but, in contrast to the younger onset pauciarticular group, the hip can also be affected. HLA B27 is present in about 50% of children. Some of these children develop enthesitis and/or sacroiliitis several years later, and some will develop ankylosing spondylitis or other spondylarthropathies. Iritis, usually acute and symptomatic, occurs in 15–25% of this group.

Polyarticular Onset JCA. Approximately 20% of children with JCA have polyarticular onset, with five or more joints involved in the first 6 months of disease. This subtype is divided into those who have persistent serum IgM rheumatoid factor (RF) and those who do not.

The RF-negative polyarticular onset JCA is often indistinguishable from the arthritis that follows systemic onset JCA. These patients may have low-grade fevers. This form of the disease occurs throughout childhood. It comprises approximately 15% of the JCA cases. The joints tend to be symmetrically involved, with the knees, wrists, and ankles being most commonly affected. The neck is often involved and occasionally patients will present with torticollis.

The RF-positive polyarticular onset JCA is very similar to adult onset rheumatoid arthritis. Most patients are female and present between 12 and 16 years of age.

Systemic Onset JCA (Still's Disease).   This subtype is most often associated with the most serious short- and long-term morbidity as well as significant mortality. It makes up 20% of the total JCA population and is defined by its extraarticular features of fever, rash, lymphadenopathy, hepatosplenomegaly, and asymptomatic pericarditis. Fever up to 40°C usually occurs late in the afternoon or evening (Fig. 4.31).

When there is fever, a characteristic evanescent salmon-colored eruption may occur on the trunk and thighs. Children with systemic onset JCA develop arthritis fairly early, i.e., within few months of the onset of the fever. The wrists, knees, and ankles are most commonly involved.

2.2.2   Late Manifestations

Growth abnormalities are common. Children with knee involvement before the age of 3 years may have a longer leg on the side of the involved knee. In children over 9 years old, local growth disturbances often result in early

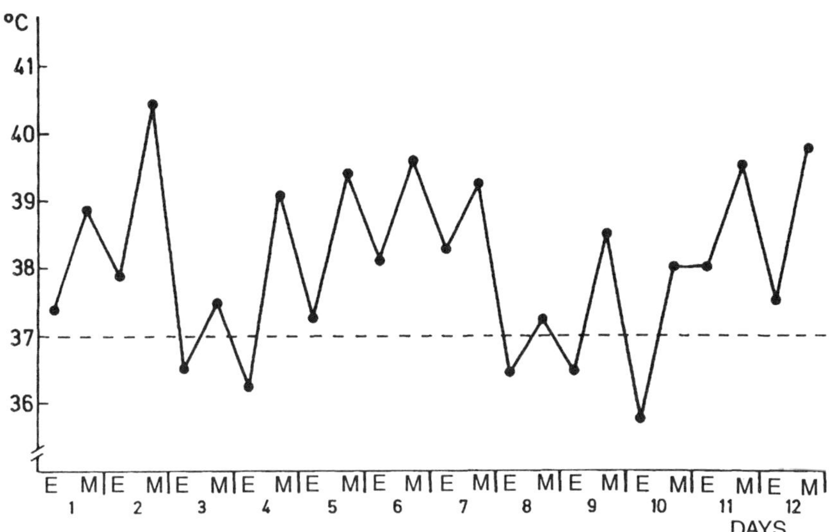

Figure 4.31   Typical fever pattern of juvenile chronic arthritis. M = morning; E = evening.

epiphyseal closure, causing a shortened leg. Bony ankylosis, more common in children with arthritis than in adults, is seen most frequently in the carpal and tarsal bones and in the cervical spine apophyseal joints, and is more characteristic of the systemic onset patients. Micrognathia is observed in 20% of children with JCA.

2.3 Confirming the Diagnosis—Investigations

As JCA is a diagnosis of exclusion, laboratory studies can only be used to support the clinical suspicion of JCA. Most of the laboratory abnormalities reflect the extent of the inflammatory response. Anemia is common in all forms of JCA and is more pronounced in the systemic onset. Leukocytosis up to 15,000–25,000/mm^3 with a neutrophilic predominance is seen in 81% of those children with systemic onset JCA. ESR is usually elevated, except in the pauciarticular patients where it is frequently normal. Serum immuno-globulins will often be elevated as will the ASO titer, even though there is no evidence for a recent streptococcal infection. The present of rheumatoid factor (RF), antinuclear antibodies (ANAs), and certain HLA antigens—in particular HLA B27—may assist in classifying patients. ANA is positive in 40–60% of pauciarticular onset JCA before age 5 years and this is associated with chronic uveitis. HLA B27 is positive in more than 50% of the adolescents with pauciarticular disease without correlation with evolution of ankylosing spondylitis. Except for epiphyseal growth plate changes, X-ray features resemble those of rheumatoid arthritis. In JCA, however, earlier bone ankylosis is more often seen.

2.4 Diagnostic Difficulties

2.4.1 Septic Arthritis

Infection must be excluded early through aspiration and culture of the affected joint. Infective arthritis is usually monoarticular.

2.4.2 Lyme Arthritis

Lyme arthritis can masquerade as JCA, particularly because it tends to be migratory over several months to years. A serologic test for *Borrelia burgdorferi* can be helpful but should be interpreted in connection with clinical findings.

2.4.3 Leukemia

In a child with painful joints and fever, acute lymphoblastic leukemia has to be excluded. Thrombocytopenia and neutropenia are not seen in systemic onset JCA.

2.4.4 Acute Rheumatic Fever

Usually rheumatic fever has a sustained fever. The migratory arthritis is exquisitely painful in contrast to systemic JCA and the rash migratory.

2.5 Epidemiology and Historical Data

The prevalence of JCA is not well established and varies from 0.40 to 1.13 per 1000, and incidence rate between 2.2 and 18.2 per 100,000. These large differences can be explained by differences in the definition of JCA, which in fact is a conglomerate of many possible rheumatic diseases.

In 1896, Georges Frederic Still of London gave for the first time a full description of juvenile rheumatoid arthritis on the basis of 21 cases. Since then his name has been associated with arthritis in children. Some people utilize Still's disease as only applying to the systemic form; others to all forms of juvenile arthritis.

2.6 Pathophysiology

In the context of the available information, any hypothesis for the etiology of chronic childhood arthritis must include major roles for infection and genetics. To date, with the exception of the reactive arthritides and Lyme disease, the evidence that any single microbial agent causes a significant proportion of chronic arthritis in childhood is largely circumstantial or indirect. An increasing understanding of the interactions between the HLA molecules on antigen-presenting cells, the T-cell receptor, and the processed antigen holds promise for establishing the identity of antigens involved in the immunopathogenesis of chronic arthritis.

2.7 Management

Early diagnosis and comprehensive therapy of JCA are important to minimize deformity and maximize normal growth and development. The immediate therapeutic goals for JCA are relief of symptoms, maintenance of joint range of motion and muscle strength in patients seen early in their illness, and rehabilitation of those seen later in the disease. Physical, emotional, and pharmacologic aspects of therapy are all important.

If JCA is incompletely responsive to aspirin or other NSAIDs after several months, intramuscular gold therapy may be added. Gold is as effective in the treatment of children as it is in adults. It is given at a dosage of 0.7–1 mg/kg each week, up to a maximum of the adult dosage of 50 mg weekly. Therapy should be monitored by blood counts, urinalysis, and physical examinations. Gold is often continued for several years. Oral weekly pulse methotrexate, started at 10 mg/M^2 or 0.3 mg/kg up to 1 mg/

kg/week, is now often substituted if gold is ineffective, or it may be started before gold.

Methotrexate should be considered early for the treatment of severe, longstanding, corticosteroid-dependent, or rapidly progressive JCA.

Hydroxychloroquine and *p*-penicillamine have been used in JCA with results less favorable than those seen in adults. Use is generally only adjunctive or is reserved for methotrexate or gold treatment failures.

Systemic corticosteroids are contraindicated in the treatment of JCA, except for patients with life-threatening systemic disease or, rarely, in low doses for short periods while awaiting response to methotrexate or gold. Oral corticosteroid therapy should begin with an alternate day regimen and must include good parent and patient education about growth suppression and other toxicities. There is no indication for systemic corticosteroids in pauciarticular or mild polyarticular JCA. Disabling pain or flexion contraction in one or a few joints may occasionally be treated by intraarticular long-acting corticosteroid injections and splinting.

Muscle weakness and atrophy, decreased endurance, and contractures are features of JCA that contribute significantly to disability. Exercises to maximize muscle strength, joint range of motion, and function are extremely valuable. Evaluations by physical and occupational therapists are important. Treatment plans should reflect the child's level of maturity; be performed daily, and be adopted by child, parents, and school as part of their normal activities of daily living.

Morning baths are excellent to relieve stiffness. An auxillary electric blanket plugged into a timer, set to activate 1 hr before the child arises, is an effective alternative. Emphasis on good posture should start at diagnosis. Wrist contractures may be reduced by the use of resting splints; a soft cervical collar may retard neck flexion deformities. Bedrest is contraindicated and children with JCA should be encouraged to be physically active, as tolerated.

Synovectomy does not benefit the course of JCA but may be helpful for pain reduction in rare instances. Total joint replacements may greatly improve function in longstanding disease but must await full bone growth near affected joints. Early closure of epiphyses, although complicated by reduced total bone size, may permit surgery by the early to mid-teenage years.

Children with JCA should be strongly encouraged to be self-sufficient and responsible to an age-appropriate extent, should attend regular schools, and should lead as normal a life as possible.

Adaptive devices may be helpful in achieving independence in some cases. Vocational and psychological counseling are often beneficial for teenagers, even in the absence of significant disabilities. The goal of all treatment for JCA is to optimize health status and functional outcomes.

2.8 Impact of Disease and Prognosis

Although JCA is often chronic, the prognosis for most children is good. At least 75% of patients eventually enter long periods of disease quiescence or remission with little or no residual disability. Many parents and children are alarmed by the diagnosis; thus effective treatment begins with detailed education of the child, parents, and community. Attention to counseling needs is important and the school should also be actively involved. Many children with objective arthritis complain little of joint pain, particularly if they are younger than 10 years old.

The prognosis varies in each group, being best in the oligoarticular patient and worst in the rheumatoid factor–positive polyarticular group.

Although in the majority of patients the long-term prognosis is favorable, several cases with longstanding polyarthritis, unremitting high ESR despite treatment, turns out to have a bad prognosis, ending up with severe joint deformities and amyloidosis.

Amyloidosis in children suffering from JCA varies greatly from country to country. Amyloidosis in children with JCA is, for example, much more frequent in Eastern Europe than in other countries. Severe hip disease may require early total hip replacement.

Blindness due to chronic uveitis is not always avoided even with careful treatment and follow-up by an ophthalmologist. Children at greatest risk are those with pauciarticular disease with onset before the age of 5 years and who are ANA-positive.

REFERENCES

1. Panayi GG. Immunology of Connective Tissue Diseases. Norwell, MA: Kluwer Academic Publishers, 1994.
2. Pinus T, Callahan LF. How many types of patients meet classification criteria for RA? J Rheumatol 1994; 21:1385–1389.
3. Pincus T, Callahan LF. Rheumatology function tests: grip strength, walking time, button test and questionnaires document and predict longterm morbidity and mortality in rheumatoid arthritis. J Rheumatol 1992; 19:1051–1057.
4. Pincus, T, Callahan LF. Early mortality in RA predicted by poor clinical status. Bull Rheumatic Dis 1992; 41:1–4.
5. Pincus T, Callahan LF. The "side effects" of rheumatoid arthritis: joint destruction, disability and early mortality. Br J Rheumatol 1993; (suppl 1)32:28–37.
6. Pincus T, Callahan LF. Reassessment of twelve traditional paradigms concerning the diagnosis, prevalence, morbidity and mortality of rheumatoid arthritis. Scand J Rheumatol 1989; (suppl)79:67–95.

5

Ankylosing Spondylitis and Related Conditions

Ankylosing spondylitis (AS) is a chronic inflammatory disease that primarily affects the axial skeleton with sacroiliac joint involvement (sacroiliitis) and strong genetic association with HLA B27. Two forms of the disease are recognized: primary (idiopathic) and secondary associated with reactive arthritis, psoriasis, or inflammatory bowel diseases (Table 5.1).

1 CLINICAL FEATURES

1.1 Early Manifestations

Pain or stiffness in the lower back, which is worse in the morning and eased by mild physical activity, usually beginning in late adolescence or early adulthood, more in men than in women. At times the pain may wake the patient from sleep. The pain is dull in character, difficult to localize, and felt deep in the gluteal, sacroiliac region or lumbar area. It may be unilateral and intermittent at first. Sometimes the first symptoms result from involvement of hips or shoulders.

Extraarticular enthesitis at the costosternal junction, iliac crest, greater trochanters, ischial tuberositis, or heels may be present or antedate the spinal features. Also intermittently, acute iritis may have occurred before the spinal inflammation. Acute iritis (anterior uveitis) occurs in 25–30% of patients at some time in the course of the disease. A family history

Table 5.1   Ankylosing Spondylitis

Chronic inflammatory disease of the spine
Sacroiliitis in young individuals
More in males than in females
HLA B27–associated
Primary: idiopathic
Secondary: to reactive arthritis, psoriasis, inflammatory bowel disease
Extraarticular feature: enthesitis, anterior uveitis — aortic insufficiency
Prognosis: bamboo-spine end stage in some
NSAID in early disease

of AS is often noted. The clinical features of ankylosing spondylitis are summarized in Table 5.2 and the 1966 New York Criteria for ankylosing spondylitis in Table 5.3.

A thorough physical examination of the axial and peripheral skeleton is critical in making an early diagnosis. Physical signs may be minimal in the early stage of the disease. Limitation of the motion of the spine should be examined and measured by fingertip–floor distance, Schober test, and chest expansion on breathing (see Chapter 1).

Direct pressure over the inflamed sacroiliac joints frequently causes pain, but sometimes the sacroiliac pain may be elicited by pressure over both anterior iliac crests with the patient lying supine; maximal flexion, abduction, and external rotation of the hip joints; compression of the pelvis with the patient lying on the side; or direct pressure over the sacrum with the patient lying prone (see Chapter 1). These signs may be negative in some AS patients because the sacroiliac joints are surrounded by strong ligaments that may allow only minimal motion or in late stages of the disease when inflammation is replaced by fibrosis and bony ankylosis.

Table 5.2   Clinical Features of Ankylosing Spondylitis

Skeletal	Extraskeletal
Axial arthritis, such as sacroiliitis and spondylitis	Eyes (acute iritis)
Arthritis of hip and shoulder joints	Heart and ascending aorta
Peripheral arthritis	Lung (apical fibrosis)
Others: enthesopathy, osteoporosis, spinal fracture, spondylodiscitis, pseudoarthrosis	Cauda equina syndrome
	Amyloidosis

Table 5.3   1966 New York Criteria for Ankylosing Spondylitis

Presence of history of pain at dorsolumbar junction or in lumbar spine
Limitation of motion in anterior, lateral flexion and extension
Limitation of chest expansion to 1 in. (2.5 cm) or less at the fourth intercostal space
Requirements:
Either positive radiographs (grade 3–4 bilateral SI) and one or more clinical criteria,
   or grade 3–4 unilateral or grade 2 bilateral SI with clinical criterion 2 or with
   clinical criteria 1 and 3

1.2   Late Manifestations

The entire spine becomes increasingly stiff after many years of disease progression, with continued flattening of lumbar spine and gentle thoracic kyphosis. Involvement of the cervical spine results in progressive limitation of neck motion and a forward cervical stoop that can be assessed by measuring the distance from occiput to wall with the patient standing with back against the wall. The chest becomes flattened, the breathing becomes primarily diaphragmatic, and the abdomen becomes protuberant. The diagnosis is readily apparent at this advanced stage because of the characteristic gait and posture (Fig. 5.1) and the way the patient sits or rises from the examining table.

Cardiac involvement is rare and includes ascending aortitis, aortic valve incompetence (3.5–10%), and conduction abnormalities (2.7–8.5%), sometimes leading to implantation of cardiac pacemaker. Risk increases with age, duration of AS, and the presence of peripheral joint arthritis. Lung parenchymal involvement is a rare and late extraskeletal manifestation and is characterized by a slowly progressive fibrosis of the upper lobes of the lungs that appears on average two decades after the onset of AS.

Neurologic involvement may occur, most often related to spinal fracture/dislocation, atlantoaxial subluxations, or cauda equina syndrome. The fracture usually occurs in the cervical spine: the resultant quadriplegia is the most dreaded complication, with a high mortality. Spontaneous anterior atlantoaxial subluxation is a well-recognized complication of AS. It occurs in about 2% of patients and presents as occipital pain with or without signs of spinal cord compression. It is generally observed in the later stages of the disease, more commonly in those with peripheral joint involvement. Slowly progressive cauda equina syndrome is a rare but significant and underdiagnosed complication of longstanding AS, manifested clinically by a gradual onset of urinary and fecal incontinence, pain, and sensory loss in the sacral distribution ("saddle anesthesia"), impotence, and, occasionally, loss of ankle jerks.

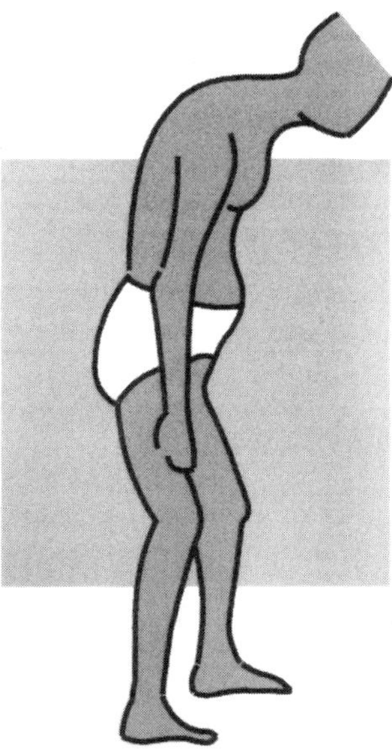

Figure 5.1 Characteristic position of advanced ankylosing spondylitis.

The marked muscle wasting seen in some patients with advanced disease results from disuse atrophy, although some ultrastructural changes and raised levels of serum creatinine phosphokinase have been observed in patients. Amyloidosis (secondary) is a rare complication; the presence of proteinuria and progressive azotemia should raise the possibility of amyloidosis with renal involvement. IgA nephropathy can cause hematuria.

2 CONFIRMING THE DIAGNOSIS—INVESTIGATIONS

The diagnosis is based on clinical features. Often the best clues are offered by the patient's symptoms, family history, articular and extraarticular physical findings, and roentgenologic evidence of bilateral sacroiliitis.

There are no diagnostic or pathognomonic tests. An elevated erythrocyte sedimentation rate is seen in up to 75% of patients, and mild to moderate elevation of serum IgA concentration is also frequently observed. There is no association with rheumatoid factor and antinuclear antibodies, and the synovial fluid does not show distinctive features as compared to other inflammatory anthropathies. A mild normocytic normochronic anemia may be present in 15% of patients.

HLA B27 typing can occasionally be used as an aid to the diagnosis of AS, but an overwhelming majority of patients can be diagnosed clinically on the basis of history, physical examination, and roentgenographic findings. It is not a routine, diagnostic, confirmatory, or screening test for AS in patients with back pain, even though the test in some ethnic and racial groups is highly sensitive for AS (90% sensitivity among Caucasians). The clinical usefulness of a test depends on the setting in which it is performed.

The characteristic radiographic changes of AS evolve over many years, and are primarily seen in the axial skeleton, especially in the sacroiliac, discovertebral and apophyseal joints. Sacroiliitis is the earliest and most consistent finding. A simple posteroanterior roentgenograph is usually sufficient for its detection, as well as for the vertebral manifestations, e.g., the T11 femoral head picture (Fig. 5.2).

The changes are bilateral and symmetric, and consist of blurring of the subchondral bone plate, followed by erosions resembling postage stamp serrations, and sclerosis of the adjacent bone. They are first noted and are more prominent on the iliac side of the joint. Progression of the subchondral bone erosions can lead to "pseudowidening" of the sacroiliac joint space, followed later by gradual narrowing due to interosseous bridging and ossification. After many years there may be complete bony ankylosis of the sacroiliac joints and resolution of the juxtaarticular bony sclerosis (Fig. 5.3).

The inflammatory lesions in the vertebral column affect the superficial layers of the annulus fibrosus, at their attachment to the corners of vertebral bodies, resulting in reactive bone sclerosis, seen roentgenographically as highlighting of the corners and subsequent bone resorption (erosions) (Fig. 5.4). This leads to "squaring" of the vertebral bodies and grad-

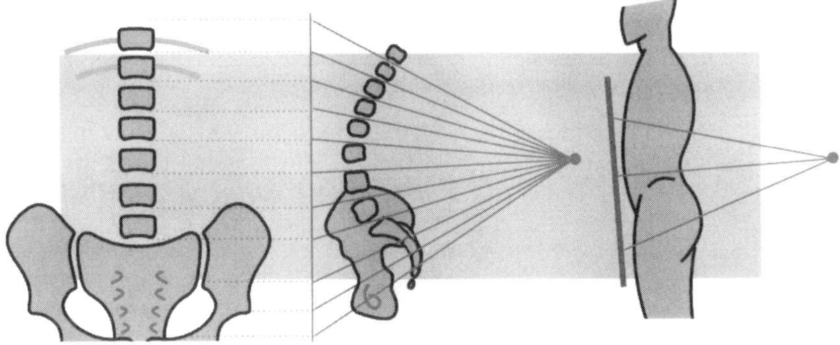

Figure 5.2 Posteroanterior X ray of lumbar spine. T11 to femoral head.

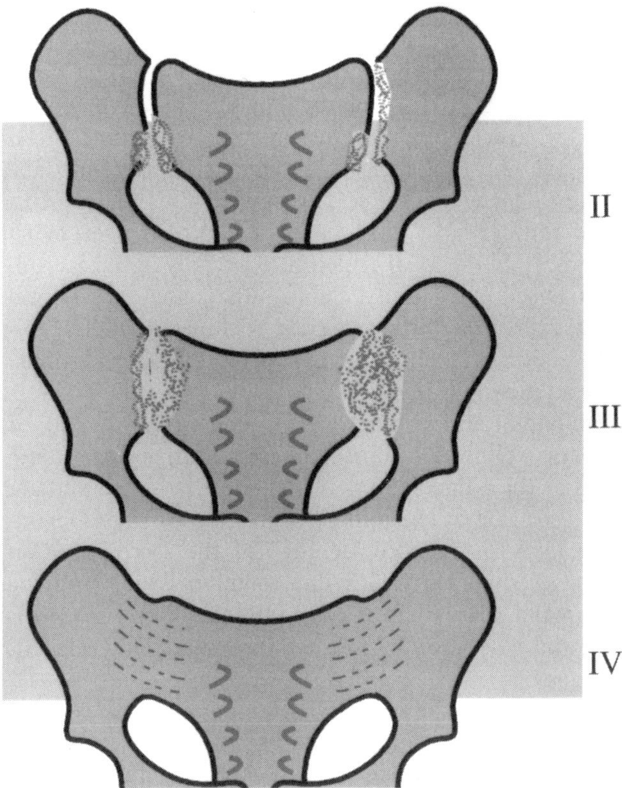

Figure 5.3   Grading sacroiliitis X ray from II to IV.

ual ossification of the superficial layers of the annulus fibrosus, which forms intervertebral bony "bridging." Before bridging occurs, *syndesmophytes* can be seen on X rays at the thoracolumbar and upper lumbar area.

There are often concomitant inflammatory changes resulting in ankylosis of the apophyseal joints and ossification of the spinal ligaments, ultimately resulting in a virtually complete fusion of the vertebral column (bamboo spine) in patients with severe AS of long duration (Fig. 5.5).

Spinal osteoporosis is also frequently observed as a result of ankylosis and lack of spinal mobility. Bony erosions and osteitis ("whiskering") at sites of osseous attachments of tendons and ligaments are frequently seen, particularly at the ischial tuberosities, iliac crest, calcaneum, femoral trochanters, and spinous processes of the vertebrae.

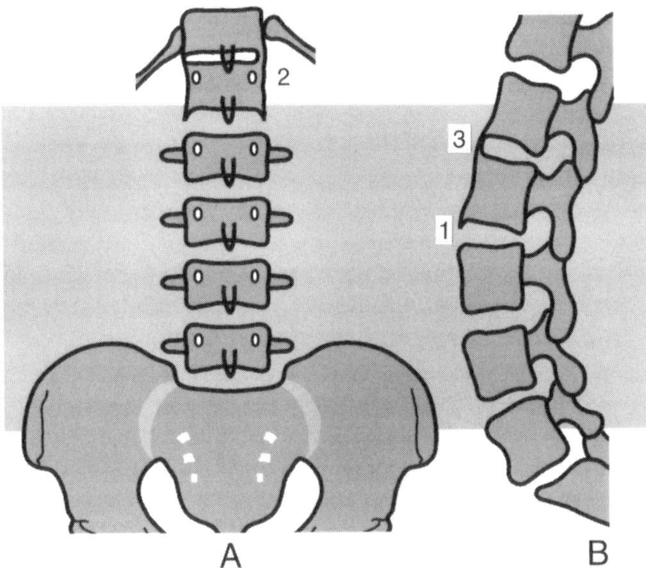

Figure 5.4 Early X-ray changes ankylosing spondylitis. (A) Lumbar spine and pelvis in posteroanterior X ray: bilateral sacroiliitis (1), enlarged joint space, irregular and vague joint margins and sclerosis. Intervertebral ligamentous ossification at the thoracolumbar area (syndesmophytes), fully calcified bridging (2). (B) Lumbar spine in profile: anterior spondylitis (Romanus sign) (1), erosion vertebral margins with sclerosis and squarring; early ligamentous ossification (2), full bridging between two adjacent vertebrae (3).

Hip joint involvement leads to symmetric concentric joint space narrowing, irregularity of the subchondral bone plate with subchondral sclerosis, and osteophyte formation at the outer margin of the articular surface, including the acetabulum and the femoral head. It may results in bony ankylosis. Shoulder joint involvement causes concentric joint space narrowing, with erosions primarily at the superolateral aspect of the humeral head.

In patients with early disease in whom standard roentgenography of the sacroiliac joints may show normal or equivocal changes, computed tomography (CT) appears to be more sensitive but equally specific. However, it is rarely needed. Magnetic resonance imaging (MRI) can produce excellent but costly imaging without ionizing radiation and is especially useful in visualizing posterior lumbosacral arachnoid diverticuli associated with cauda equina syndrome (Fig. 5.6). Quantitative radioactive bone scintigraphy is too nonspecific to be useful in detecting early sacroiliitis.

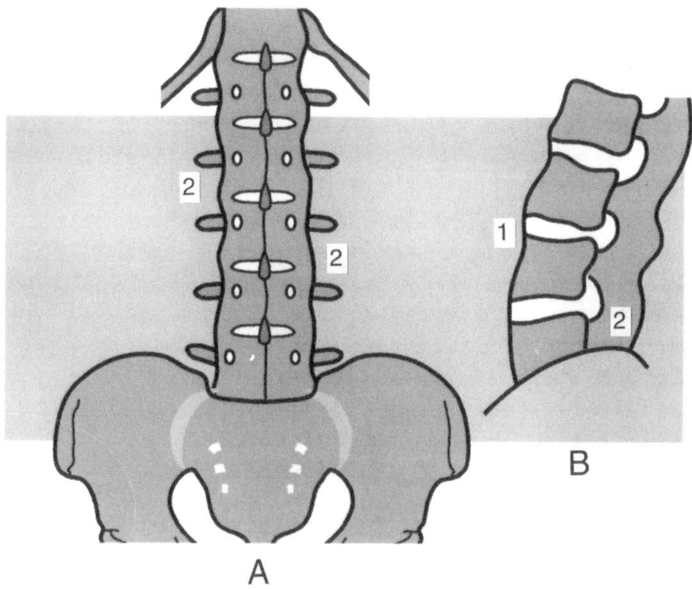

Figure 5.5 Advanced X-ray changes ankylosing spondylitis. (A) Lumbar spine in posteroanterior X ray: sacroiliacal ankylosis (1), multiple intervertebral calcified ligamentous bridges (bamboo spine), ossification of the interprocesus spinosus ligament (2). (B) Lumbar spine profile X ray: intervertebral ossification (1), ankylosans of the interapophyseal joints (2).

3   DIAGNOSTIC DIFFICULTIES

Spondylosis (degenerative backpain). However, low back pain is an extremely common symptom in the general population and is mostly due to mechanical, not inflammatory, causes. This pain is generally aggravated by activity and relieved by rest. There is no limitation of chest expansion or of lateral flexion of the lumbar spine; the erythrocyte sedimentation rate is frequently normal; and pelvic radiograph reveals absence of sacroiliitis.

Ankylosing hyperostosis (also called Forestier's disease or diffuse idiopathic skeletal hyperostosis, DISH) is a condition usually first seen at an older age and characterized by thick, layered hyperostosis affecting the anterior longitudinal ligament and bony attachments of tendons and ligaments and normal disc space (Fig. 5.7). It might be roentgenographically confused with advanced ankylosing spondylitis.

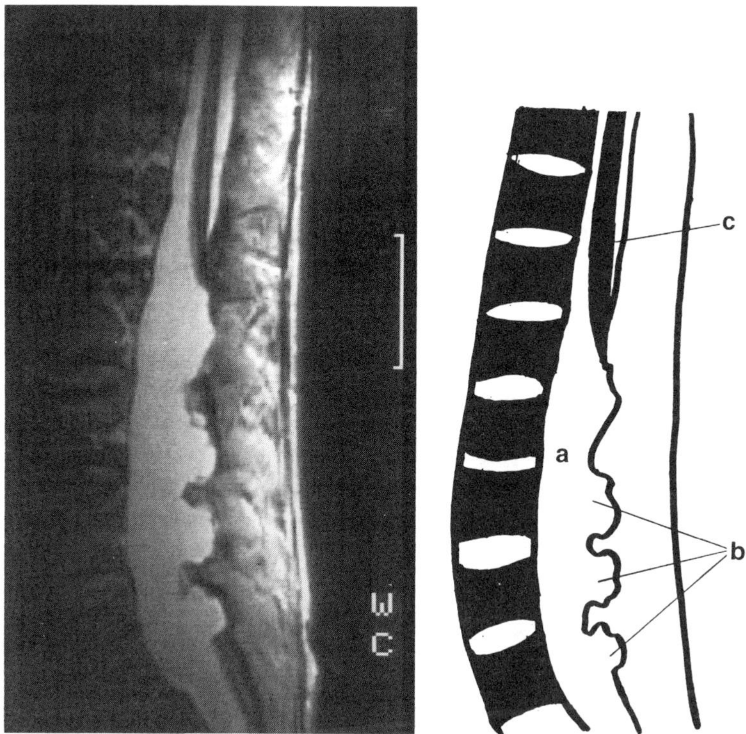

Figure 5.6 MRI cauda equina ankylosing spondylitis: (a) widened dural sac, (b) diverticula, (c) conus terminalis.

Osteitis condensans ilii is most common in young women and produces bone sclerosis limited to the iliac side of the sacroiliac joint. Osteitis condensans of the ilium is nearly always a chance radiologic observation in women who have had multiple pregnancies. Apart from nonspecific backache, which may be confined to the lower lumbar region, there are no clinical complaints. The radiologic picture, showing sclerosis of the ilium opposite the lower part of the sacroiliac joint, may disappear completely after a time.

Related spondylarthropathies. Secondary ankylosing spondylitis may occur in association with reactive arthritis, Reiter's syndrome, psoriasis, or chronic inflammatory bowel disease (see Chapter 3). Involvement of peripheral joints, other than hips and shoulders, is infrequent in primary ankylosing spondylitis and therefore the physician should search for clinical features as seen in the reactive arthritis.

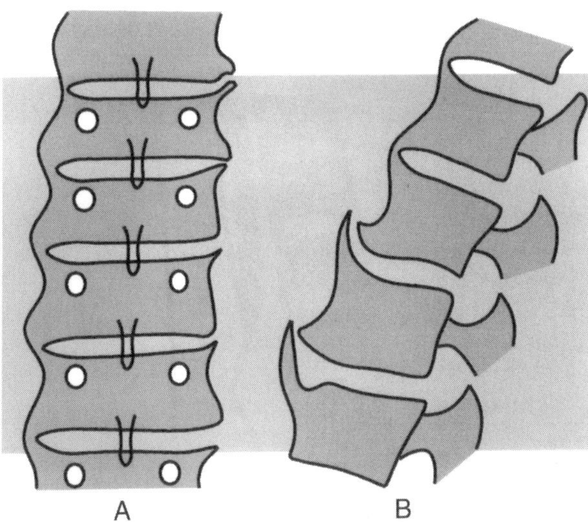

Figure 5.7 Hyperostosis vertebralis: (A) bony intervertebral bridging T7 to T12 right side, (B) pronounced osteophytosis at the L2–L3 and L3–L4 region.

4 EPIDEMIOLOGY AND HISTORICAL DATA

Ankylosing spondylitis (AS)—also called Bechterew's (1893 in St. Petersburg), Strümpell's(1897 in Berlin), or Marie's (1898 in Paris) disease for historical reasons—was for many years regarded as a severe, crippling rheumatic disease, affecting males only and occurring in perhaps less than 0.10% of the general Caucasian population. Recent studies, however, have clearly shown that the demographic and clinical spectrum of AS is much wider. The disease affects women not infrequently and is of higher prevalence than was previously appreciated. The prevalence differs according to the presence of HLA B27 in the population. The prevalence of HLA B27 in the general population does, however, show considerable geographic variation occurring in 50% of the Haidi Indians of northern Canada, but being virtually absent among black Africans and Guatamalan Indians. In Euro-Caucasians, 4–13% has prevalence in the northern Europe (Scandinavia). In Caucasian population, the prevalence of AS is about 0.5–1% and in HLA B27 individuals 5%.

5 PATHOPHYSIOLOGY

Ankylosing spondylitis and reactive arthritis are sometimes grouped under the name "spondyloarthropathies" and share a number of common features, of which the most important may be an association with the histocompatibility antigen HLA B27. Although there are significant clinical differences between these conditions, the common clinical manifestations, along with the association with HLA B27, implies that they might form a group of conditions with a related pathogenic mechanism. The spondyloarthropathies include ankylosing spondylitis, Reiter's syndrome, reactive arthritis, spondylitis associated with psoriasis and inflammatory bowel disease, and a variety of less clearly defined conditions termed undifferentiated spondyloarthropathies. In each of these conditions, there is infiltration of affected structures by inflammatory cells, including lymphocytes, plasma cells, macrophages, polymorphonuclear leukocytes, and mast cells. These findings are not unique to the spondyloarthropathies, however, but can be found in many other forms of inflammatory arthritis. The etiopathogenesis of none of these conditions is really understood, although an interaction between microorganisms and the gut or antigen derived from them and HLA B27 is likely to play a central role in most of them (see Pathogenesis of reactive arthritis, Chapter 3).

6 MANAGEMENT

There is currently no preventive measure or cure for AS. A concerned physician providing continuity of care can be most valuable. Patient education is crucial for successful management. The patient should thoroughly understand that although pain and stiffness can often be controlled by appropriate use of nonsteroidal antiinflammatory drugs (NSAIDs), regular therapeutic exercise to minimize and prevent deformity and disability is the single most important measure in medical management. The patient should walk erectly, do back extension exercises regularly, and sleep on a firm mattress, without a pillow if possible. It is better to sleep on the back or in a prone position with an extended and stretched back, and avoid sleeping curled up on one side. The patient should stop or avoid cigarette smoking and do regular deep breathing exercises to preserve normal chest expansion. Swimming is the best overall form of exercise for patients with AS, and use of snorkel and face mask can permit even those with considerable cervical flexion deformity to do free-style swimming.

NSAIDs or aspirin seldom provide an adequate response. Phenylbutazone is probably the most effective, but because of serious potential risk of bone marrow toxicity other NSAIDs, in particular indomethacin, should be tried first.

Sulfasalazine may be effective for peripheral arthritis in some AS patients, and because of its efficacy in inflammatory bowel disease as well, it appears to be especially useful in enteropathic AS, with peripheral arthritis, or for those intolerant to NSAIDs. Oral corticosteroids have no therapeutic value in the long-term management of the musculoskeletal aspects of AS because of their potential for serious side effects and they do not halt the progression of the disease. Recalcitrant enthesopathy and persistent synovitis may respond quite well to a local corticosteroid injection.

Acute anterior uveitis can be very well managed with dilatation of the pupil and use of corticosteroid eyedrops. Systemic steroids or immunosuppressives may be needed for refractory iritis. Cardiac complications may require aortic valve replacement or pacemaker implantation. Apical pulmonary fibrosis is not easy to manage: surgical resection of the apical segment of the lung may rarely be required.

Radiotherapy has little role in the modern management of patients with AS because of the high risk of leukemia and aplastic anemia.

7 ATYPICAL FORMS

7.1 Enteropathic Spondylarthropathy

7.1.1 Definition (Table 5.4)

The arthritis pattern observed in ulcerative colitis and Crohn's disease share many features—oligoarthritis, axial involvement in some, and genetic susceptibility—which are common to reactive arthritis. Therefore they will be discussed together briefly in this chapter.

7.1.2 Main Clinical Features

Peripheral Arthritis.   Peripheral arthritis occurs in 17–20% of patients, with a higher prevalence in those with Crohn's disease. The arthritis is pauciarticular, most asymmetric, and frequently transient and migratory. Large and small joints, predominantly of the lower limbs, are involved. The arthritis usually is nondestructive and many episodes subside within 6 weeks. Recurrences are common. Sausage-like fingers and toes may occur but are unusual. Enthesopathies, especially inflammation of the Achilles tendon (Fig. 5.8) or insertion of the plantar fascia, are known manifestations and may also involve the knee or other sites. The peripheral arthritis

Table 5.4 Enteropathic Spondylarthropathy

Spondylarthropathy/reactive arthritis associated with chronic inflammatory
  bowel disease
Oligoarthritis in males and females
Spondylarthropathy in males HLA B27 +

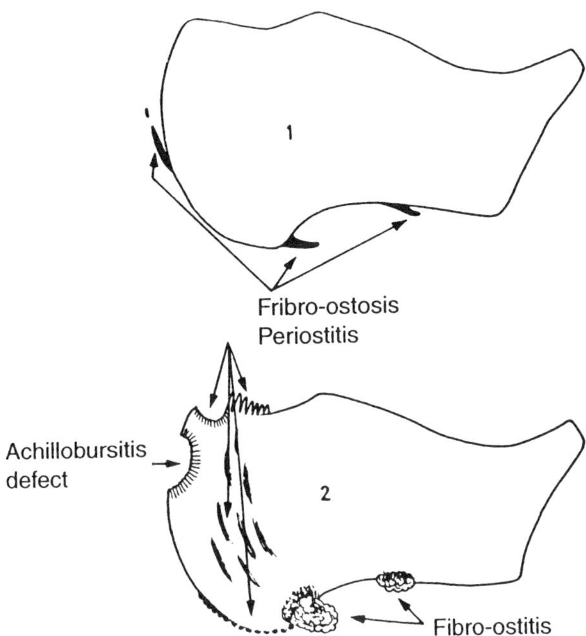

Figure 5.8 Achilles tendonitis enthesopathy.

may become chronic in some cases. Destructive joint lesions of small joints and hips have been described.

In most cases intestinal symptoms antedate or coincide with the joint manifestations, but the articular symptoms may precede the intestinal symptoms by years. There is evidence that in some cases of spondylarthropathy Crohn's disease could remain subclinical, with joint and tendon inflammation being the only clinical manifestation. In ulcerative colitis, there is a more distinct temporal relationship between attacks of arthritis and flares of bowel disease. Surgical removal of the diseased part of the colon can induce remission of the peripheral arthritis. In Crohn's disease, colonic involvement increases the susceptibility to peripheral arthritis, but surgical removal usually has little effect on the joint disease.

Axial Involvement. Axial involvement is similar in both diseases. The true prevalence of sacroiliitis is difficult to estimate because onset is frequently insidious. Prevalence rates of 10–20% for sacroiliitis and 7–12% for spondylitis have been described although the actual figures are probably higher.

The clinical picture may be indistinguishable from that of uncomplicated ankylosing spondylitis (Fig. 5.9). The patient complains of an inflammatory low back pain, thoracic or cervical pain, buttock pain, or chest pain. Limitation of motion in the lumbar or cervical region and reduced chest expansion are characteristic clinical signs. Peripheral arthritis may be associated. The onset of axial involvement does not parallel that of bowel disease and frequently precedes it. The course is also totally independent of

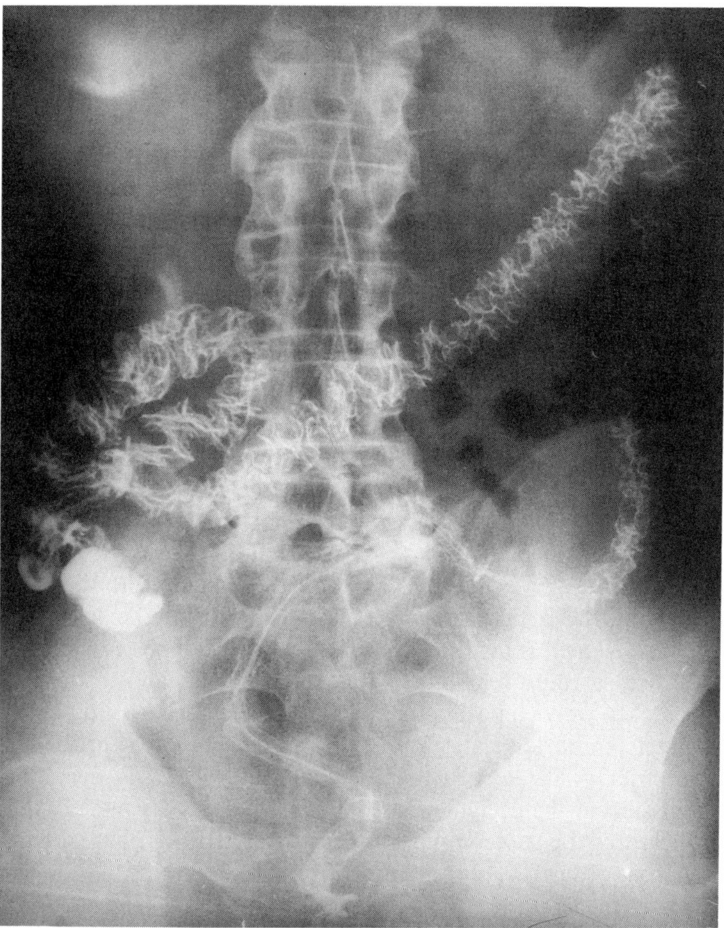

Figure 5.9 Typical X-ray features of ankylosing spondylitis, bilateral sacroiliitis, and syndesmophytes in a case with rectocolitis, abnormal pattern of intestinal mucosa, loss of sacculation.

the course of the intestinal disease. Bowel surgery does not alter the course of any associated sacroiliitis or spondylitis.

Extraintestinal and Extraarticular Features.   A variety of cutaneous, mucosal, serosal, and ocular manifestations may occur in inflammatory bowel disease. Skin lesions are most frequently associated and occur in 10–25% of patients. Erythema nodosum parallels the activity of bowel disease, tends to occur in patients with active peripheral arthritis, and is probably a disease-related manifestation. Pyoderma gangrenosum is a more severe but less common extraarticular manifestation, generally not related to the bowel and joint disease, and is probably an associated disorder. Leg ulcers and thrombophlebitis also may be seen.

Ocular manifestations, predominantly anterior uveitis, frequently accompany inflammatory bowel disease (3–11%). Uveitis is often acute in onset unilateral and transient, but recurrences are common. It generally spares the choroid and retina; however, a chronic course with lesions in the posterior part of the eye has been described. Granulomatous uveitis is rare but may be present in Crohn's disease. Acute anterior uveitis is more closely related to the axial involvement and to HLA B27. Conjunctivitis and episcleritis have also been described. Pericarditis is an uncommon complication, but secondary amyloidosis with involvement of major organs can be seen in Crohn's disease.

7.1.3 Confirming the Diagnosis—Investigations

Raised serum indicators of inflammation (especially C-reactive protein), thrombocytosis, and hypochromic anemia are common findings. The synovial fluid analysis findings are nonspecific and consistent with inflammatory arthritis, showing a cell count rating from 1500 to 50000 cells/mm^3. Cultures are negative. Synovial biopsies have been limited, but granulomas have been reported in some patients with Crohn's disease.

Sacroiliitis and spondylitis to a lesser degree than in uncomplicated ankylosing spondylitis are associated with HLA B27. The prevalence of HLA B27 ranges between 50% and 60%, although it is lower when only sacroiliitis is present. Ankylosing spondylitis patients not carrying the HLA B27 antigen are at a higher risk of developing inflammatory bowel disease than HLA B27–positive patients.

Radiologically, the axial involvement is often indistinguishable from uncomplicated ankylosing spondylitis. The frequency of asymmetric sacroiliitis may be higher than in idiopathic ankylosing spondylitis.

7.1.4 Pathophysiology

There is evidence of a genetic basis for both ulcerative colitis and Crohn's disease, as both occur in the same families. There is a genetic predisposition to both diseases, which seems to be genetically linked as well. No significant association with HLA antigens has been demonstrated, and the frequency of HLA B27 is within the normal range in patients with peripheral arthritis alone. The chapter on reactive arthritis presents more details concerning the immunopathogenesis.

7.1.5 Management

The pharmacologic and physical treatment of the peripheral arthritis and spondylitis is the same in inflammatory bowel disease as in ankylosing spondylitis. Nonsteroidal antiinflammatory drugs (NSAIDs) are the first choice, although they may cause an exacerbation of the intestinal symptoms in ulcerative colitis. Intraarticular corticosteroid injections may be beneficial in monoarticular chronic forms. Sulfasalazine, which was successfully used to treat the colonic inflammation in both diseases, has been found effective in the peripheral manifestations of the spondylarthropathies, especially if intestinal inflammation is present, and may help the peripheral arthritis of inflammatory bowel disease. Oral corticosteroids may reduce synovitis but are ineffective for the axial symptoms. They should be used systemically only if necessary to control bowel disease.

Intestinal surgery is infrequently indicated in the treatment of inflammatory bowel disease and can only influence the peripheral arthritis in ulcerative colitis.

7.2 Psoriatic Spondylarthropathy

7.2.1 Definition (Table 5.5)

Psoriatic spondylarthropathy is an inflammatory arthritis and/or spondylitis associated with psoriasis. The peripheral joints are often asymetrically involved; the rheumatologic factor and nodules are absent. Dactylitis and DIP joint involvement are seen more often than in other arthritides. In some cases, in particular the polyarticular ones, arthritis mutilans may be observed.

Table 5.5   Psoriatic Spondylarthropathy

Arthritis or spondylitis associated with psoriasis
Rheumatoid factor–negative
No rheumatoid nodules
Pauciarticular – polyarticular
Dactylitis and DIP–joint arthritis

7.2.2 Main Clinical Features

Early Manifestations.   In cases with psoriasis HLA B27 +, sacroiliitis and spondylitis can occur together with pauciarticular or polyarticular peripheral arthritis. In the majority of cases (75%) psoriasis procedes joint disease, but in a few cases (15%) the onset is synchronous and in 10% arthritis precedes psoriasis. It is worth repeating that in cases where there is asymmetric seronegative oligoarthritis (especially with the presence of dactylitis or DIP joint involvement), previously unrecognized psoriasis may be found in a flexural region, scalp, or nails (Fig. 5.10). Alternatively, there may be a history of widespread guttate psoriasis in childhood or a strong family history of psoriasis.

A common presentation is of an oligoarthritis consisting of a large joint as a knee, together with one or two interphalangeal joints and a dactylitic digit or toe. On occasion, the arthritis appears to follow an episode of trauma so that initially the condition is misdiagnosed as "mechanical." The psoriasis may consist of one or two small patches of chronic stable psoriasis vulgaris with or without nail involvement.

Psoriatic arthritis may present with a symmetric polyarthritis indistinguishable from RA involving small joints of the hands and feet, wrists,

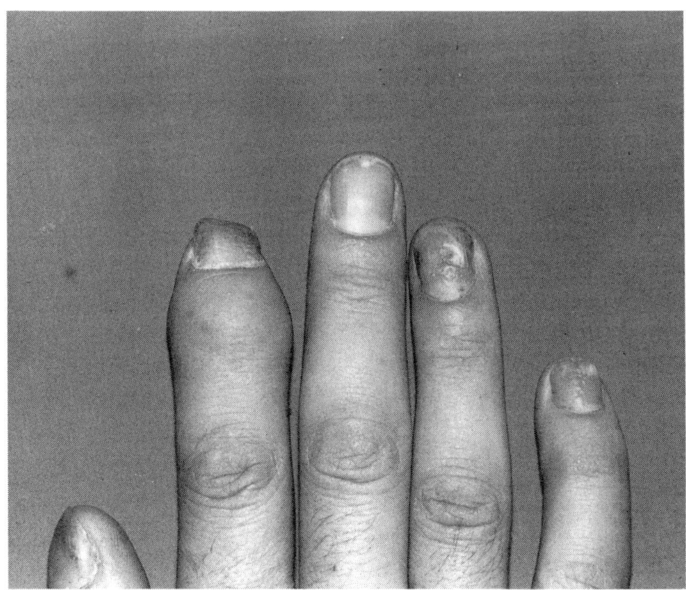

Figure 5.10 Psoriatic arthritis DIP II and nail psoriasis.

ankles, knees, and elbows. Indeed, cases of seronegative RA must occur coincidentally with psoriasis, but in the majority of cases other features suggest that the symmetric polyarthritis associated with psoriasis is a distinct clinical entity.

Dactylitis, or sausage digit, is a distinctive feature of psoriatic arthritis (Fig. 5.11). In appearance the whole digit (either toe or finger) is swollen as a result of inflammation in the digital joints and associated tendon sheaths. Dactylitic digits may also be seen in reactive arthritis.

Late Manifestations.   Arthritis mutilans, while uncommon, provides an almost characteristic late picture of this condition (Fig. 5.12). Arthritis mutilans can also be observed in other conditions with severe chronic arthritis (Table 5.6).

Radiographic features include distal interphalangeal erosive disease that can evolve into terminal whittling of the more proximal bone at the interphalangeal joints and *pencil-in-cup* appearance. In severe cases osteolysis with complete joint destruction or joint ankylosis can occur (arthritis mutilans) (Fig. 5.13).

The clinical appearance is of a severely deformed, flail hand with shortening of one or two digits, with the resulting redundant folds of skin

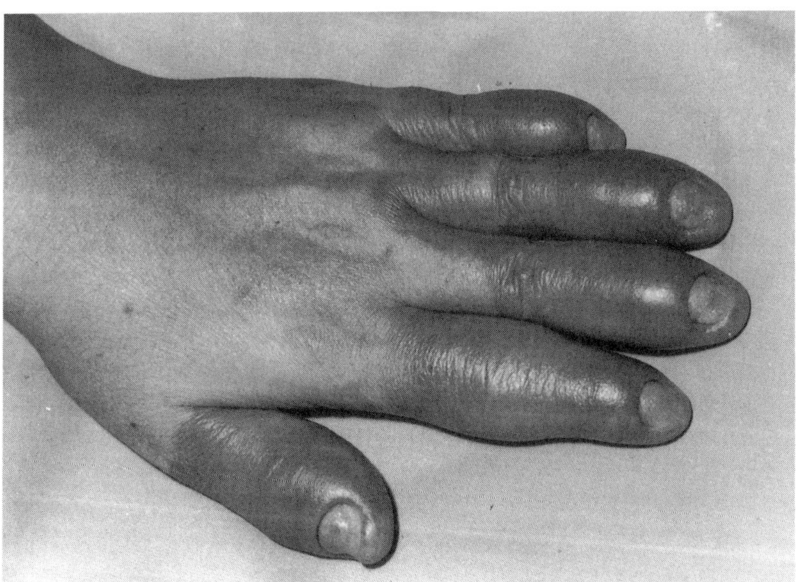

Figure 5.11   Sausage fingers.

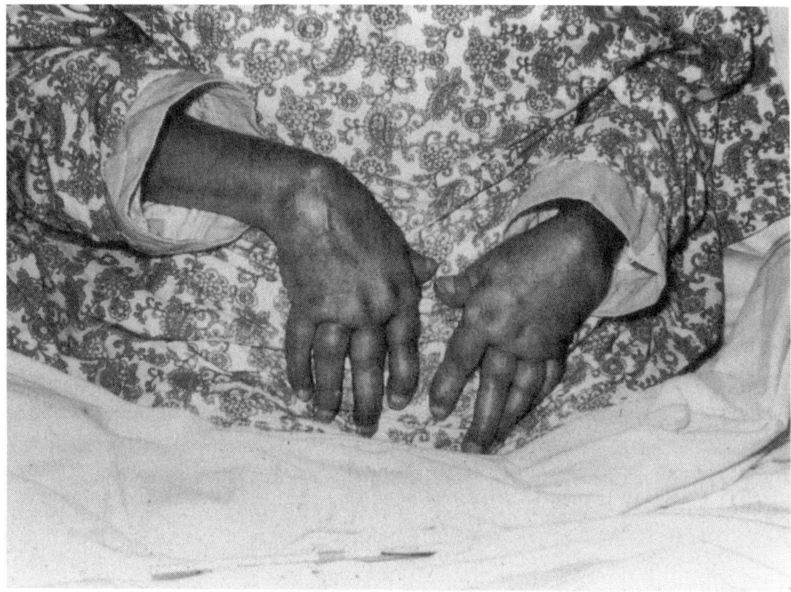

Figure 5.12 Arthritis mutilans.

enabling the examiner to extend the digit to its former length (telescoping). Similar destructive changes may appear in the feet, thus severely limiting function in the extremities.

The pattern of joint involvement varies widely. About 95% of patients with psoriatic arthritis have peripheral joint involvement. The majority of these have more than five involved joints. Others have a particular asymmetric arthritis or exclusive distal interphalangial involvement. Another 5% have exclusive spinal involvement. About 20–40% have spinal involvement with one of the forms of peripheral joint diseases. The clinical subgroups of psoriatic arthritis with destructive features are listed in Table 5.7.

Table 5.6 Differential Diagnosis Arthritis Mutilans

Arthritis mutilans: severe end stage of chronic arthritis with osteolysis at the joints

Psoriatic arthritis
Rheumatoid arthritis
Reticulohistiocytosis
Neurogenic arthritis

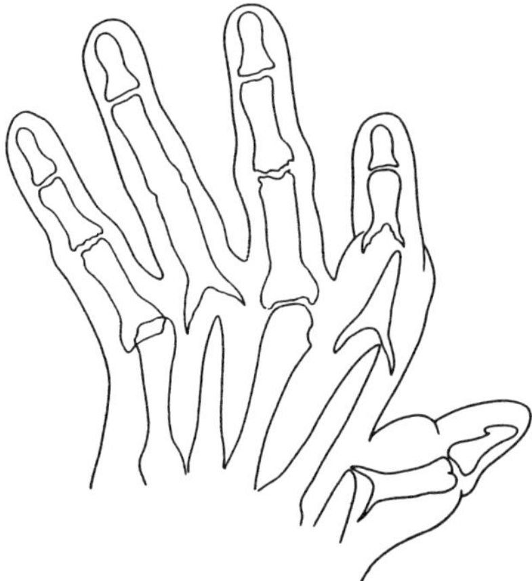

Figure 5.13 X-ray psoriatic arthritis: pencil-in cup, osteolysis, and joint anky-losis.

Spinal involvement includes sacroiliitis that is unilateral or asymmetric in the early stages but can progress to bilateral fusion. The distribution of involvement in the axial skeleton is less predictable than in AS. Isolated, sometimes unusually large and irregular, marginal or nonmarginal syndesmophytes may be seen at any level of the spine (parasyndesmophytes); rarely a bamboo spine is seen.

The peripheral arthritis is often typically located at the DIP joints and is associated with psoriatic nails.

7.2.3 Confirming the Diagnosis — Investigations

The diagnosis is based on clinical features, in particular the presence of psoriasis or positive testing of psoriasis. Laboratory abnormalities are mild and nonspecific. Rheumatoid factor is absent. The psoriatic synovium has

Table 5.7 Classification of Psoriatic Arthritis: Clinical Subgroups

Classical psoriatic arthritis confined to distal interphalangeal joints of hand and feet
Arthritis mutilans and sacroiliitis
Symmetric polyarthritis indistinguishable from rheumatoid arthritis but with
    negative serology
Asymmetric, pauciarticular, small joint involvement, with "sausage" digits
Ankylosing spondylitis with or without peripheral arthritis

Source: Ref. 1.

many similarities to the synovium in rheumatoid arthritis with lymphocyte and plasma cell infiltration.

7.2.4 Diagnostic Difficulties

Rheumatoid arthritis can coincidentally be associated with psoriasis. The presence of a positive rheumatoid factor and/or nodules direct the diagnosis to rheumatoid arthritis.

Skin lesions of *Reiter's syndrome* hyperkeratosis blenorrhagica can be confused with psoriasis pustulosa. The urethritis and conjunctivitis are helpful for the differential diagnosis.

7.2.5 Epidemiology and Historical Data

The association between arthritis and psoriasis was first made by Alibert in 1850. Five percent of psoriatic patients have one form of psoriatic arthritis. Males and females are equally affected. The prevalence rate is 50–100/ 100,000 population.

7.2.6 Management

The management of psoriatic arthritis and spondyloarthropathies is the same as for AS or rheumatoid arthritis. When peripheral joints dominate the picture and psoriasis is severe, methotrexate is the drug of choice because it may affect the skin as well as the joint changes.

7.3 Pustulotic Arthroosteitis (SAPHO)

Pustulotic arthroosteitis, also called SAPHO syndrome (*Synovitis Acne Pustulosus Hyperostosis Osteomyelitis*), is a recently described disease entity that can also be confounded with psoriasis, characterized by acne, palmoplantar pustulosis, sternoclavicular hyperostosis, and chronic osteitis of the femur or other long bones. It is also associated with sacroiliitis, spondylitis, and livido reticularis. It was first described in Japan but is now more and more recognized in the West.

8 IMPACT OF DISEASE AND PROGNOSIS

The course of AS is highly variable and characterized by spontaneous remissions and exacerbations, but it is generally favorable. Women in general have a mild disease and fewer X-ray features of AS. Earlier studies suggesting a generally unremitting course primarily involved patients with severe disease studied in hospitals. In the last decade, a number of B27-positive individuals, not previously recognized as having AS, manifested clinical features that are often relatively mild or self-limited. As a result, our understanding of what ought to be encompassed in the diagnostic entity is undergoing evolution. Good functional capacity and the ability to work are maintained in most patients, even in cases of protracted disease. Although it is difficult to predict the prognosis for an individual patient, those with hip involvement or completely ankylosed cervical spine with kyphosis are more likely to be disabled. Fortunately, the results of total hip arthroplasty in recent years are very gratifying in preventing partial or total disability. Some studies have suggested a slightly reduced life expectancy of patients with AS, but because of the selection bias for severe disease inherent in those studies, patients with relatively milder disease will likely have a normal life expectancy.

REFERENCE

1. Moll JMH, Wright V. Psoriatic arthritis. Seminars in Arthritis and Rheumatism 1973; 3:55–60.

6
Inflammatory Systemic Rheumatic Diseases

1 SYSTEMIC LUPUS ERYTHEMATOSUS

1.1 Definition (Table 6.1)

Systemic lupus erythematosus (SLE) is a relatively uncommon, chronic, inflammatory, multisystem disease that is more common in women than men and whereby a number of immunological abnormalities, especially antinuclear antibodies, may develop.

1.2 Main Clinical Features

1.2.1 Early Manifestations

SLE usually presents in a young woman with constitutional features of fever, weight loss, anorexia, fatigue, arthralgias, and arthritis (Table 6.2). The arthritis is asymmetrical and migratory. Morning stiffness lasts only minutes but joint pain exceeds the physical findings.

Blond, blue-eyed, fair-skinned individuals are more likely to develop *photosensitivity* rash usually on exposure to ultraviolet B light on exposed surfaces of the body—especially the face, on which it has the characteristic butterfly distribution (Fig. 6.1). The common, early features of SLE have been grouped together for diagnostic purposes (Table 6.3).

Table 6.1 Systemic Lupus Erythematosus

1. Multisystem autoimmune disease
2. Common in young women
3. Photosensitivity — serositis — arthralgias
4. Variability in presentation
5. Antinuclear factor positive
6. Outcome may be serious

Skin involvement is common (Table 6.4). *Alopecia* may involve any part of the body hair and can occur at any time during the illness. Various forms of *vasculitic* changes can be seen, including Raynaud's phenomenon, periungual erythema, livedo reticularis, telangiectasia, and vasculitis. The vasculitis may take several forms: urticaria, small infarcts of fingers and toes, and splinter hemorrhages of the nailfolds.

Patients may complain of chest wall pain, pleurisy, cough, or dyspnea. *Pericarditis* may be clinically manifest as a precordial rub or chest pain, or be subclinical and detected because of ECG abnormalities on echocardiography or radiology.

1.2.2 Late Manifestations

These are best grouped in terms of the organ systems involved.

Pulmonary. The *lungs* are frequently involved in SLE (Fig. 6.2). Pulmonary edema may occur secondary to cardiac or renal failure.

Cardiovascular (Table 6.5). *Myocarditis* may be suggested by disproportionate resting tachycardia and ECG abnormalities. Clinical *coronary artery disease* is becoming a problem, even in young women, and is correlated to the duration of the SLE, hypertension, and treatment with corticosteroids. *Valvular* involvement is not uncommon. Diastolic murmurs may be the result of aortic or mitral valve prolapse. Bacterial endocarditis may supervene and should be suspected if a fever and a new murmur

Table 6.2 Presenting Symptoms of SLE

Constitutional features
Skin
Renal
Pulmonary
Cardiac
Hepatosplenomegaly and lymphadenopathy
Central nervous system

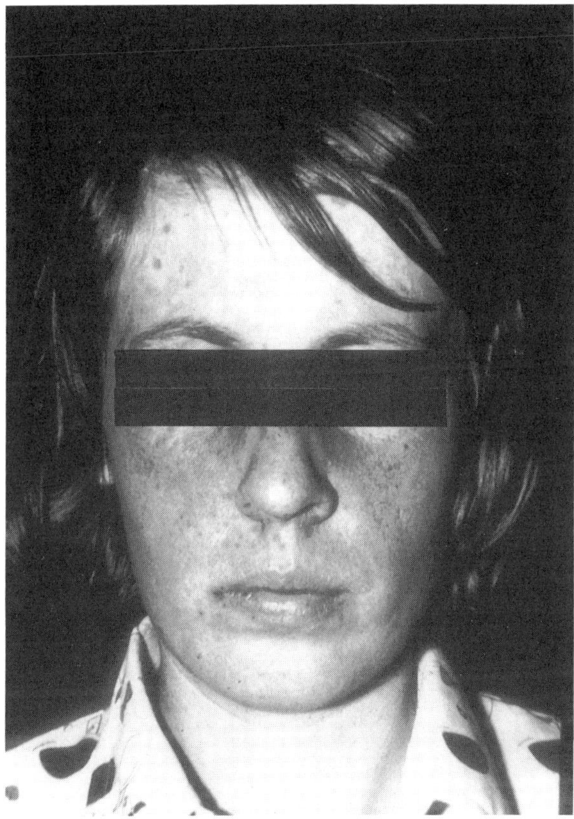

Figure 6.1 Skin involvement: lupus facies.

develop. *Conduction defects* are common as is *hypertension. Thrombo-phlebitis* usually happens in the legs and may be associated with the presence of antiphospholipid antibodies, the use of oral contraceptives, and smoking.

Renal (Table 6.6). *Urinary* abnormalities, consisting of proteinuria, as well as the presence of red and white blood cells and casts (hyaline, granular, or cellular), are a common early feature. The proteinuria may progress to *nephrotic syndrome* later in the disease. Parenchymal involvement with reduced glomerular filtration rate and the development of *renal failure* may occur. *Hypertension* is not unusual. *Urinary tract* infections are common and can occur at any time in the disease.

Table 6.3   Criteria for Diagnosis of Systemic Lupus Erythematosus

1. Malar rash
2. Discoid rash
3. Photosensitivity rash
4. Oral ulcers
5. Nonerosive arthritis
6. Pleuritis or pericarditis
7. Renal:
   persistent proteinuria > 0.5 g/day
   or
   cellular casts in urine
8. Neurologic:
   seizure with no known cause
   or
   psychosis with no known cause
9. Hematologic:
   hemolytic anemia
   or
   leukopenia $< 4000/mm^3$ on ≥ 2 occasions
   or
   lymphopenia $< 1500/mm^3$ on ≥ 2 occasions
   or
   thrombocytopenia $< 100,000/mm^3$ on ≥ 2 occasions
10. Immunologic:
    antibody to dsDNA
    or
    anti-Sm antibody
    or
    false-positive serologic test for syphilis
11. Presence of antinuclear antibody

Table 6.4   Mucocutaneous Manifestations of SLE

Early features:
   Photosensitivity
   Alopecia
   Vasculitis
Atypical forms:
   Discoid SLE
   Subacute cutaneous LE
Steroid-induced:
   Easy bruising

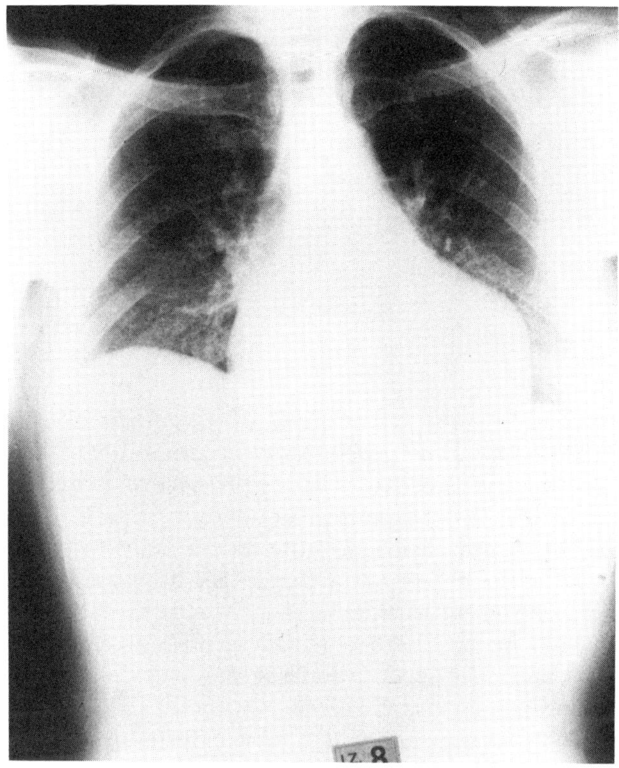

Figure 6.2 X-ray thorax: high diaphragm.

Table 6.5 Cardiovascular Manifestations of SLE

Early features:
    Pericardial involvement
    Myocarditis
    Thrombophlebitis
Late features:
    Conduction defects
    Coronary artery disease
    Valvular disease
    Hypertension

Table 6.6   Renal Manifestations of SLE

Early features:
   Urinary:
      Proteinuria
      Presence RBCs and WBC casts
Late features:
   Functional:
      Nephrotic syndrome
      Renal failure
      Hypertension
Any time:
   Urinary tract infections

Hematologic (Table 6.7). *Lymphadenopathy* occurs in about half the patients. *Thrombosis* may be associated with the presence of a circulating lupus anticoagulant and/or antiphospholipid antibody.

Neuropsychiatric. Neuropsychiatric manifestations may be functional or organic. They may be due to brain disease per se or the consequence of other organ involvement, such as uremia from renal failure or drugs, such as steroids. Functional disorders include depression, cognitive disorders, or psychosis, whereas organic manifestations include seizures, paresis, transverse myelitis, meningitis, and coma.

Gastrointestinal (Table 6.8). Gastrointestinal manifestations may be the result of the disease itself, other organ involvement, and drugs. *Dyspepsia* may be due to steroids and nonsteroidal antiinflammatory drugs. An *acute abdomen* may be the result of mesenteric or pancreatic vasculitis and is a medical emergency. Hepatitis may be due to nonsteroidal antiinflammatory drugs (NSAIDs).

Table 6.7   Hematologic Manifestations of SLE

Elevated sedimentation rate
Abnormalities of cells:
   Anemia
   Leukopenia
   Thrombocytopenia
Lymphadenopathy
Thrombosis:
   Lupus anticoagulant
   Antiphospholipid antibodies
False-positive tests for syphilis

Table 6.8   Gastrointestinal Manifestations of SLE

Dysphagia
Dyspepsia
Abdominal pain and nausea
Acute abdomen
Hepatitis

Lupus and Pregnancy. *Oral contraceptives* should be avoided as they may exacerbate lupus. *Pregnancy* is now associated with a good outcome in the majority of patients due to better management. *Miscarriage* may be a problem and linked to the presence of anticardiolipin antibodies and/or the lupus anticoagulant. *Neonatal lupus* may occur in babies born to mothers who have anti-Ro antibodies. The IgG antibody crosses the placenta and effects the development of the conduction tissue of the fetal heart, so that babies are born with a skin rash and heart block.

1.3   Confirming the Diagnosis—Investigations

The *sedimentation rate* is elevated during active disease. There are disturbances in the *formed elements* of the blood including anemia, which may be a Coomb's-positive hemolytic anemia, leukopenia ≤ 4500 mm^3, neutropenia, lymphopenia, and a mild thrombocytopenia although a severe autoimmune thrombocytopenia may supervene.

The central immunologic disturbance in patients with SLE is an autobody product against the nucleus of the cells: antinuclear antibodies (ANAs). Autoantibodies directed against components of the cell nucleus (ANAs) are the most characteristic of SLE and are found in over 95% of patients. However, ANAs are also found in other systemic connective tissue diseases. Antibody to double-stranded DNA (ds-DNA) positivity is more specific for SLE but less sensitive and is not often found in the cases with renal involvement.

If the patient is ANA-negative, then the diagnosis of SLE should be strongly questioned. A number of autoantibodies are found in the serum; they fall into two main groups. The first group is linked to the development of thromboembolic phenomena. Further analysis has shown that these antibodies are antiphospholipid antibodies or related to the presence of a circulating lupus anticoagulant. Patients may have a *false-positive VDRL* test but a negative treponema immobilization test or fluorescent treponemal antibody absorption test. Syphilis tests should only be undertaken when indicated. The second group of antibodies are the antinuclear (Table 6.9).

Table 6.9 Diagnostic Usefulness of Antinuclear Antibodies

ds-DNA, Sm	SLE
Histone	Drug-induced lupus
Centromere	CREST syndrome
Nucleoli, Scl-70	Scleroderma
RNP	Mixed connective tissue disease, scleroderma
Ro, La	Primary Sjögren's syndrome
Jo-1	Polymyositis or dermatomyositis

All of the sera are positive for ANA on screening by immunofluorescence on Hep-2 cells.

Chest X ray may show pleural effusions or infiltrates in the lung, as well as cardiomegaly. The ECG may show changes of pericarditis or myocarditis. Echocardiography helps in the diagnosis of murmurs and for the detection of Libman–Sacks vegetations on heart valves. Blood cultures should be undertaken if infection or bacterial endocarditis is suspected. Urinary abnormalities consisting of proteinuria as well as the presence of red and white blood cells and casts (hyaline, granular, or cellular) are common. Bacterial examination of the urine is mandatory if infection is suspected. *Renal parenchymal* abnormalities are invariably found on biopsy and their prevalence, pathology, and clinical outcome are shown in Table 6.10 (Figs. 6.3a,b; 6.4a,b; 6.5a,b; 6.6a,b). The question of renal biopsy should be considered on an individual basis.

Psychological and cognitive testing, CT and MRI scans, single-proton emission computed tomography (SPECT), electroencephalogram, and cerebrospinal fluid analysis may be used to establish the diagnosis. The presence of antibodies to Sm or neuronal antigens may correlate with neuropsychiatric features.

1.4 Diagnostic Difficulties

The differential diagnosis of SLE enters into many presentations involving young women as is obvious from the protean manifestations described above. The criteria for the diagnosis of SLE are particularly useful; the more criteria that a patient fulfills the more secure is the diagnosis.

1.5 Epidemiology and Historical Data

SLE is present in some 10 per 10^5 of the population but there are wide variations in the prevalence and severity of the disease in different racial groups. The disease is more prevalent and more severe in Africans, Asians, and Polynesians. Finally, SLE is overwhelmingly found in women.

Table 6.10 Pathology and Natural History of Lupus Nephritis

Type	Prevalence (%)	Clinical features	5-year mortality (%)	Pathology
Focal proliferative nephritis (Fig. 6.3)	15	Proteinuria, hematuria; renal failure rare	<10	Focal mild proliferative nephritis with Ig and C3 in mesangium
Membranous glomerulonephritis (Fig. 6.4)	15	Proteinuria; nephrotic syndrome; slowly progressive renal failure	<25	Thickened glomerular basement membrane
Minimal or mesangial nephritis (Fig. 6.5)	25	No clinical features of renal disease but may change to another type	0	Granular Ig and C3 on epithelial side of membrane Ig and C3 deposits in mesangium
Diffuse proliferative nephritis (Fig. 6.6)	45	Proteinuria, hematuria; nephrotic syndrome; renal failure	<25	Cellular proliferation with crescent formation; lumpy bumpy Ig and C3 along subendothelial aspect of glomerular basement membrane

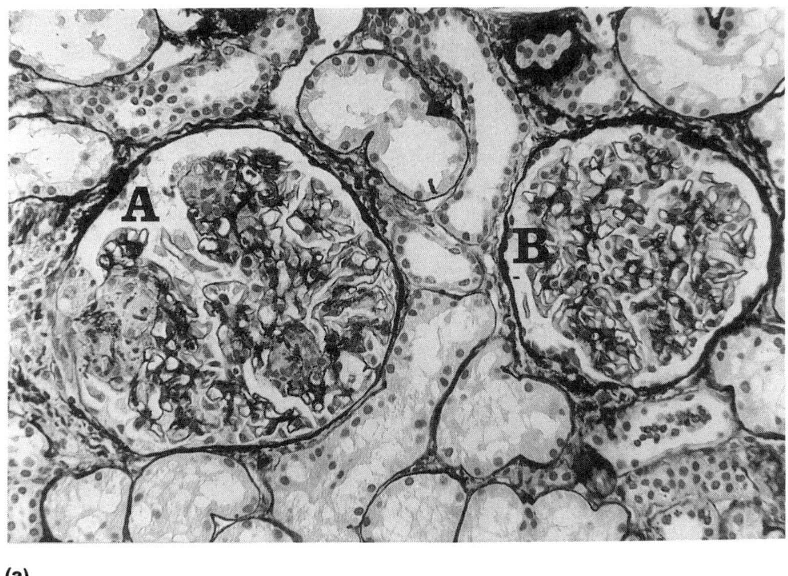

(a)

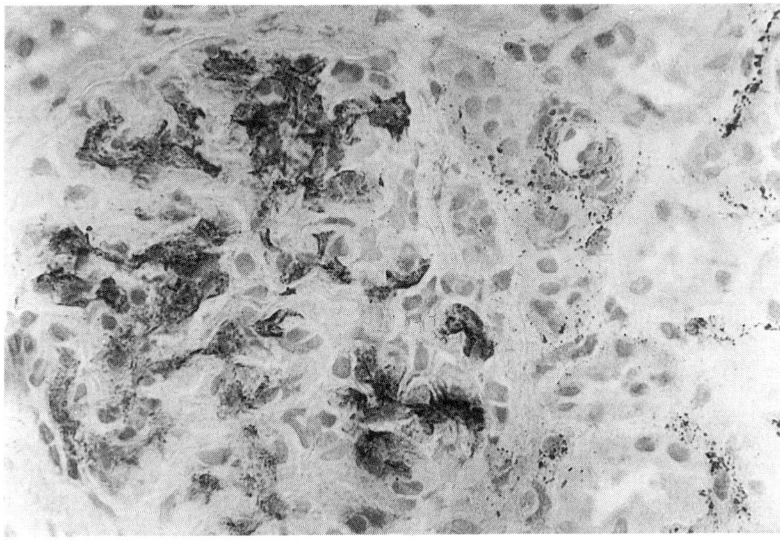

(b)

Figure 6.3 (a) Renal involvement by SLE. One glomerulus (A) involved by a proliferative focal necrotising process; (B) normal. (b) The same case showing segmental localization of C3, mainly in the mesangium.

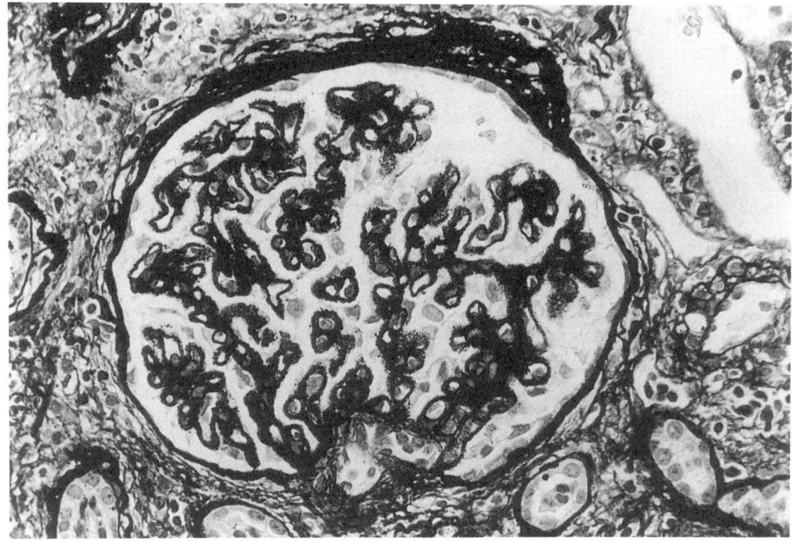

(a)

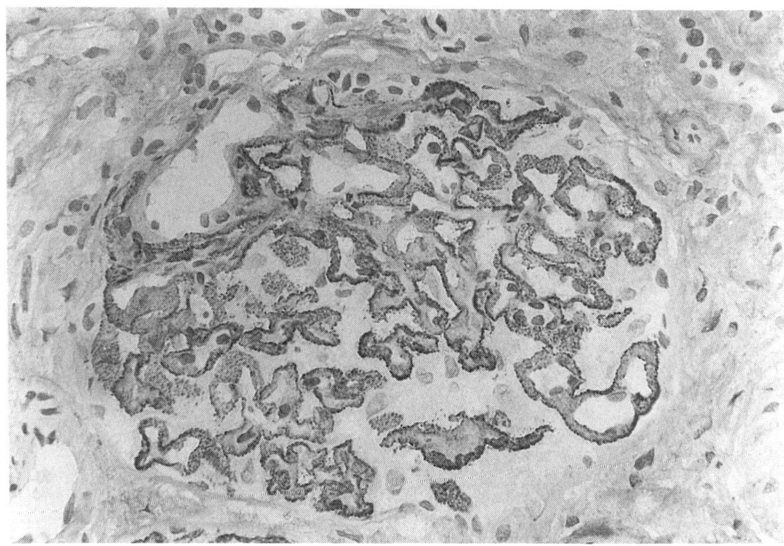

(b)

Figure 6.4 (a) Membranous nephritis in SLE. This glomerulus shows thickening of the capillary walls with the formation of spikes on the outer aspect. (b) The same case showing granular localization of IgG on glomerular capillary walls.

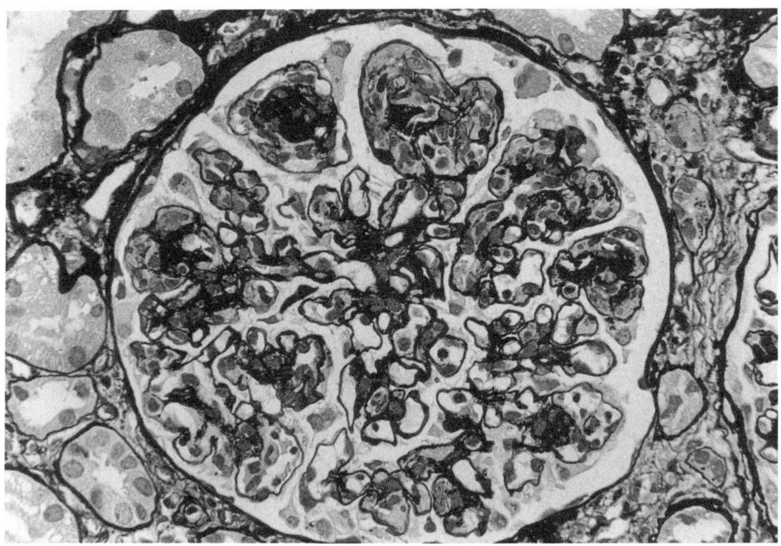

(a)

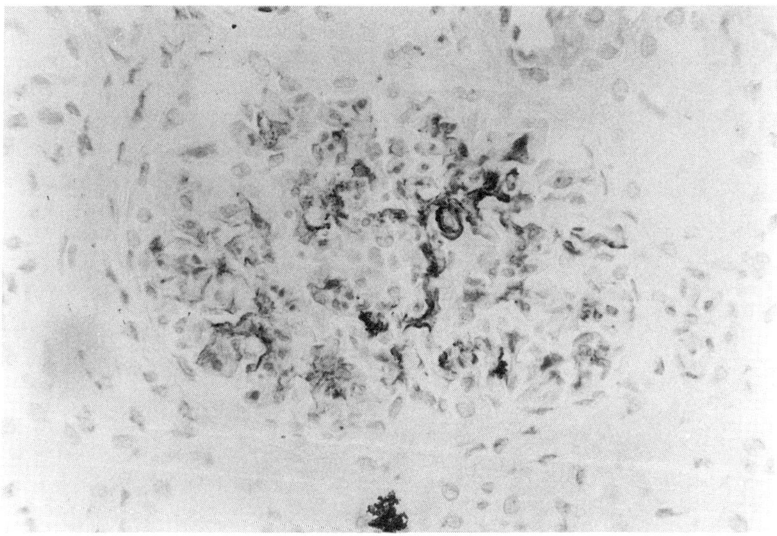

(b)

Figure 6.5 (a) Renal involvement in SLE. Glomerulus showing a mild mesangial proliferation. (b) Same case showing granular localization of a small amount of IgG, mainly in the mesangium.

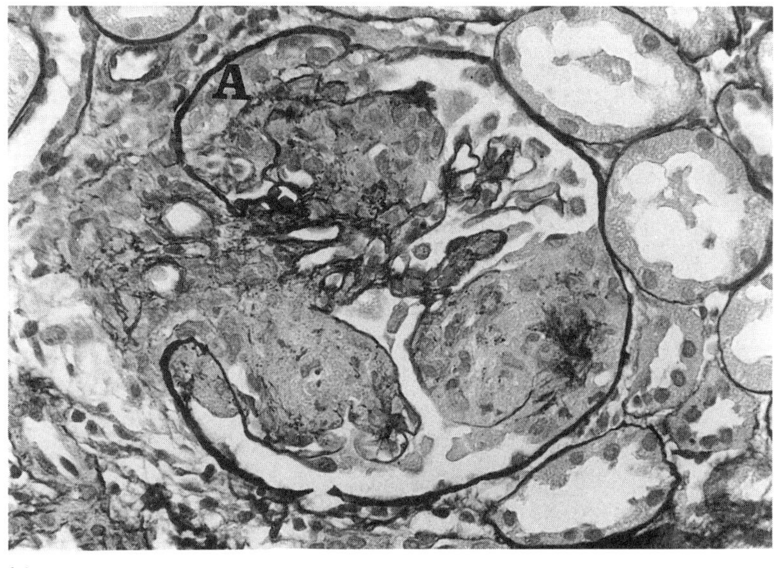

(a)

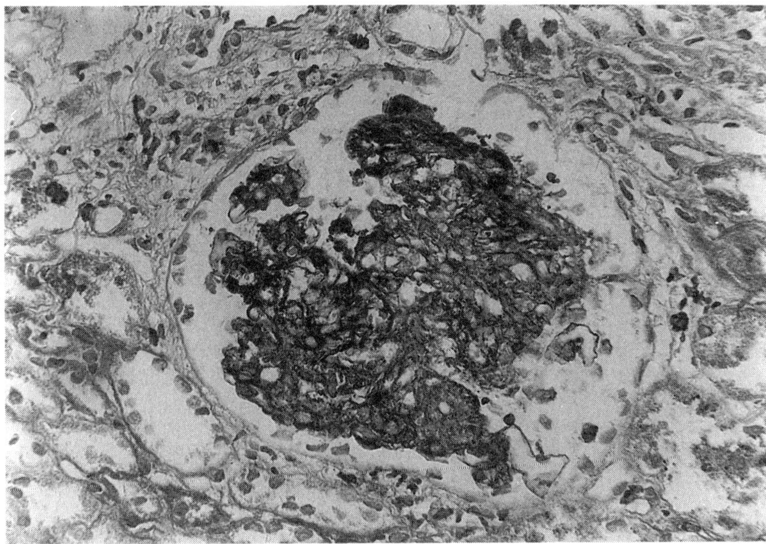

(b)

Figure 6.6 (a) Severe renal involvement in SLE. All glomeruli show similar changes of cellular proliferation and damage to capillary tufts. There is also a small cellular crescent in this glomerulus (A). (b) Same case showing granular localization of large amounts of IgG throughout the glomerulus.

1.6 Pathophysiology

The etiology of SLE is unknown. From observations in patients and mice strains that spontaneously develop SLE-like illness, it is likely that environmental, infectious, genetic, and hormonal factors are all involved.

1.6.1 Genetic

Evidence for genetic factors is found in family studies in which the prevalence of SLE is remarkably increased to up to 5% in relatives of patients. Antinuclear antibodies are present in first-degrees relatives. There is a high concordance rate in monozygotic but not dizygotic twins. SLE is linked to the histocompatibility antigens HLA A1, B8, and DR3. The HLA antigens are located on the short arm of the human chromosome 6. In the region of the chromosome located between HLA B and HLA DR loci are found genes of immunologic importance that may be involved in the pathogenesis of SLE. Thus, detection of the complement 4A null gene is found in over 50% of the HLA DR3–positive patients. This deficit of the complement component C4A may contribute to the failure to efficiently clear immune complexes. Support for this notion is provided by the finding that homozygous deficiency of C2 and C4 are frequently associated with SLE. The tumor necrosis factor–α (TNFα) gene is also located in this region and genetically determined abnormalities of its 5′ regulatory region may contribute to pathogenesis by unknown mechanisms.

1.6.2 Environmental

Although drugs such as procainamide and hydralazine may induce an SLE-like illness, this usually resolves on discontinuation of the drugs. Ultraviolet light exacerbates existing disease but does not appear to cause disease.

1.6.3 Racial

As noted above, some racial groups are more prone to develop the disease and this property may be linked to as-yet-undefined genetic factors.

1.6.4 Hormonal

Women are more prone than men to develop SLE. The exact hormonal mechanisms are unknown but may be related to excessive estrogenic activity although the influence of the X chromosome cannot be excluded.

1.6.5 Autoimmunity

There is evidence for B-cell hyperactivity and T-cell hypoactivity. The high prevalence and titer of ANA antibodies is the result of the former whereas T-cell lymphopenia and reduced T-cell activity is evidence of the latter. The antibodies form immune complexes that activate complement to induce tissue inflammation; immune complexes may be formed locally or be deposited after formation in the circulation. Immune complexes may be detected in tissue by immunofluorescence for Ig and complement components in renal and skin biopsies, for example. The renal findings have been described above. In the skin there is deposition of complexes at the dermoepidermal junction ("lupus band test") (Fig. 6.7). Pericardial, pleural, and synovial fluids and plasma contain complement degradation products as well as reduced total hemolytic complement levels.

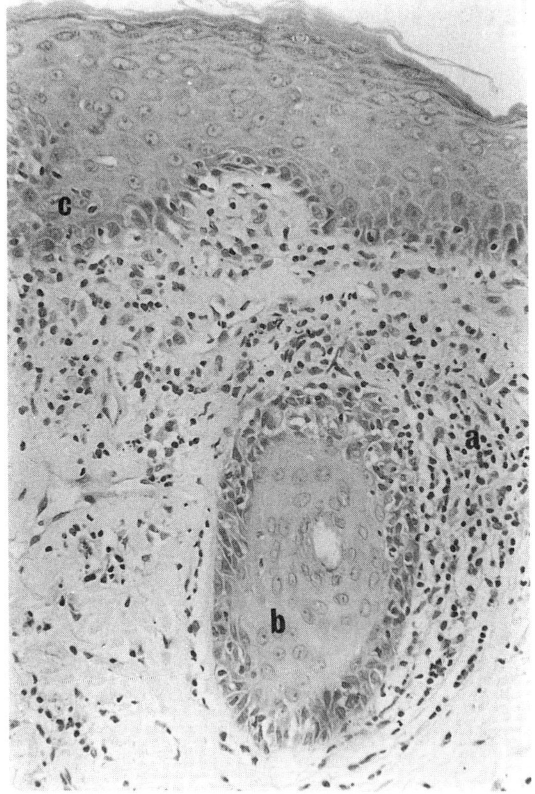

Figure 6.7 Skin involved by systemic lupus erythematosus. There is a lymphocytic infiltrate (a) in the dermis that surrounds a hair follicle (b) and involves the basal layer of the epidermis, which shows degenerative changes (c).

1.8 Management

The management of SLE is dependent on close collaboration between the general practitioner and the specialist. In mild cases of SLE without renal involvement chloroquine and NSAIDs are sufficient to control the disease.

The mainstays of the management of severe SLE are corticosteroids and cytotoxic drugs. During acute flares of the disease corticosteroids, often in doses as high as 100 mg prednisolone daily, are given. Corticosteroid dosing must be reduced to maintenance levels as soon as practicable without exacerbation of disease. Cytotoxic drugs are used for specific therapeutic effects or as steroid-sparing agents. They should be introduced and dosage adjusted by the specialist. The main cytotoxic drugs are pulsed cyclophosphamide and daily azathioprine. Infections are common in untreated SLE and are increased in frequency because of the immunosuppressive effects of treatment with steroids and cytotoxics. Hypertension, cardiac and renal failure, and focal organ deficit must be treated as indicated.

1.8 Atypical Forms

Because of the protean manifestations of SLE, atypical forms are not unusual. Thus, the disease may remain as an undiagnosed "pyrexia of unknown origin" for some time or may present as a specific dysfunction of a particular organ whose pathogenetic basis is not appreciated. Cutaneous manifestations of SLE are a good example of how this disease can present in different forms even in the same organ. *Discoid LE* can occur in the absence of systemic disease. The raised, round, erythematous, lesions occur on the face and can scar and atrophy. *Subacute cutaneous LE* begins as small, erythematous patches that can enlarge and coalesce. It occurs on the upper part of the body but spares the face. It is linked to HLA DR3 and patients are usually anti-Ro (SS-A) positive.

1.9 Impact of the Disease and Prognosis

The prognosis of SLE depends on the severity of the disease itself and complications that arise during its evolution. Renal, cardiac, and central nervous system involvement are the most important determinants of survival.

2 POLYMYOSITIS AND DERMATOMYOSITIS

2.1 Definition (Table 6.11)

Polymyositis and dermatomyositis are diseases of unknown etiology characterized by inflammatory destruction of muscle fibers and, in the case of dermatomyositis, by extensive cutaneous and vasculitic changes.

Table 6.11 Polymyositis and Dermatomyositis

Chronic inflammatory acute immune muscle disease
Morning weakness and pain: shoulders and hip girdle
Extraarticular manifestation: violaceous skin rash
Interstitial lung disease in some
Muscle enzymes elevated
Increased morbidity: aspiration pneumonitis and myocarditis

2.2 Main Clinical Features

2.2.1 Adult Polymyositis

Adult polymyositis is usually insidious in onset presenting with symmetric weakness of the shoulders and hips, particularly in the mornings, and then spreading to involve the neck flexors. The onset is accompanied with muscle pain and tenderness on palpation. There may be systemic features such as morning stiffness of the limbs, fatigue, anorexia, weight loss, and fever. The eye muscles are hardly ever involved and distal muscular involvement is uncommon.

There is a characteristic purplish rash on the eyelids, cheeks, and light-sensitive areas (Fig. 6.8). A violaceous rash may be seen on the knees, elbows, and MCP and PIP joints. Late atrophic skin lesions on the MCP and proximal interphalangeal (PIP) joints may develop (Gattron sign) (Fig. 6.9). Dysphagia may develop. Myocarditis may develop which can be clinically silent but lead to sudden death.

Examination of the lungs may reveal crackles on auscultation suggestive of lung fibrosis. Weakness of the oropharyngeal muscles may cause aspiration pneumonia. There is occasional heart involvement with arrhythmias.

2.3 Confirming the Diagnosis—Investigations

Laboratory investigation shows that muscle enzymes such as creatine phosphokinase, aldolase, LDH, SGOT, and SGPT may be elevated but are absent in the late stage. The sedimentation rate may also be elevated during the early active phase of the disease.

Electromyographic investigation of the muscles during active phases of the disease shows the characteristic triad of (1) increased insertional activity, fibrillation, sharp positive waves; (2) spontaneous high-frequency discharges; and (3) polyphasic potentials of low amplitude and short duration.

Muscle biopsy shows necrosis of muscle fibers with concomitant re-

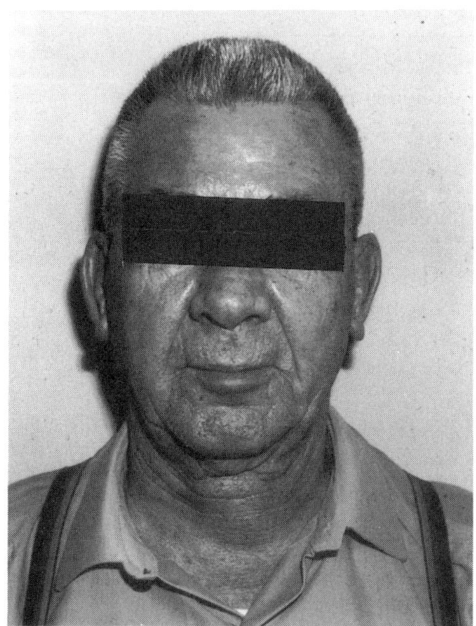

Figure 6.8 Polymyositis: characteristic facies.

generation. Muscle fiber nucleoli may be centrally located and possess prominent nucleoli. Intact fibers vary in size. There is a very prominent inflammatory cell infiltrate around muscle fibers that consist predominantly of activated CD8 cytotoxic T cells and macrophages (Fig. 6.10). These T cells are thought to be cytotoxic to the muscle fibers and it is of interest to note that such cytotoxic T cells kill target cells through class I major histocompatibility complex (MHC) molecules such as HLA B8. There is increased expression of this HLA antigen on the muscle of the fibers of patients with polymyositis. Specific autoantibodies, such as Jo-1, may be found in the serum.

Wide field capillaroscopy reveals the capillary nailbed changes similar to those seen in scleroderma. The chest X ray may show pulmonary fibrosis.

Lung function testing includes DLCO diffusion capacity and is useful for staging and early detection and monitoring of lung fibrosis.

2.4 Diagnostic Difficulties

Polymyositis and dermatomyositis may be linked with other diseases (Table 6.12) as mixed connective tissue disease, polyarteritis nodosa, scleroderma, and SLE.

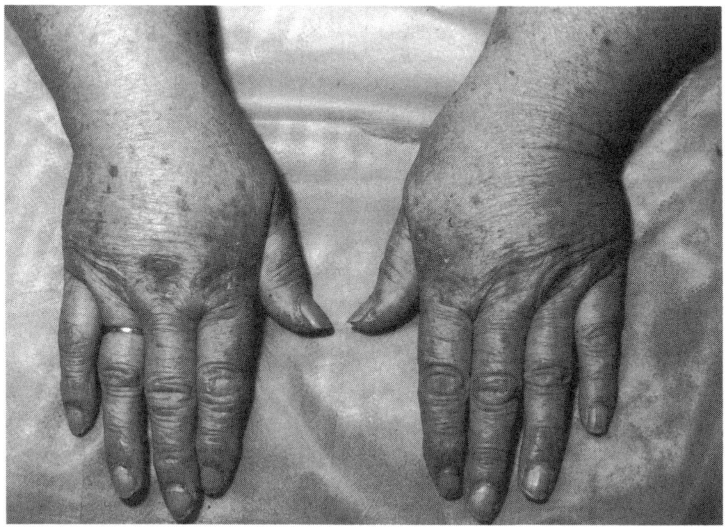

Figure 6.9 Purplish rash and atrophic skin lesion at the hand in polymyositis (Gottron sign).

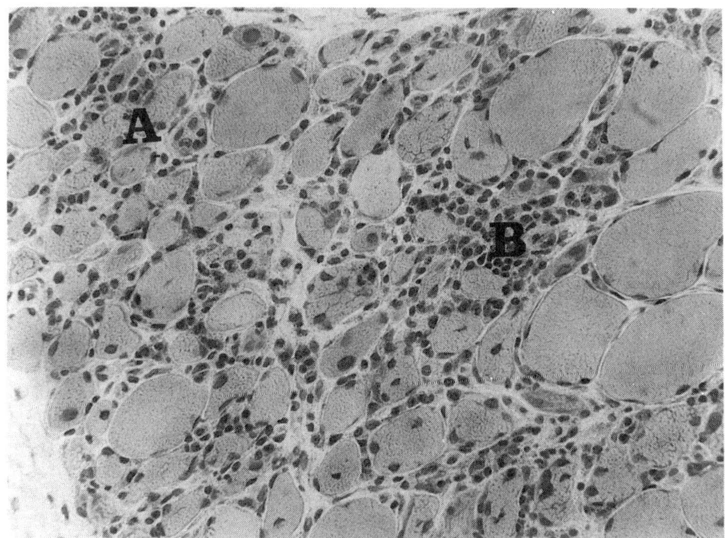

Figure 6.10 Polymyositis showing destruction of muscle bundles (A) associated with infiltrating lymphocytes (B).

Table 6.12 Connective Tissue Diseases Associated
with Inflammatory Myopathy

Mixed connective tissue disease
Polyarteritis nodosa
Scleroderma
Systemic lupus erythematosus

There may be an increased incidence of malignancy in adult patients
with dermatomyositis although there is still a matter of some debate as
to whether neoplastic disease can manifest itself by myositis. However, a
time-consuming, expensive, and invasive search for malignancy should not
be carried out as a routine in patients with dermatomyositis.

The differential diagnosis with polymyalgia rheumatica is not difficult
as long as corticosteroids have not been given. In polymyalgia muscle enzymes are not disturbed.

2.5 Epidemiology and Historical Data

Both polymyositis and dermatomyositis are relatively rare diseases with a
maximum incidence of approximately 8 cases per 10^6 of the population. It
has been described in all racial groups and geographic areas but with some
variations. Thus, adult polymyositis has the lowest incidence in Japan and
the highest in blacks in the United States. Childhood dermatomyositis has a
higher incidence in Asians and Africans and the lowest in Europeans. The
peak incidence is between the ages of 10 and 15 in children and 45 to 54
years in adults. There is a 2:1 higher prevalence in women as compared to
men.

Familial cases are described and there is a higher than expected concordance in monozygotic twins. The disease is linked to HLA B8 and HLA
DR3.

2.6 Pathophysiology

It is believed that both polymyositis and dermatomyositis may be triggered
by viruses but that they also have an autoimmune component possibly
triggered by virus (Table 6.13). As already noted, in polymyositis there is
evidence that the muscle destruction is carried out by activated CD8 cytotoxic T lymphocytes, whereas in dermatomyositis, in both the adult and
juvenile form, there is evidence of involvement of humoral immunity with
invasion of B lymphocytes as well as CD4 helper T cells, the deposition of
immunoglobulin and evidence of complement activation, and in particular

Table 6.13 Immunologic Changes in Polymyositis and Dermatomyositis

Polymyositis
    CD8 T-cell cytoxicity of muscle
Dermatomyositis
    Immunoglobulin and complement deposition, CD4 T cells
Circulating antibodies
    Directed against transfer RNA

the membrane attack complex C5-9. There are at least 10 circulating auto-antibodies characterized in these diseases, most of which are directed against proteins involved in protein synthesis and against transfer RNA. The different autoantibodies may define different clinical subgroups. Thus, patients who are Jo-1 (an antibody directed against histidyl-tRNA) are characterized by pulmonary fibrosis, arthritis, and Raynaud's phenomenon.

2.7 Management

Adequate controlled clinical trials of therapies used in the treatment of polymyositis and dermatomyositis have not been carried out. The mainstay of treatment for active disease is steroids given either intravenously as bolus doses during severe forms of the disease or in large doses by mouth. Treatment should be continued until muscle weakness has regressed or has stabilized and the muscle enzymes have returned to nearly normal levels. In steroid-resistant cases, or in an effort to reduce the steroid dose and thus reduce steroid complications, cytotoxic drugs have been used. The two main ones are azathioprine and methotrexate. Azathioprine has been shown to have a beneficial effect but this may take a year or more to manifest itself. Methotrexate should be used in the same way as it is used for the treatment of rheumatoid arthritis. On occasion none of these treatments have an impact on the skin changes of dermatomyositis, which can be troublesome. It is reported that hydroxychloroquine may be of benefit. A recent controlled study has shown that high-dose, intravenous gammaglobulin infusions may be beneficial in resistant cases of dermatomyositis. Adjunctive therapies should not be forgotten. Patients with severe respiratory muscle paralysis may require intubation and mechanical ventilation while muscle recovery is awaited. Physical therapy to maintain muscle strength and prevent joint contractures is mandatory during the recovery phase. In the event of neck muscle weakness, a soft collar may support the head.

2.8 Atypical Forms

2.8.1 Adult Dermatomyositis

This condition is polymyositis characterized by a rash over the upper part of the body; pink or violaceous scaling areas over the metacarpal phalangeal joints of the hands, elbows, and knees (Gottron sign); periungual erythema and darkened horizontal lines on the lateral and palmar aspects of the fingers ("machinist hands"). A significant proportion of patients have Raynaud's phenomenon. Patients may have a cutaneous vasculitis characterized by livedo reticularis, digital infarcts, or palpable, white-centered petechiae.

Biopsy of the muscle of patients with adult dermatomyositis shows a picture that is somewhat different from that of the muscle in polymyositis. There is an invasion of B cells and CD4 helper T cells particularly in a perivascular distribution. The skin may show an inflammatory cell infiltrate in the dermis. Both in the muscle and in the skin there is deposition of immunoglobulin and of complement components.

2.8.2 Juvenile Dermatomyositis

Early in the course there is a rash, muscle weakness, as well as vasculitis that can cause gastrointestinal ulceration with bleeding or perforation. Late in the disease, ectopic calcification and lipodystrophy may occur. The calcified tissues may ulcerate through the skin and may reduce mobility through muscle involvement. Finally, in the end stages of the disease, flexion contractures of joints may occur.

The muscle changes seen on biopsy are similar to those in adult dermatomyositis and in the skin there is a perivascular accumulation of inflammatory cells in areas involved with vasculitis.

2.8.3 Inclusion Body Myositis

This is a recently recognized condition that may affect up to 30% of patients with inflammatory myopathy. It requires histochemical examination of frozen section and electron microscopy for diagnosis, which show the characteristic intracellular lined vacuoles and tubular and filamentous inclusions, respectively.

2.8.4 Myositis Ossificans

This can occur in two forms: localized, which invariably follows trauma, and widespread (myositis ossificans progressiva), which is an inherited autosomal dominant condition appearing in childhood in which the muscles are involved with a hard mass of ossified muscle restricting function.

2.9 Impact of Disease and Prognosis

There is an increased mortality during the first 2 years of the disease, particularly from aspiration pneumonitis and myocarditis. Later the problems of rehabilitation from muscle loss and lung fibrosis are the most important determinants of the quality of life.

3 SCLERODERMA: SYSTEMIC SCLEROSIS

3.1 Definition (Table 6.14)

Scleroderma, or systemic sclerosis (SS), is an infiltration of the connective tissues of the skin and of internal organs by increased connective tissue, particularly collagen and mucopolysaccharides.

3.2 Main Clinical Features

The main clinical features of organ involvement are shown in Table 6.15. Sclerodermatous change can involve the skin and internal organs such as the heart, lungs, kidney, and gastrointestinal tract.

3.2.1 Early Manifestations

About 70% of patients present with Raynaud's phenomenon, i.e., finger and hand swelling with carpal tunnel syndrome due to median nerve compression being not unusual (Fig. 6.11). The skin involvement usually begins in the fingers and the hands, which have a shiny, taut, and swollen appearance with limitation of fist closure and finger extension.

Gradually the transverse lines of the skin at the DIP joint disappear, and the involvement spreads to the upper arms, neck, face, chest, abdomen, back, and legs. Arthritis may also be a presenting manifestation. The patients can have generalized arthralgias with morning stiffness and loss of

Table 6.14 Scleroderma–systemic sclerosis

Chronic infiltrative connective tissue diseases
Sclerodactyly and tight skin
Arthralgias with finger deformity
Dysphagia and interstitial lung disease
Raynaud's — telangiectasis
Calcinosis of the skin
    Diffuse disease: anti Scl-70: 40% +
    Limited disease: anticentromere antibodies 90% +
Lung, heart, or renal disorders: poor prognosis

Table 6.15 Organ Involvement in Systemic Sclerosis

Calcinosis and skin thickening
Lung
    Pulmonary fibrosis
    Loss diffusing capacity
  Pulmonary hypertension
Kidney
    Renal crisis
    Hypertension
    Renal failure
Gastrointestinal: malabsorption
Heart: conduction defects
Endocrine: hypothyroidism
Secondary Sjögren's syndrome
Entrapment neuropathies
Malignancy

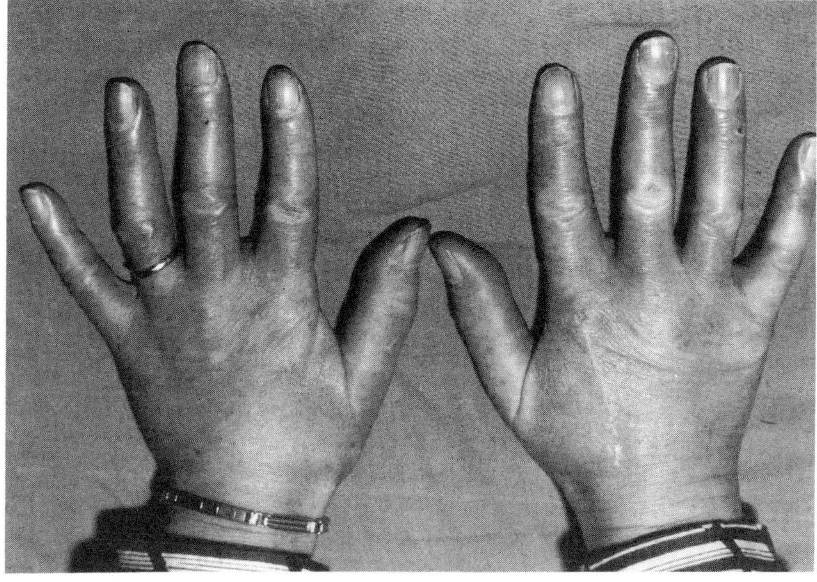

Figure 6.11 Scleroderma: early manifestations.

hand function but joint erosions are rare. Muscle weakness may be present due to disuse atrophy but a primary myopathy may occur. Internal organ involvement either can be presenting manifestation or can arise at a variable time after skin involvement.

Esophageal involvement is frequent and can present as heartburn and dysphagia. Small bowel involvement is frequent with bloating, abdominal cramps, diarrhea, and malabsorption.

3.2.2 Late Manifestations

In the late phases the face has a pinched look with poor mouth opening and radial furrowing of lips and telangiectasias. The skin may be tightened or pigmented, with atrophic changes, fragility, and hyper- or hypopigmentation (Fig. 6.12).

Acroosteolysis (resorption of the digital tuffs) is common. Subcutaneous calcinosis occurs in about half patients involving the fingers, the forearms, the anterior compartment of the knees, and the tendons (Fig. 6.13).

The calcinotic deposits may become inflamed, infected, and be extruded through the skin causing considerable pain and discomfort. There may also be pulmonary hypertension with an increased and palpable pulmonary component of the second heart sound, right ventricular gallop, murmurs of pulmonary and tricuspid valvular incompetence, jugular venus distention, and leg edema.

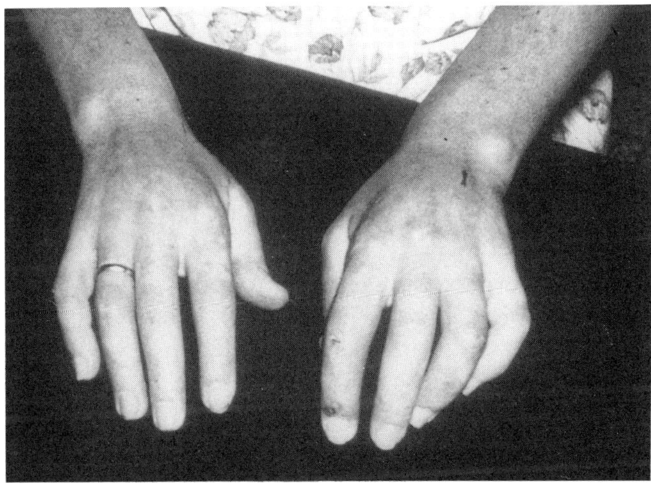

Figure 6.12 Scleroderma: late manifestations.

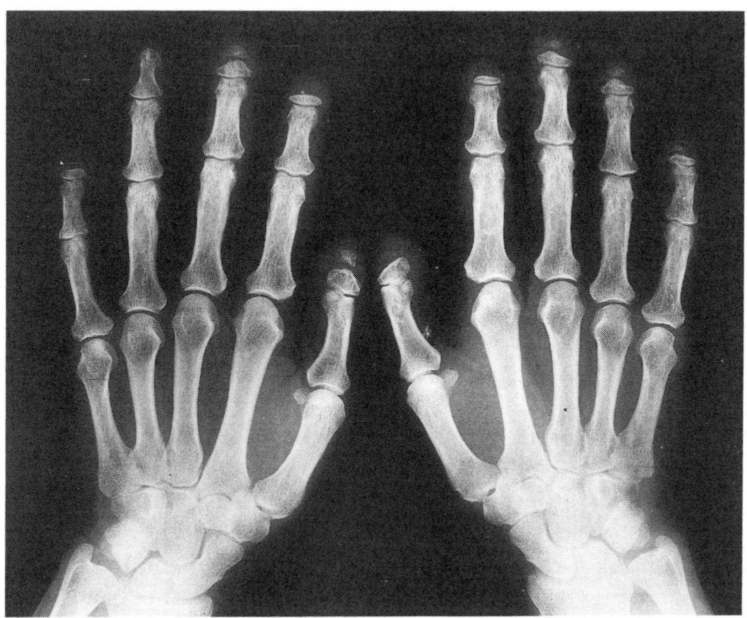

Figure 6.13 Acroosteolysis.

Hypothyroidism is often present but is clinically occult and is best diagnosed by an elevated thyroid-stimulating hormone in the serum.

Secondary Sjögren's syndrome occurs in 20–30% of patients and is due to fibrosis of the salivary, parotid, and lachrimal glands. Only half of these patients have the characteristic antibodies of primary Sjögren's, namely, SSA and SSB. The clinical presentation is that of dry eyes and dry mouth.

Entrapment neuropathies are not infrequent because of fibrosis and can involve the median nerve, meralgia paraesthetica involving the lateral cutaneous nerve of the thigh, trigeminal neuropathy with facial pain, and a facial nerve palsy.

Pregnancy does not worsen scleroderma and there are no adverse effects on the pregnancy by scleroderma.

Malignancy may be increased, particularly of the lung.

3.3 Confirming the Diagnosis—Investigations

Raynaud's phenomenon is not unusual, particularly in women. When a person presents with Raynaud's phenomenon the possibility of scleroderma should be borne in mind and other suspicious features looked for: capillaroscopic abnormalities of the nailbed, clinical features of scleroderma, serologic abnormalities, and evidence of internal organ involvement.

A variety of antibodies can occur in the serum of patients with scleroderma (Table 6.16). Over 90% of patients have ANAs as detected by Hep-2 immunofluorescence. Anti-Scl-70 antibody is very specific for scleroderma, particularly of the systemic type, but is only found in some 40% of patients. This antibody has been characterized as being the enzyme DNA topoisomerase 1.

Investigations show decreased motility and abnormal manometry of the esophagus. The chest X ray shows increased interstitial lung markings. Diagnosis is made easier by high-resolution computerized axial tomography (Fig. 6.14).

Investigation shows a restricted defect with decreased vital capacity, compliance, and diffusing capacity. The condition is usually progressive.

3.4 Diagnostic Difficulties

Scleroderma may occur as a diffuse disease with systemic organ involved or as a localized skin disease. It may occur as an overlap disease with SLE, polymyositis, rheumatoid arthritis, Sjögren's syndrome, and organ-specific autoimmune diseases such as Hashimoto's thyroiditis and primary biliary cirrhosis. The overlap disease has also been called mixed connective tissue disease.

A particular variant of scleroderma, also called the limited form, CREST, is characterized by the presence of anticentromere antibodies. This is the condition of calcinosis (C), Raynaud's (R) phenomenon, esophageal (E) involvement, scleroderma (S), and telangiectasia (T).

Table 6.16 Autoantibodies Found in Systemic Sclerosis

Antinuclear	90%
Anticentromere	
Limited disease	90%
Diffuse disease	< 10%
Anti-Scl-70	40%
Anti-RNP	20%
Rheumatoid factor	30%
Absent	
Anti-double-stranded DNA	
Anti-Sm	
Anti-cardiolipin	

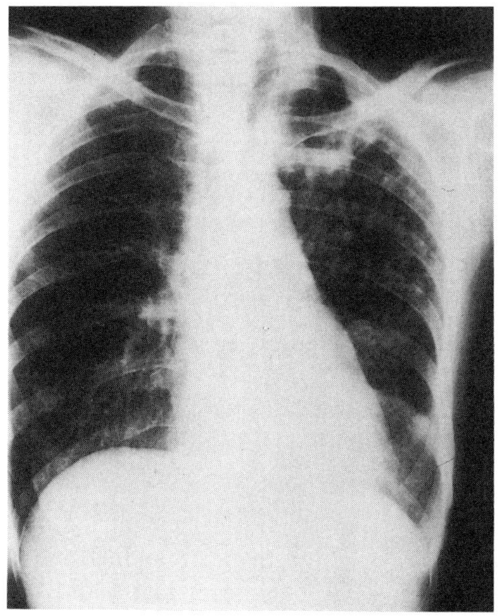

(a)

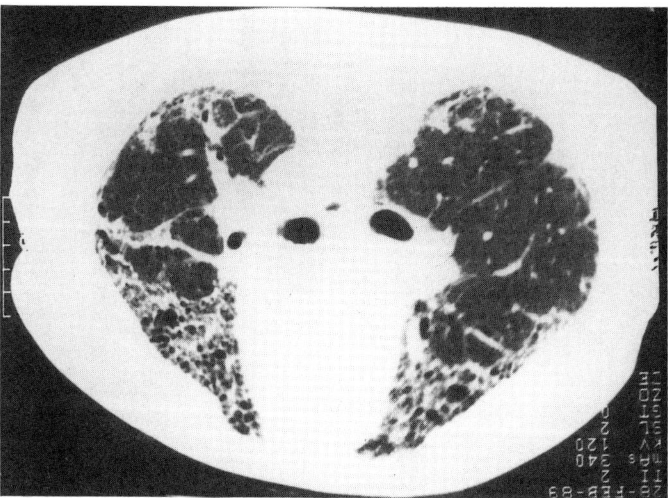

(b)

Figure 6.14 Lung involvement in systemic sclerosis: (a) X-ray thorax; (b) high-resolution CT.

3.5 Epidemiology and Historical Data

The incidence of scleroderma is about 4–12 cases per million persons per year. It is likely that it is still being underdiagnosed. It has been described in all geographic areas of the world and in all races although the prevalence may be higher in blacks. Maximum disease onset is between 30 and 50 years and there are 4 times as many females involved as males. The cause is unknown but in some cases toxins are involved such as vinylchloride and epoxy resins. There is only a very weak family history and there is no clear-cut HLA association.

3.6 Pathophysiology

The pathogenesis of scleroderma may be ascribed to three factors that may be interacting in an unknown manner one with the other: viral, vascular, and immunologic. The evidence for viral involvement is meager but there is substantial evidence for vascular and immunologic mechanisms operating in the disease. Biopsy of the early skin lesion shows an inflammatory cell infiltrate consisting of mast cells and CD4+ helper T lymphocytes. These cells, and probably the involved vascular endothelium, release a number of cytokines such as TNFα and TNFβ, platelet-derived growth factors, and transforming growth factor β which activate skin and organ fibroblasts to increased metabolism to produce more type I and III collagens. There is also increased production of type V collagen, which is normally found in the basement membrane, and increased secretion of glycosaminoglycans in the skin. In the late stages of the disease the collagens are crosslinked to give the unyielding characteristic of the skin.

At the very early stage of scleroderma the puffy and swollen appearance of the hands is due to the deposition of glycosaminoglycans, water retention, and the inflammatory changes themselves. The associated early changes in the vessels are microvascular in nature and consist of enlargement and tortuosity of capillary loops with areas of capillary loop dropout as seen by wide field capillaroscopy of the nail fold capillary bed.

Later in the disease there is intimal hyperplasia due to collagen and ground substance deposition in the blood vessels of the fingers and internal organs. Raynaud's phenomenon is characterized by undue intolerance to environmental cold causing vasopasm. The mechanism is multifactorial and not fully understood. Raynaud's phenomenon can also occur in internal organs such as lungs, heart, and kidneys and can be demonstrated by appropriate imaging techniques. The gradual encroachment on the vascular lumen eventually leads to organ atrophy and ischemia.

Malabsorption is due to bacterial overgrowth of a blind loop formed by the aperistaltic bowel and can be treated with antibiotics. In a small proportion of patients there may be coexistent primary biliary cirrhosis.

3.7 Management

Complete, spontaneous remission of the disease is extremely rare. No drugs are of proven value in either preventing extension of the disease or improving existing disease. A number of drugs have been used not always with good evidence for their benefit.

Steroids are particularly useful for inflammatory changes in the joints, skin, muscle and in the early phase of lung disease. They may be helpful during the painful process of extrusion of calcinotic deposits.

D-Penicillamine is the mainstay of treatment of scleroderma. It may improve or retard deterioration in the skin and reduce the incidence of new visceral manifestations. There is some evidence that it may increase the survival of patients with internal organ involvement. It requires constant monitoring toxic effects because of the possible development of which may be hematologic, renal, and cutaneous.

Antibiotics should be given in the presence of intestinal malabsorption in order to eradicate bacterial overgrowth in a blind loop.

Other therapies are more questionable. Cytotoxic drugs are of no value. Although cyclosporin may be of some benefit, it is associated with unaccepted renal toxicity. Physical therapies such as plasmapheresis, lymphocytapheresis, or photopheresis have been tried but their exact role in the management of patients is questionable. Different drugs have been used for the treatment of the vascular phase of the disease including captopril, ketanserin, nifedipine, and iloprost with variable success. A particularly important advance has been the use of angiotension-converting enzyme (ACE) inhibitors.

The management of patients with scleroderma requires a number of supportive measures that should be used as the situation demands, e.g., the appropriate management of renal crisis and cardiac problems.

3.8 Atypical Forms

3.8.1 Localized Scleroderma
Linear.   This is the involvement of a single upper arm extremity or the face (coup de sabre). This is particularly commoner in children and in young adults. Involvement leads to atrophy of half the face or a limb with major cosmetic and/or functional disability. During the active phase there may be eosinophilia, hypergammaglobulinemia, and positive antinuclear antibodies. Biopsy reveals the changes of scleroderma. Treatment is unsatisfactory.

Morphea. Morphea can occur at any site and at any age. Small spot (guttate morphea) or larger patches (morphea en plaque) are characterized by a central hypopigmented area with a violaceous or erythematous border. These spots may enlarge, thicken, and become tethered to the underlying tissue. The problem is usually one of cosmetic appearance but may rarely lead to joint contracture. Treatment is unsatisfactory.

Toxic Oil Syndrome. Toxic oil syndrome developed after the consumption of adulterated olive oil in Spain. The pathogenesis is not understood.

Eosinophilic Myalgia Syndrome. Eosinophilic myalgia syndrome developed after the excessive ingestion of contaminated L-phenylalanine by body building enthusiasts.

Eosinophilic Fasciitis. Eosinophilic fasciitis is inflammation of the fascii with eosinophilia after unaccustomed exercise. It usually responds well to steroids.

3.9   Impact of the Disease and Prognosis

Lung involvement is a leading cause of morbidity and mortality in scleroderma.

The degree and severity of myocardial involvement is one of the principal factors determining survival. In about 50% of patients there are electrocardiographic abnormalities including conduction defects.

Renal involvement is also one of the important determinants of survival. Especially in early diffuse scleroderma, scleroderma "renal crisis" may mean a significantly shortened life if not adequately treated. It is characterized by accelerated or malignant hypertension, rapid progression to renal failure, hyperreninemia, and microangiopathic hemolysis. Renal biopsy shows the characteristic intimal proliferative lesion of the renal arteries (Fig. 6.15).

4   VASCULITIC DISEASES

4.1   Definition

The definition of vasculitic diseases or syndromes is difficult. There is considerable overlap in terms of clinical presentation and manifestations; classification on the basis of histologic findings is also extremely variable. Part of the problem may relate to the evolutions of the lesions themselves and the variability of expression of the disease depending on the size of the vessel involved. Veins may also be involved to cause thrombophlebitis. A simple but convenient classification of this group of diseases is shown in

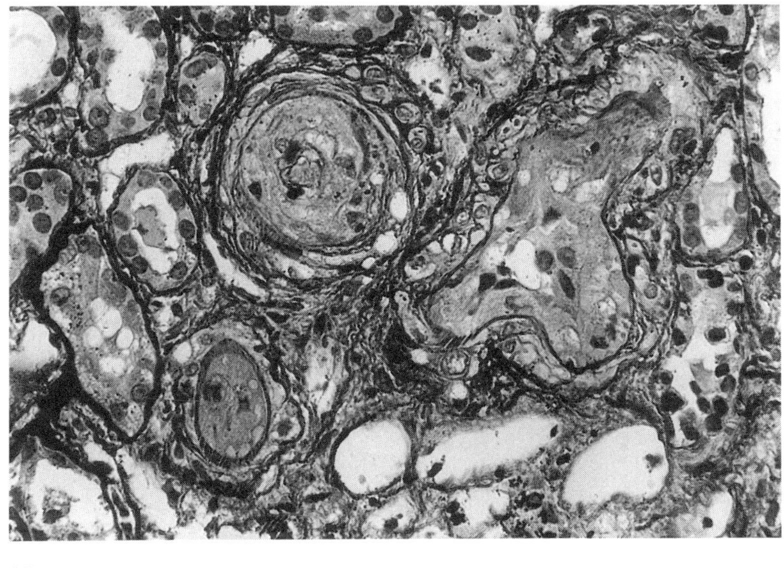

(a)

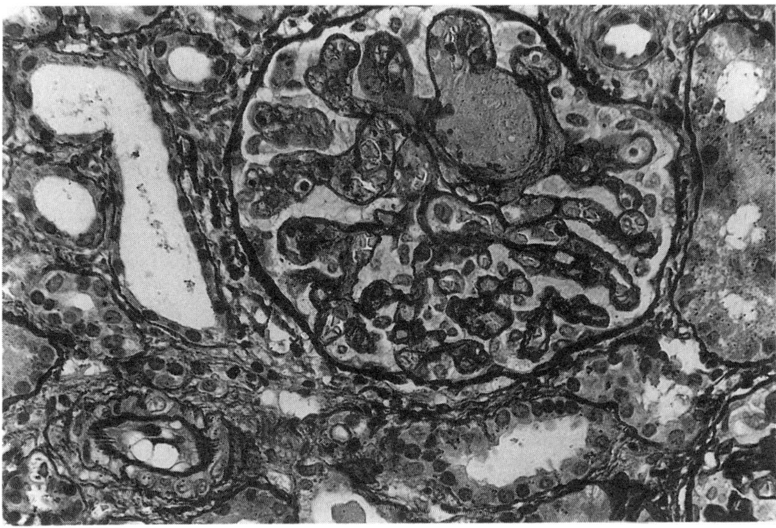

(b)

Figure 6.15 Intimal proliferative lesion of renal arteries in systemic sclerosis.

Table 6.17 Classification of Vasculitic Disorders

Primary:
    Polyarteritis nodosa
    Wegener's granulomatosus
    Hypersensitive vasculitis
    Takayasu's arteritis
   Adamantiades — Behçet's disease
    Giant cell arteritis
Secondary:
    Systemic lupus erythematosus
    Rheumatoid arthritis
    Drug-induced
    Virus-induced

Table 6.17, but a classification based on the size of the vessels involved can also be made (Table 6.18).

The ideal classification would be one based on etiology or even pathogenesis, but these goals seem far distant at present.

A particularly interesting development has been the discovery that viruses and other infectious agents may be involved in the etiology of these diseases.

5 POLYMYALGIA RHEUMATICA/GIANT CELL ARTERITIS

5.1 Definition (Table 6.19)

Polymyalgia rheumatica (PMR) and giant cell arteritis (GCA) are chronic inflammatory diseases of unknown etiology that particularly affect people over the age of 55 years.

Table 6.18 Classification of Vasculitic Disorders According to the Size of the Vessels Involved

Large vessel vasculitis (aorta and its largest branches)
    Giant cell arteritis
    Takayasu's arteritis
Medium vessel vasculitis (main visceral arteries)
    Polyarteritis nodosa
    Kawasaki's disease
Small vessel vasculitis (venules, arterioles and capillaries)
    Wegener's granulomatosus
    Microscopic polyangiitis (microscopic polyarteritis)
    Hypersensitivity vasculitis
    Adamantiades — Behçet's syndrome

Table 6.19 Polymyalgia Rheumatica and Giant Cell Arteritis

Occurs in the elderly
Pain and stiffness in the muscles of the pelvic and shoulder girdles in the morning
Constitutional features: weight loss, fever
Arterial features:
    Tender scalp arteries
    Blindness
    Strokes
Elevated ESR and C-reactive protein
Good to very good response to corticosteroids

5.2 Main Clinical Features

In GCA, the patients may complain of feeling unwell, having a poor appetite, loss of weight, and a fever. The typical presentation is of headache, especially severe temporal or occipital headaches. Some patients may experience painful jaw muscles during chewing (jaw claudication). Involvement of arteries may lead to blindness or even strokes if not promptly and effectively treated (Fig. 6.16).

PMR is a disease of sudden onset. The patient frequently complains of difficulty in getting out of bed in the morning because of severe and

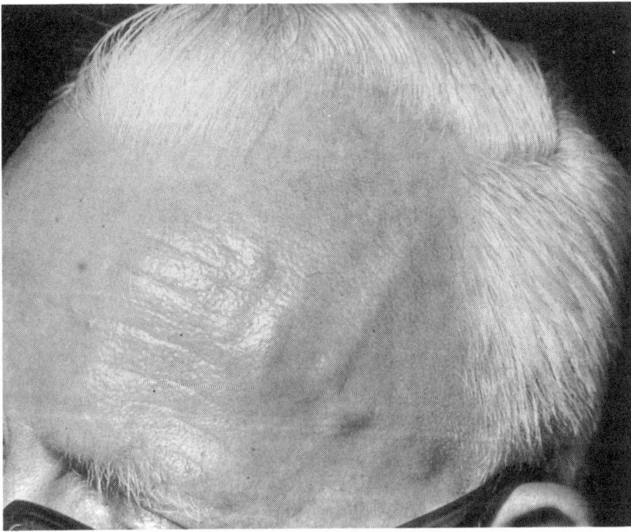

Figure 6.16 Inflamed and enlarged temporal artery.

prolonged stiffness of the muscles of the shoulder and pelvic girdles. Clinical examination of a patient with PMR shows restriction of bilateral shoulder movement with tender muscles on palpation of the shoulder and pelvic girdles. Passive movement is full and unrestricted. There is no obvious wasting. Some patients present with overlapping features, so that these two diseases are frequently classified together. Some patients have symptoms of pauciarticular synovitis especially of the knee joints.

5.3 Confirming the Diagnosis—Investigations

In both PMR and GCA investigation reveals an acute phase response with an elevated sedimentation rate and increased concentration of serum C-reactive protein. There is an associated anemia of chronic disease. Investigations for myositis, such as estimations of serum creatine phosphokinase, are negative. Electromyographic studies are normal in the majority of patients and do not show any evidence of myositis or myopathy. The diagnostic test is temporal artery biopsy but this is frequently negative even in patients with the characteristic symptoms and signs of GCA. This may be due to the fact that the arteries are involved in an intermittent manner with "skip" lesions. Patients with a typical PMR history and clinical findings may also have a positive temporal artery biopsy.

5.4 Diagnostic Difficulties

Since these diseases occur in an elderly population with loss of weight and pyrexia, the presentation could be evidence of serious underlying disease. Patients should be investigated for the exclusion of rheumatoid arthritis, multiple myeloma, infection, and malignant disease. This, however, is not a justification for indiscriminate and expensive tests. Hence, serum electrophoresis and a rheumatoid factor test and X rays of the hands and chest are reasonable standard investigations. Takayasu's disease should be considered in younger women presenting with features of GCA.

5.5 Epidemiology and Historical Data

Exact estimates of the prevalence of PMR and GCA are not available. The prevalence of polymyalgia rheumatica has been calculated to be approximately 500 per 100,000 persons aged 50 and older. It is relatively common in Europe and the United States but it is in fact of worldwide distribution. The prevalence of GCA is less than that of PMR.

Historically PMR and GCA have been described under many different names: *senile rheumatic gout, periarhrosis humeroscapularis, periextraarticular rheumatism, myalgic syndrome of the elderly with systemic reaction, pseudopolyarthrite rhizomélique, arthritic rheumatoid disease,* and *polymyalgia arteritica*. GCA is in many countries also named Horton's disease.

5.6 Pathophysiology (Table 6.20)

Involved arteries in GCA are characterized by an infiltration of T lymphocytes and macrophages. The T cells are of the helper subset being CD4+. These infiltrates are found in the region of the internal or external elastic lamina or adventitia. There is disruption of all layers of the vessel wall. Characteristic multinucleated giant cells, which give the disease its name, may be found (Fig. 6.17).

The inflammatory cells synthesize and secrete inflammatory cytokines, such as interleukin-1 and TNFα, which may be responsible for the clinical symptomatology. It is important to remember that these changes affect a vessel in a segmental or patchy fashion. The pathophysiology of PMR is a mystery. In a proportion of patients, biopsy of the temporal artery reveals the characteristic changes of GCA. It is believed that the shoulder and pelvic girdle symptoms of PMR are due to a synovitis or capsulitis of the shoulder and hip joints.

Both diseases are linked to HLA DR4 suggesting that they are driven by antigens, presented in the context of HLA DR4, stimulating CD4+ T cells in the lesion. It is important to note that the molecular form of HLA DR4 is different from that associated with rheumatoid arthritis. The triggering agents for both of these diseases is unknown. Possibilities include viral infection of the endothelial cells as well as stimulation by superantigens of unknown origin.

5.7 Management

The treatment of both diseases is with corticosteroids. The characteristic treatment pattern for PMR is the use of 15–20 mg of prednisolone daily,

Table 6.20 Pathologic Features of PMR and GCA

Associated with HLA DR4
In GCA:
   Destructive granulomatus lesion of cranial arteries with multinucleate cells
In PMR:
   Synovitis shoulder and hip joints
Release of inflammatory cytokines

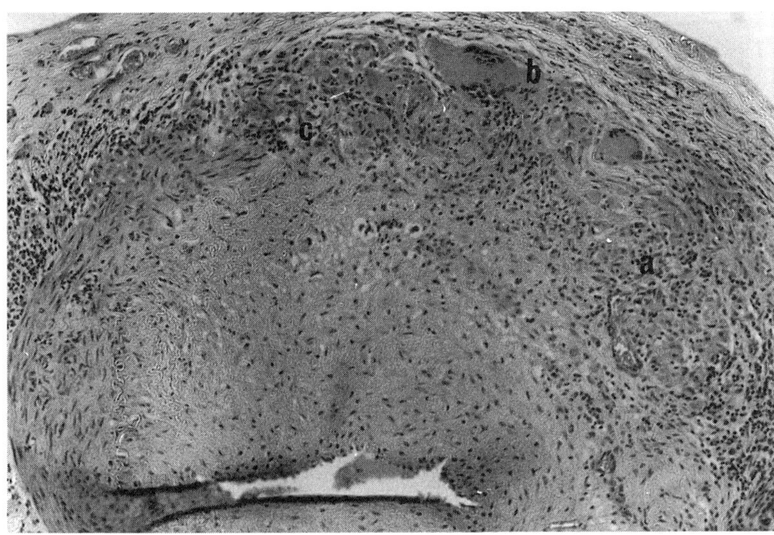

Figure 6.17 A portion of temporal artery in temporal (giant cell) arteritis. The media of the vessel is infiltrated by lymphocytes (a) and associated multinucleated giant cells (b). This is accompanied by destruction of the muscle and elasticity of the vessel wall (c).

gradually reducing this to the minimum maintenance dose, which usually lies somewhere between 5 and 10 mg daily. The reduction from 20 mg should be gradual and take place over the space of 3 months. In the event of recrudescence of the disease the steroid dose should be increased to the one prior to the exacerbation.

GCA is a more serious disease because of the possibility of blindness and stroke. Most rheumatologists would initiate treatment with 40 mg daily and gradually reduce this to maintenance doses by about 4–6 months. A close check should be kept on symptoms, signs, and the acute phase response. Steroids should be increased if there is clinical evidence of return of the disease or elevation of the sedimentation rate or the concentration of serum C-reactive protein. It is unfortunately documented that even with apparent excellent control of the disease blindness can still occur.

Patients with prolonged disease have been treated with azathioprine as a steroid-sparing agent in order to prevent the usual adverse effects of corticosteroids experienced by 20–50% of patients (Table 6.21).

Table 6.21 Adverse Effects of Corticosteroids in PMR and GCA

Peptic ulceration
Diabetes mellitus
Thin skin and easy bruising
Osteoporotic fractures

5.8 Atypical Forms

Patients with PMR may present without an elevated erythrocyte sedimentation rate (ESR), although in a proportion of these C-reactive protein may be increased in the serum. Occasionally, patients with GCA may present with organ involvement such as blindness, myocardial infarction, cholecystitis, or a pyrexia of unknown origin.

5.9 Impact of the Disease and Prognosis

Both PMR and GCA are important treatable diseases of the elderly. It is said that both of them will spontaneously remit after some 2 years of therapy with corticosteroids but a significant proportion are still receiving these drugs even at 5 years of treatment. Continued treatment with corticosteroids leads to osteoporosis which, when added to the osteoporosis of old age or of postmenopausal origin, provides an additional morbidity and mortality to this elderly population. The prevalence and severity of osteoporosis is directly related to the total dose of corticosteroids. Thus, treatment should be as effective as possible for the shortest possible time. It seems not unreasonable to give concomitant calcium and vitamin D supplements in order to stabilize bone calcium mass.

6 TAKAYASU'S ARTERITIS

6.1 Definition (Table 6.22)

Takayasu's arteritis (TA) is characterized by an arteritis of medium-sized arteries in children and young women particularly involving the aorta and its primary branches.

6.2 Clinical Features

In the prepulseless phase the predominant features are those of a systemic illness with fatigue, fever, weight loss, and arthralgias. During the later, pulseless phase, there is vascular inflammation with tenderness, decreased

Table 6.22 Takayasu's Arteritis

Arteritis of aorta and its primary branches
Pulseless disease
Young women and children
Positive response to corticosteroids

pulsation, and bruits of the brachial, subclavian, or carotid arteries. Decreased circulation leads to a cool extremity or even ischemic ulcers. There may be the development of a collateral circulation, e.g., around the shoulders. Involvement of renal vessels may lead to hypertension. Decreased cerebral blood flow may cause vertigo, syncope, convulsions, dementia, headaches, and loss of visual acuity.

The clinical diagnostic criteria for Takayasu's arteritis is shown in Table 6.23.

6.3 Confirming the Diagnosis—Investigations

During active phases of the disease there may be anemia, elevated sedimentation rate, elevated immunoglobulins, and hypoalbuminemia. Arteriography reveals the characteristic narrowing or total occlusion of the aorta and its proximal branches.

6.4 Diagnostic Difficulties

Computed tomography and magnetic resonance angiography (MRA) studies show luminal narrowing and mural thickening in vessels and may be useful to support initial arteriographic findings and in follow-up monitoring.

Because of the size of the vessels affected, biopsies are rarely obtained. The differential diagnosis includes carotid artery dissection that is

Table 6.23 Diagnostic Criteria for Takayasu's Arteritis

Age at onset $\leq$ 40 years
Claudication of extremities
Decreased brachial artery pulse
BP difference > 10 mm Hg between the arms
Bruit over subclavian arteries or abdominal aorta
Arteriographic abnormality

Three or more criteria must be present.

usually localized, early arteriosclerosis in the setting of risk factors, heritable connective tissue disorders such as Ehlers–Danlos syndrome, and giant cell arteritis.

6.5 Epidemiology and Historical Data

Takayasu's arteritis predominantly affects young women between 15 and 25 years of age, with a female/male ratio of 9:1. It is rare. It is commoner in Japan. The cause is unknown.

6.6 Management—Impact of the Disease and Prognosis

The mainstay of therapy is oral corticosteroids (prednisone) in a dose of 1 mg/kg/day followed by maintenance dose of 5–10 mg/day.

Takayasu's arteritis tends to be chronic. The 5-year survival rate has been reported to be over 90%.

7 POLYARTERITIS NODOSA

7.1 Definition (Table 6.24)

Polyarteritis nodosa (PAN) is a disease characterized pathologically by intense inflammation of all three layers of medium sized arteries and clinically by systemic features and multiple organ involvement.

7.2 Main Clinical Features

Patients with PAN may present with different clinical patterns involving most tissues and organs of the body, so that the diagnosis may be difficult to make particularly in the early stages. The diagnostic criteria for PAN are shown in Table 6.25.

Despite its name, nodules are uncommon and the most common presentation is that of an urticarial rash, livedo reticularis (Fig. 6.18), or palpable purpura. Raynaud's phenomenon is rare. There may be localized small digital infarcts.

Table 6.24 Polyarteritis Nodosa (PAN)

Intense inflammation of medium-sized arteries: involving all segments of the arteries
Multiple organ involvement (heart–liver–kidneys)
Livedo reticularis — palpable purpura
Mononeuritis multiplex
Fever — malaise
Prognosis improved with corticosteroids and cytotoxic drugs

Table 6.25 Diagnostic Criteria for Polyarteritis Nodosa

Weight loss ≥ 4 kg
Livedo reticularis
Testicular pain or tenderness
Myalgias, weakness, or leg tenderness
Mononeuropathy or polyneuropathy
Diastolic BP > 90 mm Hg
Elevated urea or creatinine
Hepatitis B virus surface antigen or its antibody in the serum
Arteriographic abnormality
Biopsy of small or medium-sized artery containing granulocytes or granulocytes plus mononuclear leukocytes in the vessel wall

Three or more criteria must be presented.

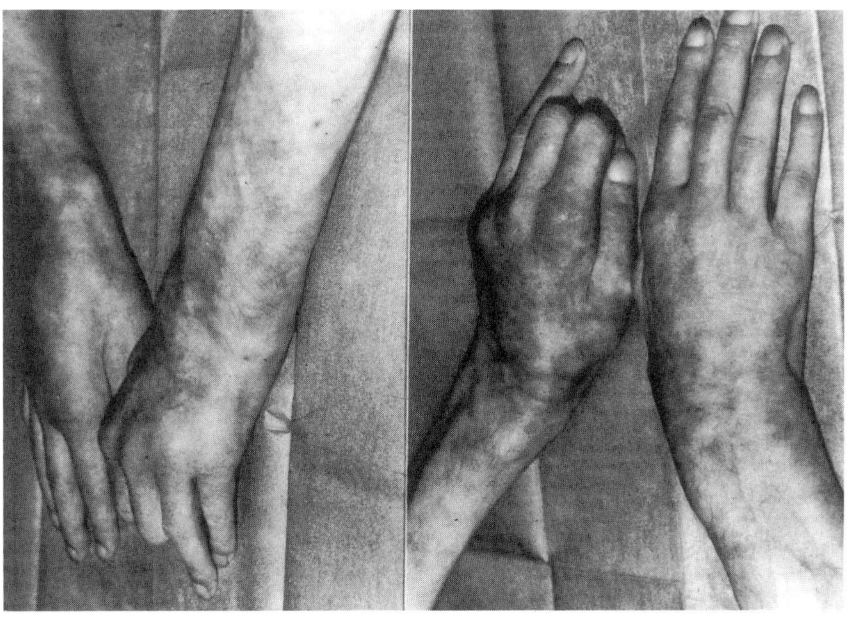

Figure 6.18 Livedo reticularis.

An asymmetric nondeforming arthritis may be present in the disease. Abdominal pain may be a presenting feature. It is due to infarction and hemorrhage in any of the abdominal viscera including the pancreas, liver, gallbladder, and gut.

There is frequently a peripheral neuropathy, which usually presents as a mononeuritis multiplex in the form of a pure motor neuropathy. Central nervous system involvement with seizures and hemiparesis may occur. Heart involvement is more commonly found pathologically than clinically. Tachycardia may be present and is a poor prognostic sign. Pericarditis is found. Heart failure may be due to the heart involvement itself or to the renal hypertension. It is the next most common cause of death after renal involvement. Primary eye involvement may be due to arteritis, which can lead to loss of vision, visual field defects, and amaurosis fugax, or there may be secondary eye changes due to hypertension. Pulmonary infiltrates may be seen on the chest X ray but clinical involvement is rare in classical PAN. Muscle pain, tenderness, and wasting may be prominent features. Muscle spasm may be particularly marked in the legs and may be exacerbated by walking. Renal involvement occurs in some 80% of patients with proteinuria and hematuria being the commonest manifestations. Attacks of renal pain with hematuria, due to infarction, and acute and rapidly progressive glomerulonephritis and renal failure are rarer features.

The clinical features of PAN are summarized in Table 6.26.

7.3 Confirming the Diagnosis—Investigations

Patients have an elevated sedimentation rate, an anemia, a leukocytosis with neutrophils typically above $11,000/mm^3$ thrombocytosis, and elevated immunoglobulins in the serum. The number of neutrophils may be useful in following disease activity as is the sedimentation rate. Autoantibodies are usually absent, although there may be low-titer antinuclear antibodies and rheumatoid factors.

Angiography of involved organs may show either thrombosed vessels or the characteristic aneurysms that are particularly found at the bifurcation of blood vessels. In descending order of efficacy, angiography should be carried out in the kidney, liver, or gut (Fig. 6.19).

Biopsy of a cutaneous lesion or an involved organ, usually muscle, may provide the diagnosis.

7.4 Diagnostic Difficulties

Similar angiographic changes may be present in other forms of vasculitis including Wegener's granulomatosis, Churg–Strauss syndrome, vasculitis in SLE, or other illnesses such as infective endocarditis, atrial myxoma, and

Table 6.26 Clinical Features of Polyarteritis Nodosa

Constitutional
Skin:
    Palpable purpura
    Livedo reticularis
    Rashes
Arterial:
    Digital gangrene
    Intermittent claudication
Heart:
    Tachycardia
    Myocardial infarction
    Pericarditis
Renal:
    Hypertension
    Proteinuria, haematuria
Gastrointestinal:
    Acute abdomen
    Visceral infarction
Nervous:
    Central: seizures, hemiplegia
    Peripheral: neuropathy
    Mononeuritis multiplex
Lung:
    Infiltrates

noninflammatory connective tissue disorders such as fibromuscular dysplasia.

7.5 Epidemiology and Historical Data

Polyarteritis nodosa is uncommon and estimates of its incidence in the general population have ranged from about 5 to 220 per million persons per year. The disease is twice as frequent in men. It may be observed in children and the elderly but is more common in middle-aged persons.

7.6 Pathophysiology

There is a granulomatous infiltration with mononuclear cells and giant cell formation in the adventitia and the outer part of the media of arteries. There is thickening of the intima with narrowing or obliteration of the lumen leading to thrombosis or dissection or aneurysmal formation (Fig.

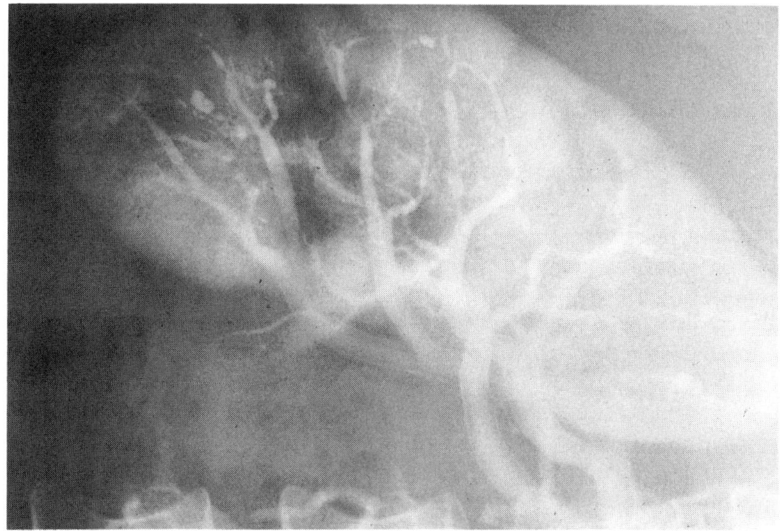

Figure 6.19   Angiography findings in the kidney in polyarteritis nodosa.

6.20). These changes are commonest in the kidneys, muscles, peripheral nerves, and gastrointestinal tract.

This was probably the first human disease in which direct evidence for the deposition of immune complexes containing a virus, hepatitis B, was obtained. Although circulating immune complexes are present in the majority of patients with PAN, no viral component has been described.

7.7   Management

The mainstay of treatment is steroids, which may have to be given in large doses of more than 50 mg/day. Ideally, the diagnosis should be made early before there are irreversible changes in blood vessels. Steroids should be reduced to a maintenance dose. Cytotoxic drugs should probably only be used as steroid-sparing agents. Complications should be treated as they arise.

7.8   Impact of the Disease and Prognosis

Prior to the use of corticosteroids, the 5-year survival of polyarteritis was reported to be less than 15%. In recent years survival has improved; studies now indicate a 5-year survival of 60% or more. The prognosis of polyarteritis nodosa is worse in older persons and those with more extensive visceral or central nervous system involvement.

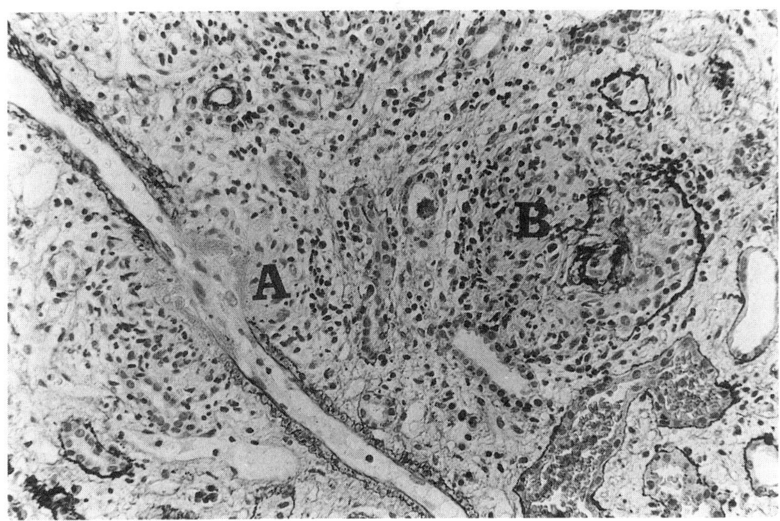

Figure 6.20 Pathologic features of polyarteritis nodosa: (A) granulomatous infiltration with mononuclear cells and (B) giant cell formation in the adventitia and outer part of the median of arteries. There is thickening of the intima with narrowing of the lumen.

Most deaths in PAN occur during the first year of the disease due to vasculitis or infectious complications of treatment. Deaths after the first year depend primarily on complications and especially renal failure, heart failure, or cerebrovascular ischemia.

The cutaneous form of PAN is less aggressive and carries a better prognosis.

8 WEGENER'S GRANULOMATOSUS

8.1 Definition (Table 6.27)

Wegener's granulomatosus (WG) is a necrotizing granulomatous disease involving various internal organs, but in particular the upper and lower respiratory tract and kidneys.

8.2 Main Clinical Features

Because of multiple organ involvement the diagnosis of WG may be difficult. Table 6.28 shows the criteria developed to aid in diagnosis.

WG may present as a chronic sinusitis, chronic rhinitis, nasal ulcer-

Table 6.27 Wegener's Granulomatosus

Necrotizing granulomatous disease of upper and lower respiratory tract and kidneys
Chronic sinusitis – nasal ulceration
Dyspnea – hemoptysis
Proteinuria
Vasculitis of the skin
ANCA (anticytoplasmic antibodies)–positive
Cyclophosphamide + corticosteroids improve serious prognosis

---

ation, or a serous otitis media accompanied by the systemic features of fever, anorexia, and weight loss.

Cough, hemoptysis, and dyspnea may be features. The chest X ray shows characteristic transient pulmonary infiltrates occasionally with cavitation which, however, may be asymptomatic. Renal involvement is late in the disease but can occur in 85% of patients with proteinuria, hematuria, and red blood cell casts. Renal failure and hypertension are uncommon. Palpable purpura may occur.

Early in the course of the disease joint pains are not infrequent but resolve with no sequelae. Conjunctivitis, scleritis, episcleritis, or extension of the sinusitis into the orbit are all various aspects of eye involvement. Nervous involvement is uncommon but may consist of cranial nerve paresis and a multiple mononeuropathy or asymmetric polyneuropathy.

8.3 Confirming the Diagnosis—Investigations

Patients during the active phase of the disease have anemia, leukocytosis, and thrombocytosis. There is elevated sedimentation rate and C-reactive

Table 6.28 Clinical Features of Wegener's Granulomatosus

Lung:
    Infiltrates
Paranasal sinuses:
    Sinusitis, infection
Nasopharynx:
    Mucosal ulceration, saddle nose, serous otitis media
Renal:
    Nephritis
Joints:
    Polyarthralgia
Skin:
    Vasculitis

---

protein. Immunoglobulins are elevated but particularly immunoglobulin A. Rheumatoid factor is present to a variable degree in about 50% of patients. There may be proteinuria and a urinary sediment if there is renal involvement. The chest X ray may reveal pulmonary infiltrates with cavitation. Biopsy of the nasal mucosa, the paranasal sinuses, and the vasculitic lesions may reveal the diagnosis.

One of the most important developments in the diagnosis and management of WG has been the description of anticytoplasmic antibodies (ANCAs) in the serum of these patients. There are two forms of ANCAs, namely, cANCAs and pANCAs referring to cytoplasmic or perinuclear distribution, respectively. In 90% of patients with WG cANCAs are found. They are also in cases of systemic necrotising small vessel vasculitis (microscopic polyarteritis nodosa) and in those of isolated rapidly progressive nephritis. These conditions may represent different parts of the WG spectrum. Disease activity can be monitored by following the titers of the antibody.

Biopsy of the lesions show neutrophil infiltration with granuloma formation and fibrosis in the late stages involving arteries and adjacent veins (Fig. 6.21).

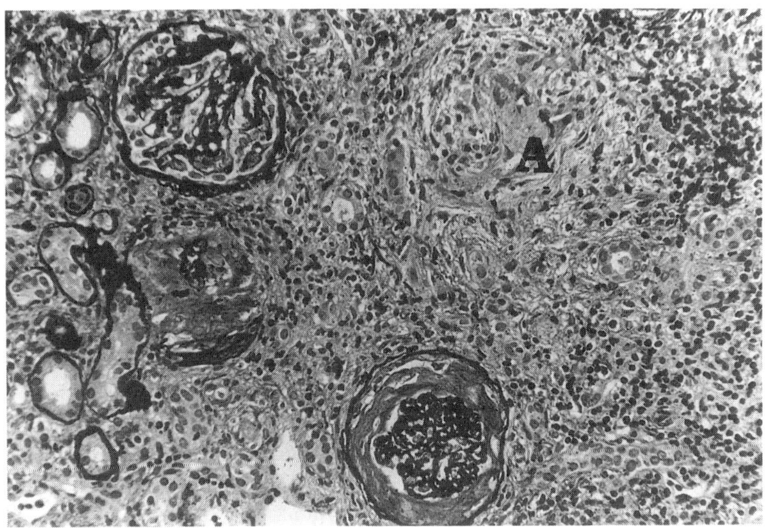

Figure 6.21 Pathologic features of Wegener's granulomatosus.

8.4 Diagnostic Difficulties

Patients with Churg–Strauss syndrome, allergic granulomatous angiitis, may present with a similar triad of organ involvement. Eosinophilia is present in almost all patients with Churg–Strauss syndrome but resolves in response to treatment. ANCAs are found in a minority of patients with polyarteritis nodosa and other forms of vasculitis.

8.5 Epidemiology and Historical Data

WG is rare but has been described in all racial groups and in all parts of the world. Males are slightly more commonly involved than females. The age of diagnosis is 41 years (range 5–78 years), with the majority patients being adults.

8.6 Pathophysiology

The cause of WG is unknown, but it is suspected that it may be triggered by viruses. Evidence of immunologic involvement is provided by the fact that there may be elevated levels of IgE in the serum, particularly where there is lung involvement, the response to cyclophosphamide treatment, and the association with HLA DR2.

ANCAs recognize a 29-kD molecule found in the azurophilic granules of neutrophils that is probably a serine protease. The antibodies may be involved in the pathogenesis of the disease by causing the release of enzymes and other inflammatory mediators that damage blood vessels.

8.7 Management—Impact of the Disease and Prognosis

WG can be a serious and lethal disease (20% of one large series). When death occurs during the first year it is mainly due to renal involvement and after that time to lung involvement. The mainstay of treatment is cyclophosphamide given as 2 mg/kg orally on a daily basis. Azathioprine may be used as a maintenance medication once remission has been induced with cyclophosphamide. In the event of failure to respond to cyclophosphamide or azathioprine, the addition of trimethoprim-sulfamethoxazole may bring about remission but it has to be continued almost indefinitely. Steroids are useful when there are significant systemic features but should not be used on their own but in association with the above-cited drugs. Finally, the complications should be treated as they arise.

Table 6.29 Hypersensitivity Vasculitis

Leukocytoclastic vasculitis: small vessels, skin
Palpable purpura: legs, buttocks, back
Allergy to drugs, bacteria, parasites, virus
Corticosteroid treatment
Prognosis excellent

---

9 HYPERSENSITIVITY VASCULITIS

9.1 Definition (Table 6.29)

Hypersensitivity vasculitis is a leukocytoclastic vasculitis of the small vessels of the skin that may be a hypersensitivity reaction to agents such as drugs.

9.2 Main Clinical Features

Hypersensitivity vasculitis is of sudden onset with a maculopapular rash of the skin. It usually comes on within a few days of the putative inciting agent. The rash progresses to a palpable purpura (Fig. 6.22).

It involves the legs, buttocks, back, and, on occasions, the forearms

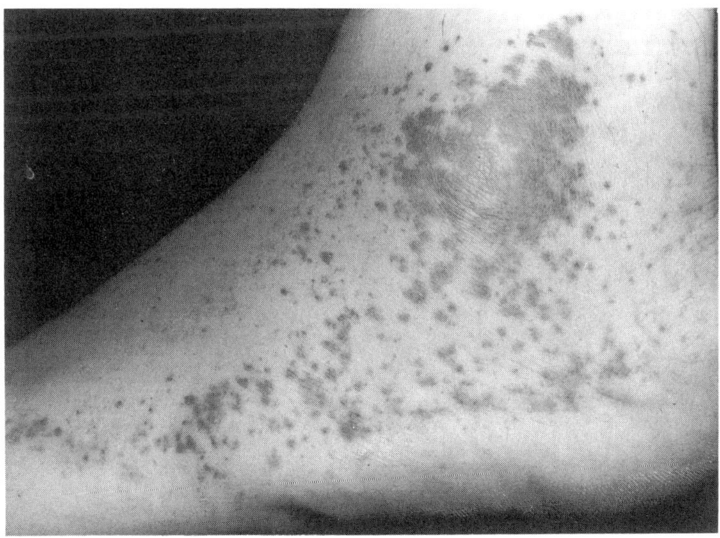

Figure 6.22 Hypersensitivity vasculitis.

and hands. The vasculitic rash comes in crops. The lesions can ulcerate. Constitutional symptoms may be present during active phases. Only rarely is there involvement of the kidney, lung, or gastrointestinal tract.

9.3 Confirming the Diagnosis—Investigations

There is deposition of immunoglobulins and complement components in involved blood vessels. The lesions are full of infiltrating polymorphs with evidence of leukocytoclasis consisting of nuclear fragmentation ("nuclear dust"), vessel wall necrosis, and fibrinoid necrosis. There is an acute phase response with elevated ESR and C-reactive protein.

9.4 Diagnostic Difficulties

Clinical manifestations in hypersensitivity vasculitis are not distinctive, and similar clinical pictures may be associated with a variety of other disorders such as Henoch–Schönlein purpura, rheumatic disorders, cryoglobulinemia, and infections. Cases of so-called microscopic polyarteritis nodosa and cutaneous polyarteritis nodosa may be difficult to distinguish from hypersensitivity vasculitis other than the chronic course in the former. Other less common forms of vasculitis such as hypocomplementemic urticarial vasculitis and certain infections, such as bacterial endocarditis, need to be differentiated.

9.4.1 Henoch–Schönlein Purpura

Henoch–Schönlein purpura (HSP) is a distinct syndrome within the hypersensitivity vasculitides. A distinctive feature is IgA deposition in cutaneous and renal lesions. It is commoner in the spring and may follow an upper respiratory tract infection. There is palpable purpura over extensor surfaces of the distal parts of the upper and lower limbs and over the buttocks. During the acute episode there may be gastrointestinal and renal involvement.

9.5 Pathophysiology

Allergy to drugs (especially penicillin and its derivatives and sulfa drugs), bacteria, parasites, and viruses have all been implicated.

9.6 Management

The offending substance should be discontinued. Steroids may be used if there is extensive skin or internal organ involvement. Any infection should be appropriately treated.

Table 6.30 Adamantiades–Behçet Syndrome

Multisystem vasculitic disease
Arterial and venous involvement
Orogenital ulceration
Uveitis + hypopyon
Meningitis — encephalitis
More common in Japan and Turkey
Corticosteroids and cytostatics
Outcome may be serious

9.7 Impact of the Disease and Prognosis

The prognosis is usually excellent. The prognosis in Henoch–Schönlein purpura depends on the extent and duration of renal involvement.

10 ADAMANTIADES–BEHÇET'S SYNDROME

10.1 Definition (Table 6.30)

Adamantiades–Behçet's syndrome (A-BS) is a multisystem vasculitic disease, both arterial and venous, with recurrent orogenital ulceration.

10.2 Main Clinical Features

The syndrome is characterized by recurrent painful, 2- to 10-mm aphthous ulcers in the mouth (cheeks, tongue, palate, pharynx) and genitals (penis, scrotum, vulva, cervix, and vagina) (Table 6.31).

Mucosal ulcerations can be found anywhere in the gastrointestinal tract but favor the terminal ileum, cecum, and ascending colon. Clinically they may present as abdominal pain, bleeding, or perforation. Vasculitic

Table 6.31 Diagnostic Criteria for Adamantiades–Behçet's Syndrome

Recurrent oral aphthous ulcers plus two of the following:
    Recurrent genital ulceration
    Uveitis or retinal vasculitis
    Cutaneous pathergy
    Large vessel vasculitis
    Meningoencephalitis
    Cerebral vasculitis

involvement of many organs and tissues is common. Their onset is episodic. *In the eye* there may be hypopyon and anterior or posterior uveitis. *The skin* is usually mildly involved with pustular lesions and, occasionally, erythema nodosum–like lesions. A *mono-* or *oligoarthritis* may involve large joints with recurrent synovitis and/or effusions but is nondestructive. Involvement of *veins with thrombophlebitis* of the extremities and of the venae cavae and its tributaries with a variety of clinical manifestations can occur. *Central nervous system* involvement with meningoencephalitis may occur with headache, fever, and stiff neck (meningitis) and signs and symptoms referrable to the corticospinal tract and cerebellum (encephalitis) with paresis, ataxia, or pseudobulbar palsy.

A summary of the principal organ involvement in BS is shown in Table 6.32.

10.3 Confirming the Diagnosis—Investigations

Laboratory investigation shows an acute phase response. The *pathergy test* has been proposed as a diagnostic test. This is the development of a nodule or pustule up to 10 mm in diameter developing 24–48 hr after pricking the skin with a sterile 20-gauge needle.

10.4 Diagnostic Difficulties

During the evolution of the disease distinction from other multisystem vasculitic diseases may be difficult. Differential diagnosis can be complex and includes other more common diseases such as Crohn's disease, cicatrical pemphigoid, lichen planus, herpes simplex, and somatization disorders, which can all have ulcerating lesions.

Table 6.32 Organ Involvement in Adamantiades–Behçet's Syndrome

Orogenital ulceration
Skin:
Pustules
Thrombophlebitis
Arthritis
Eye
Central nervous system

10.5 Epidemiology and Historical Data

A-BS has an equal sex incidence. It is particularly common in the Mediterranean and in Japan, being rare in northern Europe.

The complete syndrome was described by Hippocrates; its ocular complications by Adamantiades and then by Behçet.

10.6 Pathophysiology

The etiology of A-BS is unknown although infectious and autoimmune causes have been suggested. Involved tissues show variable degrees of vasculitis with a mononuclear and neutrophil infiltrate with deposition of IgM and complement C3. HLA B51, a split of HLA B5, is more common in severely affected patients, especially among these from Japan and the eastern Mediterranean.

10.7 Management

The response to steroids is disappointing except when used as a gargle for relief of pain of oral ulcers or as a cream for genital ulcers. Antifungal gargles can also help alleviate painful oral ulcers. The mainstay of treatment is cyclophosphamide but chlorambucil is also used. It may be worth trying azathioprine as a first cytotoxic drug but not for eye disease. Ocular inflammation may require the use of cyclosporin A but a careful watch on the development of renal toxicity needs to be maintained. Other treatments that have been used include colchicine and thalidomide. Intramuscular gold injections may control troublesome joint involvement.

Complications must be treated with appropriate medical, physical, and surgical means.

10.8 Impact of the Disease and Prognosis

The dreaded complications of A-BS are eye inflammation and meningoencephalitis, which if not adequately treated can lead to blindness and central nervous system deficits, respectively.

7

Crystal-Induced Arthritis

Acute joint inflammation may result from the presence within the synovial cavity of microcrystals such as those of urate or calcium pyrophosphate. Acute articular or periarticular inflammation may occur from the presence of hydroxyapatite crystals in structures outside the joint such as tendons or in the synovium within the joint. Massive deposits of crystals in and around joints (such as in gouty tophi) can cause destruction of articular structures and so lead to deforming arthritis.

1 GOUT

1.1 Definition (Table 7.1)

Classical or urate gout is a crystal-induced arthritis caused by the presence within the joint of microcrystals of monosodium urate monohydrate.

1.2 Main Clinical Features

1.2.1 Early Manifestations

In the early stages of the disease the patient, usually a young man, suffers from recurrent self-limited attacks of acute monoarticular arthritis. The first metatarsophalangeal is the most frequently affected joint (podagra),

Table 7.1 Gout

Urate crystal-induced arthritis
Usually monoarthritis
Incapacitating lasting ± 10 days
Often big toe involved (podagra)
Young/middle-aged males
Postmenopausal women: diuretics
Untreated develop tophi
Curable (!) with urate-lowering drugs

followed by the knee (gonagra), the ankle, other foot joints, wrist, or elbow. Involvement of the hip, shoulder, or spinal joints is distinctly uncommon. The arthritis may spread to adjacent joints, and a polyarthritis can also occur, giving rise to diagnostic confusion. Bursae (e.g., the olecranon bursa) may also be affected. Attacks may be precipitated by trauma, stress, or dietary and/or alcoholic overindulgence and last for up to a week unless aborted by treatment. The pain and tenderness is often excruciating, but may be deceptively unobtrusive in the early stages or in mild attacks. Involvement of weight-bearing joints limits or precludes standing or walking. The affected joint is swollen, red, and hot (Fig. 7.1). Any attempt at palpation or active or passive movement is strenuously resisted.

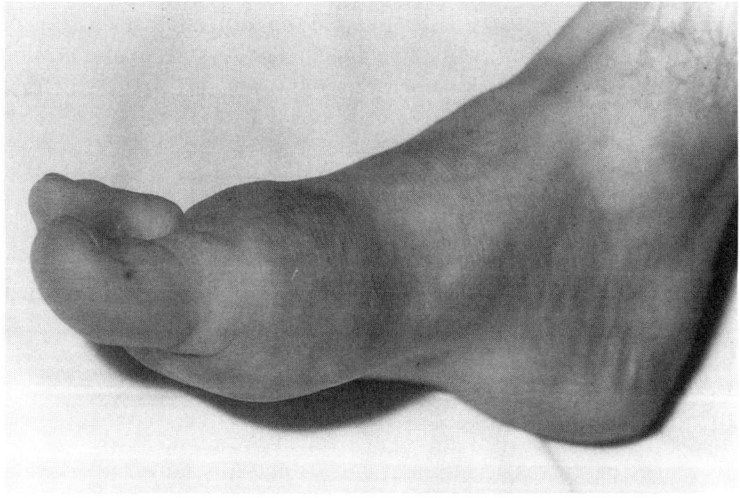

Figure 7.1 Gout arthritis of first metatarsal phalangeal joint.

1.2.2 Late Manifestations

As the months or years go by, the frequency of acute attacks increases and deposits of urate crystals called tophi appear either subcutaneously or within or adjacent to joints or in juxtaarticular bone causing significant destruction. Tophi may be observed on the pinna of the external ear, the olecranon, the hands, or the big toe (Fig. 7.2). Occasionally, severe chronic deforming arthritis occurs, notably in the hands.

1.3 Confirming the Diagnosis—Investigations

1.3.1 Early Phase

A raised plasma urate is to be expected in most instances (see below, "Diagnostic Difficulties"). Where possible a specimen of synovial fluid from the affected joint should be examined under polarized light. The finding of intraleukocytic negatively birefringent needle-shaped crystals (of sodium urate monohydrate) is diagnostic of urate gout (Fig. 7.3). At the time of the first acute attack, the X ray is normal. With recurring episodes bony tophi are seen as cyst-like areas (often with clearly defined margins) within the

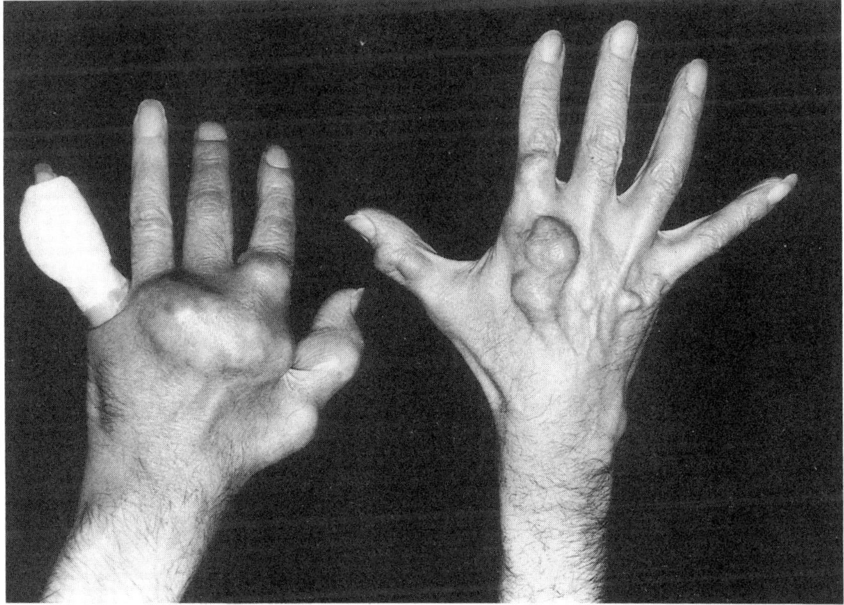

Figure 7.2 Tophi on the hands.

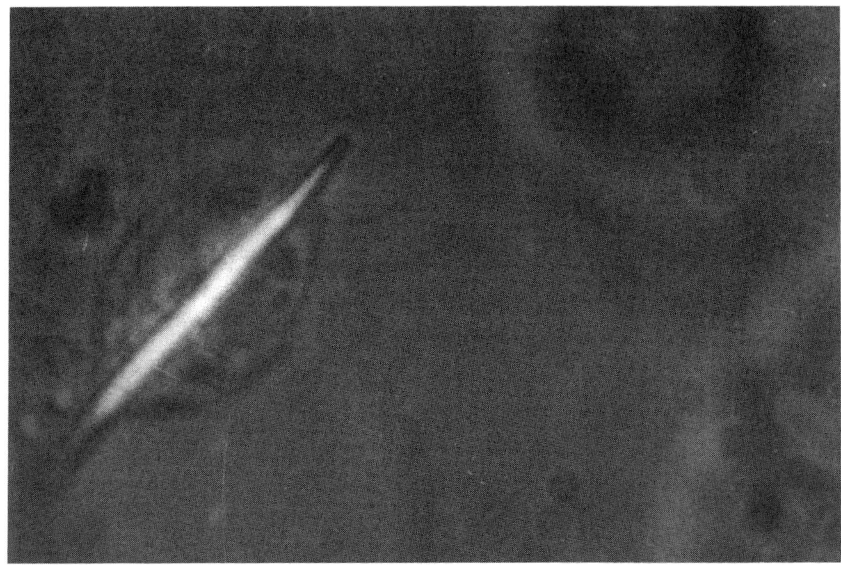

Figure 7.3   Intraleukocytic needle-shaped urate crystals in synovial fluid.

articulating bones and adjacent to (but usually not abutting) the articular surfaces (Fig. 7.4).

1.3.2   Late Phase

Extraosseous tophi are seen as soft tissue swellings around joints or bursae. They may calcify, which helps to distinguish them from other swellings. Biopsy of a tophus shows heavy deposition of urate crystals (identified in situ by polarizing microscopy) within a fibrous stroma. It is important to fix the specimen in alcohol rather than in formalin if the crystals are to be preserved. The most helpful aids for differentiation are (1) plasma urate (hyperuricemia = Pl urate > 0.5 mmol/L or 0.7 mg/L); (2) polarizing microscopic examination of synovial fluid or tissue for urate microcrystal identification in situ; (3) X-ray examination of the affected joints for evidence of radiologic tophi; (4) needle aspiration or biopsy of tophi to confirm the presence of urate crystals.

1.4   Diagnostic Difficulties

The differential diagnosis includes all forms of acute mono- or oligoarticular arthritis. Of particular importance is septic arthritis, which may mimic gout and should always be suspected and excluded in a *first* attack of acute

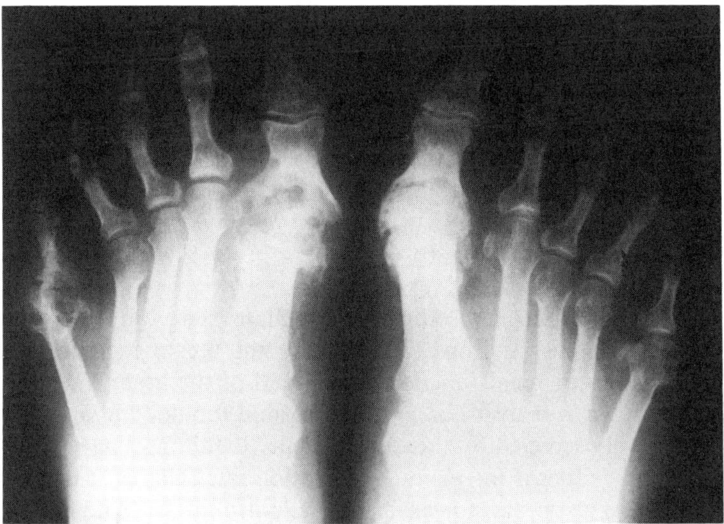

Figure 7.4   X-ray changes in chronic gouty arthritis.

gouty arthritis, if necessary, by joint aspiration and culture of the extracted synovial fluid. In the presence of a past history of gout, known hyperuricemia, visible tophi, or characteristic big toe involvement, it is permissible to forego arthrocentesis and proceed to a therapeutic trial.

Major pitfalls in diagnosis include assuming (1) that all arthritis in the presence of hyperuricemia is gout; (2) that gout never occurs in the presence of a normal plasma urate (the latter may occasionally transiently dip into the normal range around the time of an acute attack). Asymptomatic hyperuricemia (often diuretic-induced) is probably three times more common than hyperuricemia with gout. In cases of doubt intrasynovial crystals should be sought by polariscopy; and (3) that gout is the source of all afflictions of the first metatarsophalangeal joint (the most commonly affected joint in osteoarthritis).

1.5   Epidemiology and Historical Data

Gout occurs throughout the world and in all races. However, certain ethnic groups such as the Maories in New Zealand and the Pima Indians in the United States are more prone because of their tendency to hyperuricemia (high plasma levels of urate). In Western countries gout is rare in the first two decades of life and the peak age of onset in males is in the fifth decade and in females in the sixth. There is a statistical association with obesity, hypertension, hypertriglyceridemia, and vascular occlusive diseases. It has been known since Hippocrates that gout is rare in women before the menopause. Overall the male/female ratio is 10:1. The risk of gouty arthritis occurring is directly proportional to the height of the plasma urate level. Throughout the centuries the agonies of podagra have been documented from Hippocrates to Sydenham, and the sight of gout stools and crippling arthritis is part of our medical heritage.

1.6 Pathophysiology (Figure 7.5)

Urate is the endpoint of purine metabolism in humans. Two thirds of urate excretion is via the kidney and one third via the gut. Renal excretion depends on the integrity of renal function because all of the urate is filtered by the glomerulus, all is reabsorbed by the proximal tubule, and approximately 8% is actively secreted by the distal tubule. It follows that urate is retained in the body either if the glomular filtration rate falls, or if tubular secretion is inhibited as occurs, for example, with alcohol and with certain drugs, such as pyrazinamide or oral diuretics. The concentration of plasma urate is governed by urate production, which may increase as a result of de novo purine synthesis, from excessive ingestion of high-purine foods, or from the excessive catabolism of nucleoproteins as occurs in myeloproliferative diseases such as leukemia or polycythemia rubra vera especially during cytotoxic chemotherapy. Increased de novo synthesis may rarely be caused by an enzyme defect involving purine metabolism as in the Lesch–Nyhan syndrome, an X-linked heritable disorder characterized by the absence (or partial absence) of hypoxanthine-glutamylphosphoribosyltransferase (HG-PRTase). If the balance between production and excretion of urate is tipped

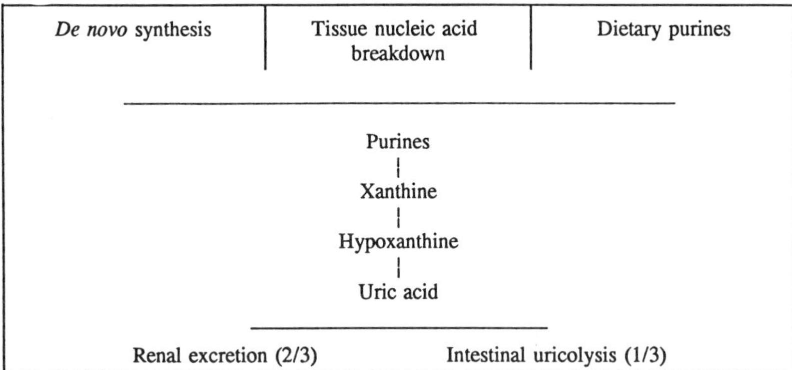

Figure 7.5 Pathophysiology of hyperuricemia.

in favor of urate retention, the plasma urate rises (hyperuricemia is said to occur when the plasma urate exceeds 0.5 mmol/L or 0.7 mg/L). Since the solubility of sodium urate in plasma and other body fluids is limited, precipitation of crystals of monosodium urate monohydrate is likely to occur within synovial joints, thereby initiating a cascade of inflammation (Fig. 7.6), which we recognize as gout. It may precipitate in the renal tract causing calculi.

1.7 Management

The aims of treatment are twofold: (1) to abort the acute attack and (2) to reduce the frequency of attacks and hopefully abolish them altogether by pharmaceutical and/or dietetic means. In the treatment of the acute attack the choice lies between (1) colchicine, (2) NSAIDs, and (3) corticosteroids. Colchicine (originally an extract of the autumn crocus) is the transitional and specific treatment for acute gout, which has withstood the test of time. It is administered orally in tablets containing 0.5 mg 2-4 hourly until the attack comes under control (or until the patient develops diarrhea which is, unfortunately, a common event). In either case the dose is reduced to twice or thrice daily after 24 hr until the attack has subsided. Most NSAIDs are effective in this situation, although a large initial loading dose (perhaps double the normal one) is recommended. Indomethacin, naproxen, and diclofenac are the most effective. Corticosteroids, in the form of oral prednisolone, intramuscular depot methylprednisolone, or ACTH, are effective in intractable cases of acute gouty polyarthritis. Depot methylprednisolone (e.g., 40-80 mg for a knee) given intraarticularly is an effective form of therapy for gouty monoarthritis resistant to oral therapy (Table 7.2).

The likelihood that gout will develop is directly proportional to the level of the hyperuricemia. It follows that reducing the plasma urate level will reduce the frequency of acute attacks and eventually (perhaps over 6-12 months) abolish them altogether. Reduction of de novo urate synthesis can be achieved by adopting a low-purine diet (avoiding liver, kidney, brains, sweetbread, fish roes, tinned fish, and red meat as well as alcoholic beverages), thereby lowering the plasma urate to a modest degree (0.05-0.1 mmol/L). More impressive and effective reduction can be achieved by therapeutic means. Uricosuric drugs, e.g., probenecid (1-1.5 g/day) or sulfynpyrazone (200-400 mg/day), act by inhibiting urate reabsorption from the distal renal tubule, thereby promoting its excretion. They are ineffective in the presence of renal failure (if no urate is filtered at the glomerulus, no amount of tampering with tubular reabsorption will affect excretion) and are contraindicated in the presence of urate kidney stones because uricosurica will only aggravate the renal obstruction problem.

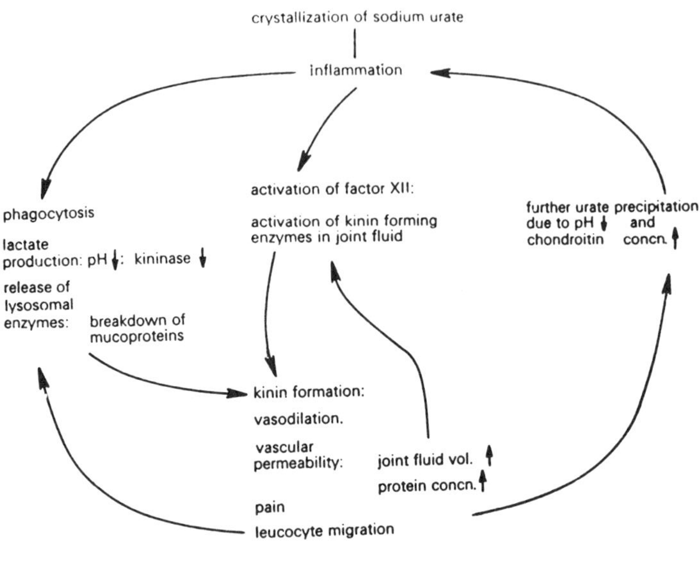

(a)

(b)

Figure 7.6 Pathophysiology of crystal-induced inflammation. (a) Cascade of inflammation; (b) granulocyte-crystal (CPPD) interaction.

Table 7.2 Gout Therapy

Lifestyle correction
Colchicine, NSAIDs for acute attacks
Xanthine oxidase inhibitors (e.g., allopurinol)
Uricosuric agents (e.g., probenecid, sulfynpyrazone)

For the same reason, uricosuric drugs should be avoided in "overexcreters of urate." In such cases (and many would recommend it in all cases of gout requiring urate-lowering therapy) allopurinol is indicated. This drug, available since the 1960s, acts by inhibiting xanthine oxidase, the enzyme responsible for promoting the last two stages of urate synthesis, namely, that from xanthine to hypoxanthine and from hypoxanthine to uric acid. The result is a reduction in plasma and tissue fluid urate levels, which in the presence of hyperuricemia results in a gradual reduction in the size of tophi and in the frequency of occurrence of acute gouty arthritis, as well as a reduced tendency to urate stone formation. The consequent rise in plasma and urinary levels of xanthine and hypoxanthine has no clinical sequelae.

The introduction of urate-lowering drug therapy is attended by an increased tendency to acute gouty attacks for the first 6 months or so (or until the miscible pool of urate is stabilized at a lower level). This effect can be minimized by avoiding starting during an acute attack, by raising the dose in stages (100 mg/day increasing at weekly intervals by 100 mg/day to 300 mg/day or more until the plasma urate is within the normal range), by coprescribing a prophylactic dose of colchicine (0.5 mg 2 times daily) or an NSAID (e.g., indomethacin 25 mg 3 times daily) for the first 6 months (longer if gout attacks continue). In patients with renal impairment or if given with azathioprine the dose should be reduced accordingly (Table 7.3).

The most common cause of failure to control gout by these means is failure of compliance. Patients should understand the need to follow instructions carefully if therapeutic success is to be achieved. Urate-

Table 7.3 Indications for Allopurinol

Gout with overproduction of uric acid
Intolerance to uricosuric drugs
Gout with urate kidney stones
Gout with chronic renal impairment
Chronic tophaceous gout
Pre-(cytotoxic) treatment of myeloproliferative disorders

---

lowering drug therapy is usually required for life and so should not be undertaken lightly. It should be reserved for those patients who suffer repeated acute attacks and whose hyperuricemia cannot be controlled by dietetic means alone. Surgical removal of tophi is rarely required nowadays as a result of improved drug treatment.

1.8 Atypical Forms

Diagnostic confusion may arise if the urate level dips into the normal range as it may do if sudden gross crystallization occurs as in severe attacks or when a widespread polyarthritis develops, often in the form of an *arthritis migrans*, mimicking rheumatoid arthritis.

1.9 Impact of Disease and Prognosis

Of all the chronic rheumatic diseases gout is the most effectively treatable, thanks to the success of treatments currently available. However, gout has not disappeared, and severe cases that have eluded correct diagnosis or have been denied (sometimes by the patient) modern therapy are still encountered. Gout and hyperuricemia are associated with obesity, hypertension, and coronary artery disease, and it is important that these aspects be adequately treated in their own right. Overindulgence in alcohol and rich food is traditionally linked to gout. This, together with drug compliance, is an area in which patient collaboration is essential for best results.

2 PSEUDOGOUT

2.1 Definition (Table 7.4)

Pseudogout, also known as pyrophosphate arthropathy, is an acute or chronic joint disease associated with the deposition within the joint of crystals of calcium pyrophosphate dihydrate (CPPD).

Table 7.4 Pseudogout-Chondrocalcinosis

Calcium pyrophosphate dihydrate (CPPD)–induced crystal arthropathy
Recurrent self-limiting attacks of monoarthritis
Knees, wrist, and hip most involved
Occurs most often in the elderly
Intraleukocytic rod-like crystals in synovial fluid
On X-ray chondrocalcinosis
May be associated with metabolic disease

2.2 Main Clinical Features

2.2.1 Early Manifestations

CPPD deposition per se is asymptomatic and probably remains so in the majority of subjects affected. However, the release of CPPD microcrystals from cartilaginous deposits near to the surface into the joint cavity may evoke recurrent brisk though self-limiting attacks of inflammatory synovitis (akin to classical urate gout). Hence its name "pseudogout" or "pyrophosphate arthropathy." Most commonly affected joints are large ones such as the knee, wrist, and hip. Acute episodes are precipitated by trauma, physical stress, or infection. They are liable to occur in the elderly during the course of another acute illness or after surgical operation. They are short-lived lasting from 2 to 7 days, intensely painful as the attack reaches its climax. The joint is tender, painful on attempted movement, and warm to the touch. Fever may be present.

2.2.2 Late Manifestations

In the late phase more chronic changes such as diminution of joint range of motion and deformity are seen, mimicking polyarticular osteoarthritis or neuropathic arthropathy.

2.3 Confirming the Diagnosis—Investigations

2.3.1 Early Phase

Aspiration of synovial fluid for examination under polarizing microscopy is an essential diagnostic procedure. The finding of intraleukocytic weakly positively birefringent rod-like crystals is pathognomonic of pyrophosphate arthropathy. In most cases radiopaque calcification (representing accumulations of CPPD) can be seen on plain radiographs with the help of a bright light, particularly at the wrist ulnar side, MCP joints, knees, and pubis (Fig. 7.7).

Caution is required in diagnosing pyrophosphate arthropathy on the basis of chondrocalcinosis alone because it may be coincidental and hence unrelated to the true cause of the arthritis. It is important to confirm the diagnosis by polarizing microscopy. Biopsy is not particularly helpful in this condition.

2.4 Diagnostic Difficulties

Pyrophosphate arthropathy may mimic septic arthritis and may resemble many other forms of acute arthritis as urate gout or septic arthritis (see Chapter 3).

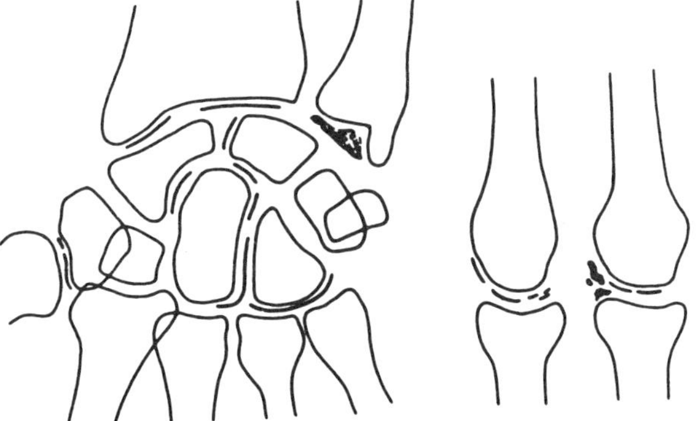

(a)

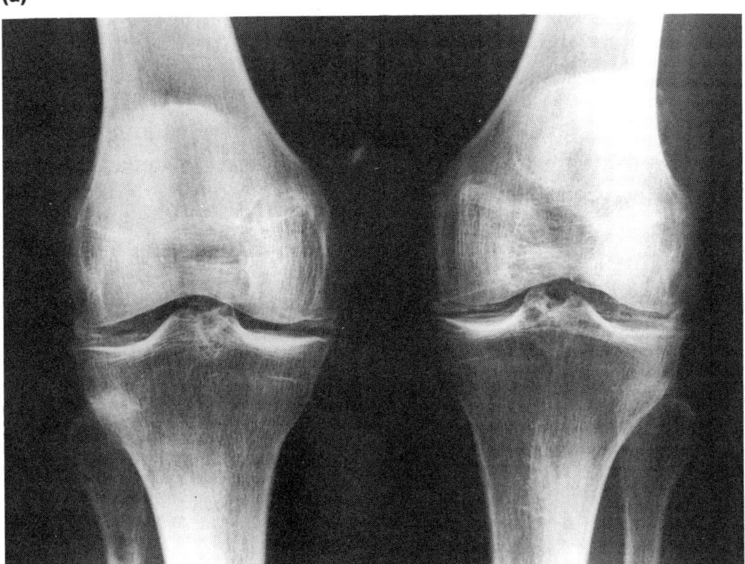

(b)

Figure 7.7 X-ray changes seen in chondrocalcinosis (a) at the metacarpophalangeal joints and wrist; and (b) at the knee.

2.5 Epidemiology and Historical Data

This is largely a disease of advancing years. CPPD deposition is a gradual process, which commences in middle life, increasing in prevalence and intensity in the latter years. It affects 5% of the adult population. The male/female ratio is 1. Families with CPPD have been described from all over the world. Its true identity and significance was not established until the early 1960s by McCarty.

2.6 Pathophysiology

The prerequisite is the CPPD deposition in articular structures, notably the hyaline cartilage of the joint surface and intraarticular fibrocartilaginous structures (chondrocalcinosis) such as the menisci of the knee, the triangular ligament of the wrist, and the pubic symphysis. Such deposition may arise in a minority of cases as the result of metastatic calcification in chronic hypercalcemia states as occurs in primary hyperparathyroidism. It also occurs typically in hemochromatosis, in which it may antedate organ involvement by up to 20 years. It then constitutes an indication for early treatment, which may successfully prevent subsequent organ deterioration.

In most cases, however, there is no underlying disease and the chondrocalcinosis is merely seen as a feature of aging (Table 7.5).

2.7 Management

There is no known means of eradicating the calcium pyrophosphate crystals from the cartilage. Once the process is initiated it tends to progress slowly but relentlessly. The use of prophylactic colchicine 0.5 mg twice daily may prevent attacks. Even the removal of an underlying parathyroid adenoma is incapable of slowing down or reversing the process.

Acute arthritic episodes may be treated by colchicine or NSAIDs in short courses. However, the efficacy of these drugs in this situation is difficult to evaluate owing to the brief duration and spontaneous recovery of the attacks. In some cases the act of joint aspiration is therapeutic and promotes resolution. Physical therapy may be helpful in the more chronic

Table 7.5   Diseases Associated with Chondrocalcinosis

Hyperparathryoidism
Hemochromatosis
Hyperuricemia and gout
Diabetes mellitus
Familial (genetic) form

Table 7.6   Atypical forms of CPPD Disease

Pseudorheumatoid arthritis
Pseudoosteoarthritis
Pseudoneuropathic joint
Idiopathic CPPD disease

phases where joint function is impaired through deformity and/or muscle wasting. Surgery may be required for associated osteoarthritis.

2.8 Atypical Forms

A chronic destructive polyarthritis is occasionally seen that is virtually indistinguishable from rheumatoid arthritis. Another variant occurs in association with osteoarthritis in weight-bearing joints resulting in unusually severe joint destruction (Table 7.6).

2.9 Impact of Disease and Prognosis

While acute attacks can cause severe pain and disability, this is usually short-lived. Frequently recurring bouts are distressing, though fortunately they are uncommon and rarely end up in a Charcot-like (pseudoneuropathic) joint.

3 HYDROXYAPATITE ARTHRITIS

3.1 Definition (Table 7.7)

Hydroxyapatite arthritis is a crystal-induced arthritis caused by the presence within or around the joint of microcrystals of hydroxyapatite, a complex crystalline salt of calcium and phosphate $[CA_{10}(PO_4)_6OH]$ similar to that found in normal bone. When deposited in soft tissues (a process known as calcinosis), it can lead to an acute or chronic form of crystal-induced inflammation or calcific periarthritis. The most commonly affected tissue is

Table 7.7   Hydroxyapatite arthritis

Hydroxyapatite-induced crystal arthritis
Calcific tendonitis
Recurrent self-limiting periarthritis
Soft tissue calcinosis
Associated with severe osteoarthritis and Milwaukee shoulder

the tendon, resulting in calcific tendonitis, and the most frequently affected group of tendons that which constitutes the rotator cuff of the shoulder. However, it may also be deposited in various soft tissues throughout the body, giving rise to more widespread and recurrent episodes of soft tissue inflammation. Hydroxyapatite is also found in articular structures where it is believed to play a part in the pathogenesis of destructive forms of osteoarthritis in weight-bearing joints, and also in a particularly aggressive shoulder arthropathy known as "the Milwaukee shoulder" or "apatite-associated destructive arthropathy." Other joints (knee, ankle, hip) have also been implicated. Hydroxyapatite has also been found in normal joints, but its prevalence and significance here is not known.

3.2 Main Clinical Features

3.2.1 Early Manifestations

Calcinosis per se is asymptomatic, and only when inflammation occurs does the patient become aware of a problem. A common presentation is sudden onset of severe pain in the shoulder associated with marked (sometimes total) loss of shoulder movement. This is a self-limiting condition that subsides spontaneously within a week in most cases, irrespective of treatment. As long as the calcinosis persists there remains the likelihood of recurrences. For further details of clinical manifestations, see the section on soft tissue lesions in Chapter 8.

3.2.2 Late Manifestations

The reader is referred to the section on clinical features of osteoarthritis in Chapter 8.

The Milwaukee shoulder presents as an uncommon chronic painful and restricted shoulder arthropathy in elderly persons.

3.3 Confirming the Diagnosis—Investigations

3.3.1 Early Phase

Calcific tendonitis is confirmed by the finding of the clinical features of an acute rotator lesion in association with extraarticular calcification on the shoulder radiograph (Fig. 7.8). This is usually seen in the position of the supraspinatus tendon. Serial X rays may show progressive calcium deposition or, alternatively, disappear altogether. Aspiration of the lesion may yield a paste-like material shown on microscopy to contain masses of hydroxyapatite crystals.

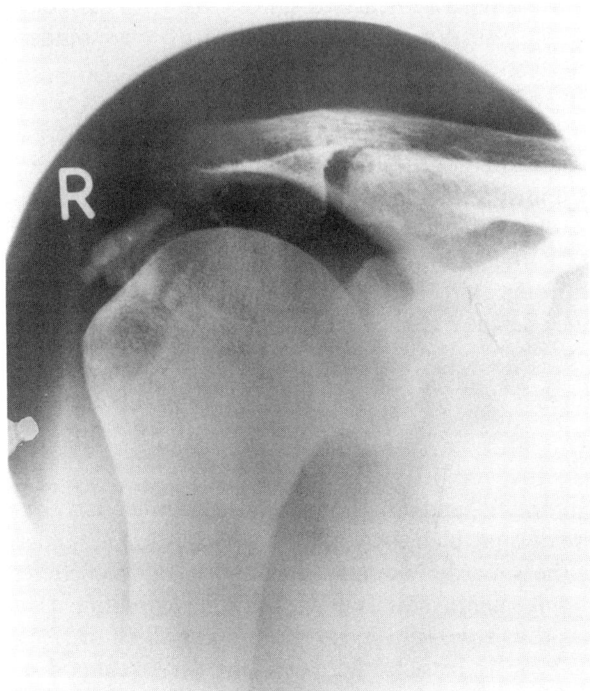

Figure 7.8   X-ray changes in calcific tendonitis.

3.3.2 Late Phase

In the Milwaukee shoulder, aspiration of the effusion may also yield hydroxyapatite crystals. The radiographic appearances are striking with gross destruction of the joint surfaces impinging on the humeral neck and proximal shaft.

3.4 Diagnostic Difficulties

Calcific tendonitis may be confused with noncalcific tendonitis, which is a simple overuse lesion (see Chapter 8). Milwaukee shoulder may be confused with a neuropathic arthropathy of the shoulder.

3.5 Epidemiology and Historical Data

There are no epidemiologic data available for hydroxyapatite diseases. Calcific tendonitis has been recognized since the early days of radiology.

3.6 Pathophysiology

The mechanism for the induction of inflammation by hydroxyapatite or for the gross destruction in Milwaukee shoulder is unknown.

3.7 Management

Treatment of acute calcific tendonitis is the same as for other forms of rotator cuff lesions. The only effective form of treatment for Milwaukee shoulder is total shoulder replacement.

3.8 Atypical Forms

3.8.1 Hydroxyapatite Disease

Some patients have recurrent attacks of hydroxyapatite at multiple locations such as the shoulder, elbow, base of the thumb, greater trochanter region, etc. Apatite deposition at multiple joints, including small joints, is seen in patients with disturbances of calcium and phosphorus metabolism, in particular those on dialysis. This may mimic rheumatoid arthritis. Typical X-ray appearances reveal calcification at the site of insertion of ligament into bone (Fig. 7.9).

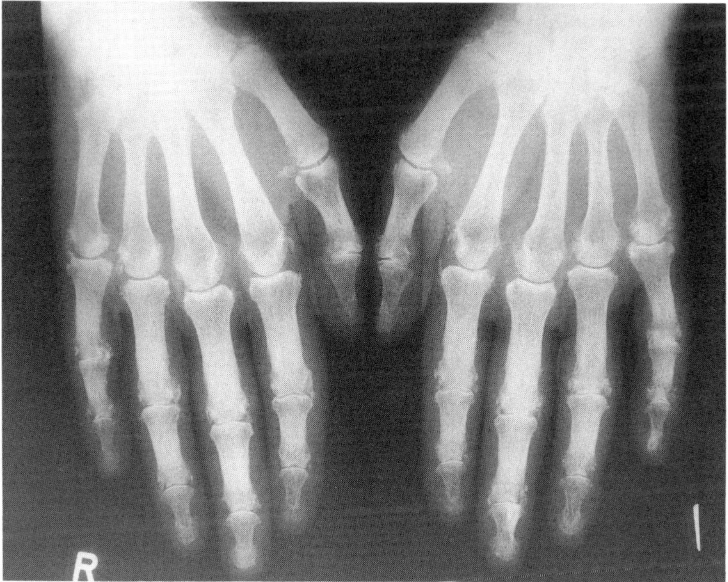

Figure 7.9 X-ray changes in hydroxyapatite disease in a renal dialysis patient.

Calcinosis also occurs as a feature of scleroderma and dermatomyositis (Chapter 6), or as an isolated phenomenon in calcinosis circumscripta.

3.9   Impact of Disease and Prognosis

Acute calcific tendonitis is a distressingly painful condition. Fortunately, it is a self-limited condition.

4   ALKAPTONURIA-OCHRONOSIS

4.1   Definition (Table 7.8)

Alkaptonuria is a chronic degenerative condition of hyaline and fibrocartilage caused by the deposition of homogentisic acid.

4.2   Clinical Features

4.2.1   Early Manifestations

The early phases of crystal deposition are asymptomatic.

4.2.2   Late Manifestations

As the articular cartilage undergoes progressive degeneration in the larger joints, they develop changes identical to those of advanced osteoarthritis (see Chapter 8). In the spine the fibrocartilaginous intervertebral discs gradually disintegrate and literally disappear, leaving a spine that is rigid, deformed (kyphotic), and considerably shorter. Loss of height and flexibility are the most prominent symptoms. Pain is either absent or minimal. Bluegray discoloration (due to deposits of homogentisic acid) of fibrocartilaginous structures, such as the pinnae or the nose, may be visible.

4.3   Confirming the Diagnosis

4.3.1   Early Phase

Confirmation may be possible by observing the black discoloration of the urine on standing. Laboratory confirmation by chromatography is advisable.

Table 7.8   Alkaptonuria-Ochronosis

Homogentisic acid deposition in hyaline and fibrocartilage
Kyphosis
Multiple disc calcifications
Hereditary absence of homogentisic acid oxidase enzyme

4.3.2 Late Phase

The late phase is as for the early phase. Radiographs of the spine reveal a characteristic appearance, namely, multiple disc calcifications with disappearance of the disc spaces throughout the spine, which is pathognomonic (Fig. 7.10).

4.4 Diagnostic Difficulties

The spinal rigidity may be confused with ankylosing spondylitis (Chapter 5). However, the X-ray appearances in the spine are quite distinctive. Furthermore, in alkaptonuria sacroiliitis is absent.

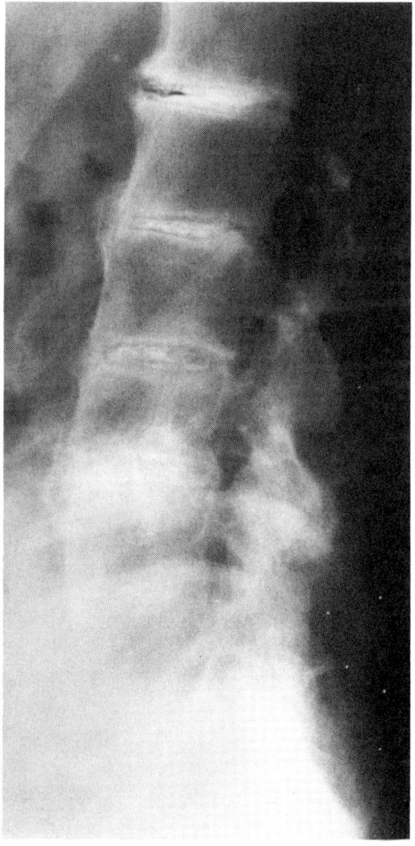

Figure 7.10 Multiple disc calcification is characteristic for ochronosis.

4.5   Epidemiology and Historical Data

Alkaptonuria is a rare hereditary disease. The pattern of inheritance is autosomal recessive. Cases tend to occur in isolated pockets in association with affected families.

4.6   Pathophysiology

The basic defect is an absence of the enzyme homogentisic acid oxidase, which plays a key role in the metabolism of tyrosine, whose metabolism is blocked with the resultant accumulation of homogentisic acid. The black color is caused by its polymerization.

4.7   Management

Only symptomatic treatment is available for this condition. Pain control is by the use of analgesics. Restoration-impaired spinal and joint mobility can be helped and spinal deformities minimized by physiotherapy. Total hip replacement may sometimes be required.

4.8   Impact of Disease and Prognosis

This is a progressively disabling disease as a result of the loss of spinal and peripheral joint mobility.

8

Localized Painful Conditions

1 OSTEOARTHRITIS-OSTEOARTHROSIS

1.1 Definition (Table 8.1)

Osteoarthritis or osteoarthrosis (OA) is a multifactorial, age-dependent, degenerative disease of synovial joints leading to a loss of articular cartilage, refashioning of the articular surfaces. The result is a progressive loss of joint movement, deformity, and impairment of function. OA may be "localized" and affect a single joint or may be "generalized" and attack a large number of joints in sequence or simultaneously. Weight-bearing and non-weight-bearing joints can be involved. OA of the facetal joints of the spine, which is invariably associated with degenerative changes in the intervertebral discs, is termed spondylosis. It will be considered in the section on back pain (see below).

1.1.1 Terminology

There is a worldwide confusion on the terminology for this degenerative joint disease. The term osteoarthritis is mainly used in the English-speaking countries, whereas in the others osteoarthrosis is the term most commonly used. Although in this degenerative disease group there are signs of inflammation at some time of the development of the disease (primary or second-

Table 8.1 Osteoarthritis-Osteoarthrosis

Multifactorial degenerative disease leading to a loss of articular cartilage
Generalized (primary OA) or localized (secondary)
Age-dependent and sometimes unnoted
Pain: intermittent and mechanical
Knee, hip, and spine the most invalidating localizations
Heberden and Bouchard nodes the hallmark of primary generalized OA
Usually a well-nourished middle-aged or elderly person
X-ray typical but not related with complaints
No specific therapy: weight reduction, muscle training, NSAID intermittent, braces,
    joint replacement

arily), clinical features all over are dominantly noninflammatory and this makes the big difference with the other rheumatic diseases that have dominantly inflammatory signs such as rheumatoid arthritis, gout arthritis, etc.

1.2 Main Clinical Features

1.2.1 Early Manifestations

The early years of OA may pass entirely unnoticed by the patient or they may be punctuated by episodes of pain after unaccustomed physical activities. The patient is usually a well-nourished middle-aged or elderly person. As time goes by there is an increasing loss of the range of motion in the affected joint(s). In OA of the hip, for example, the patient finds it difficult to bend down to put on socks or tights, or to climb on to a high step, because of a significant loss of hip flexion. With OA of the knee the complaint may be one of anterior knee pain on climbing or going down stairs. If the hand is involved the pain is in the thumb base (trapeziometacarpal) or in the distal interphalangeal joints of the fingers. Joint pain is a very variable feature and tends to occur after particularly strenuous use. It may be entirely absent until the disease is advanced. Pain and tenderness at the distal interphalangeal joints (DIPs) in females at around the time of the menopause may herald the development of Heberden's nodes—the classic hallmark of primary generalized osteoarthritis (PGOA). Other features include pain in the thumb base (trapeziometacarpal) joint or the first metatarsophalangeal joint of the foot (bunion joint) and involvement of the proximal interphalangeal joints (PIPs), termed "Bouchard nodes" (Fig. 8.1) (Table 8.2).

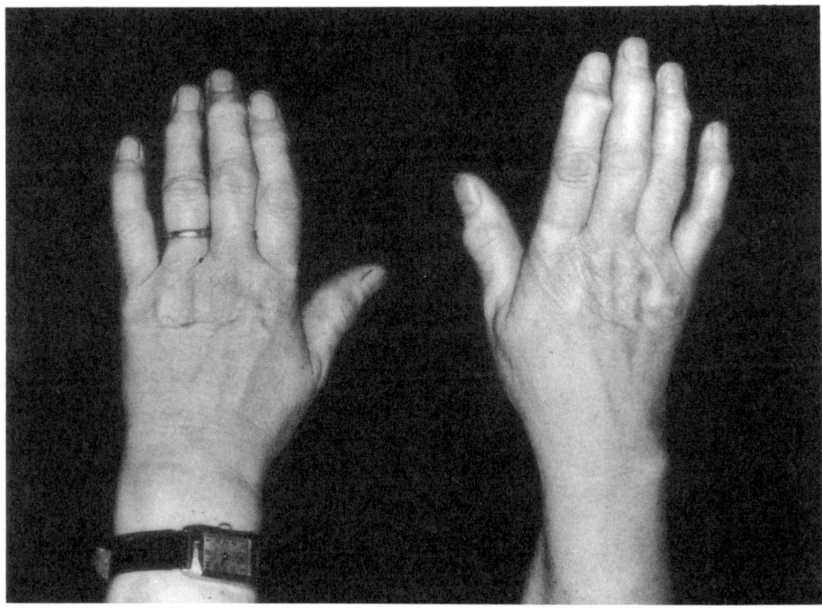

Figure 8.1 Heberden nodes at the distal interphalangeal joints and Bouchard nodes at the proximal interphalangeal joints of the hands.

1.2.2 Late Manifestations

Advanced OA of the hip or knee brings about progressive impairment of walking. Upper limb function may be similarly impaired by OA involvement of the shoulder, elbow, or wrist.

1.3 Confirming the Diagnosis and Investigations

1.3.1 Early Phase

The clinical picture of PGOA is recognized by ascertaining the distribution of joints involved, the typical bone swellings that constitute Heberden and

Table 8.2 Features of Osteoarthritis

Pain on exercise or use
Monoarticular or polyarticular
Bony swelling
Little or no signs of inflammation
Crepitus
Reduction of joint range

Bouchard nodes, and the radiographic appearances, comprising loss of joint space, flattening and sclerosis of the articular surfaces, and marginal projection of new bone (osteophytes) (Fig. 8.2). Laboratory tests for inflammatory joint disease—raised erythrocyte sedimentation rate (ESR)/ C-reacting protein (CRP) tests for rheumatoid factor—are negative.

Magnetic resonance imaging (MRI) can disclose in a noninvasive way

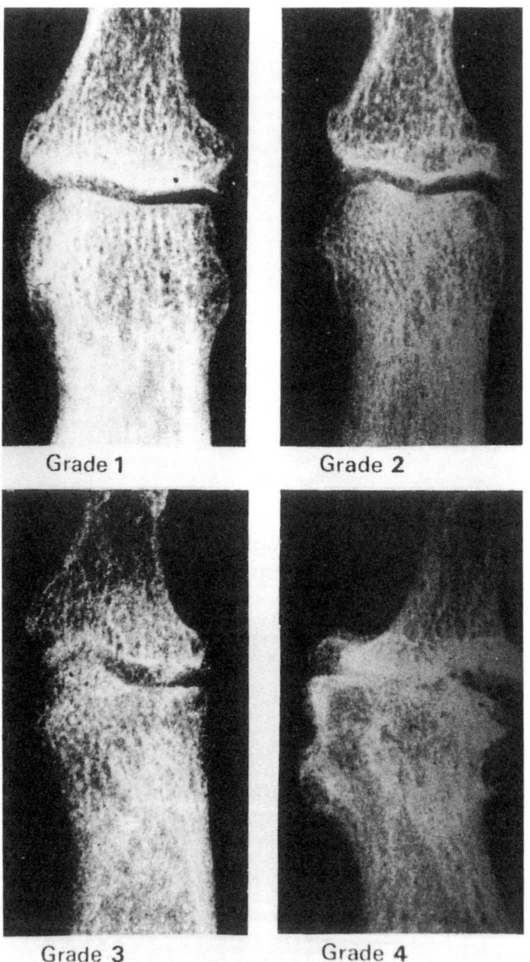

Figure 8.2 Radiographic changes and Kellgren grades in osteoarthritis (DIP joints): asymmetric loss of joint space, flattening and sclerosis of articular surfaces, marginal osteophytes.

menisc tears and therefore can be useful in the early diagnosis of knee derangement before operation is considered.

Arthroscopy Biopsy. An experienced arthroscopist can detect and observe chondromalacia of the patella and exclude menisc and ligament lesions and synovitis. However, this is an invasive procedure that has complications and may provoke reflex algoneurodystrophy. As a preoperative procedure, arthroscopy is indicated in particular when menisc tears are suspected.

Scintigraphy is not useful because it will show hot spots in the region of osteophyte formation. However, it might be useful in the differential diagnosis with osteonecrosis or osteochondritis dissecans in unilateral knee or hip pain (see diagnostic difficulties) (Table 8.3).

1.3.2 Late Phase

The combination of loss of joint range of motion (usually) in the absence of significant inflammation is likely to denote OA. In the knee genu varum deformity or a fixed flexion deformity is commonly seen. In the OA of the hip a painful limp may develop partly due to shortening of the limb, which results from disintegration of the femoral head and neck. Again, the radiographic appearances are highly suggestive and the lab tests negative, so that the diagnosis is seldom in doubt.

1.4 Diagnostic Difficulties

Diagnostic difficulties may arise in distinguishing between OA and inflammatory joint disease such as rheumatoid arthritis. This is most commonly a problem in primary generalized osteoarthritis (PGOA), where the polyarticular pattern may confuse the unwary. In PGOA, however, the wrists are not involved, whereas in rheumatoid arthritis the wrist is involved in most patients. Attention to the points mentioned above should obviate diagnostic

Table 8.3 Investigations in Osteoarthritis

X-ray:
    loss of joint space
    sclerosis of bone
    remodeling of joint surface
    osteophyte formation
Blood tests:
    sedimentation rate normal
    autoantibody tests negative

errors of this nature. Formation of Heberden's nodes may cause confusion with psoriatic arthritis, which also affects the distal interphalangeal joints.

1.4.1 Osteonecrosis-Osteochondritis Dissecans

In mechanical unilateral knee, hip, and other joint pain, osteoarthritis has to be differentiated from osteonecrosis. Osteonecrosis, also called osteochondritis dissecans (knee), occurs at sites where bone vascularization is fragile and easily interrupted, in particular at the head of the femur and humerus and at the medial condyle of the femur.

Osteonecrosis has been described in a variety of clinical settings associated with a disease (Gaucher's disease, SLE, and rheumatoid arthritis), a medication (corticosteroids), a physiologic process (pregnancy), a pathologic process (embolism), or in the absence of any apparent predisposing factor or condition (truly idiopathic). Osteonecrosis occurs in individuals of both sexes and all age groups. It occurs, for the most part, in the epiphysis of long bones such as the femoral and humeral heads, but other bones can also be affected. The femoral head is the most common site of osteonecrosis. It can occur in more than one bone, with the multiple bones affected sequentially or simultaneously. The availability of better imaging techniques, particularly MRI, permits diagnosis of osteonecrosis at a very early stage before radiographic changes occur, and even before scintigraphic signs or clinical manifestations are present (Fig. 8.3).

1.5 Epidemiology and Historical Data

OA is a common disorder in all parts of the world especially affecting those in middle and advancing years. There is a strong hereditary tendency, particularly in respect of PGOA. It is the most highly prevalent of all chronic arthropathies. OA of one joint is seen in Western Europe in about 50% of the population. Paleopathologic studies suggest that OA dates back to prehistory and was present in skeletons of Neanderthal man.

1.6 Pathophysiology

Osteoarthritis results from an imbalance between cartilage synthesis and its degradation. The precise sequence of events is still a mystery, but several studies have shown that changes in the area of cartilage, just below the surface, lead to flaking and "fibrillation" of the surface with clustering of chondrocytes around clefts. Deep clefts then appear that allow digestion of the cartilage by synovial enzymes. The changes in OA cartilage are distinct from senescent changes. Whereas with advancing years the water content of cartilage is reduced, in OA it is increased in the early stage. An abnormal

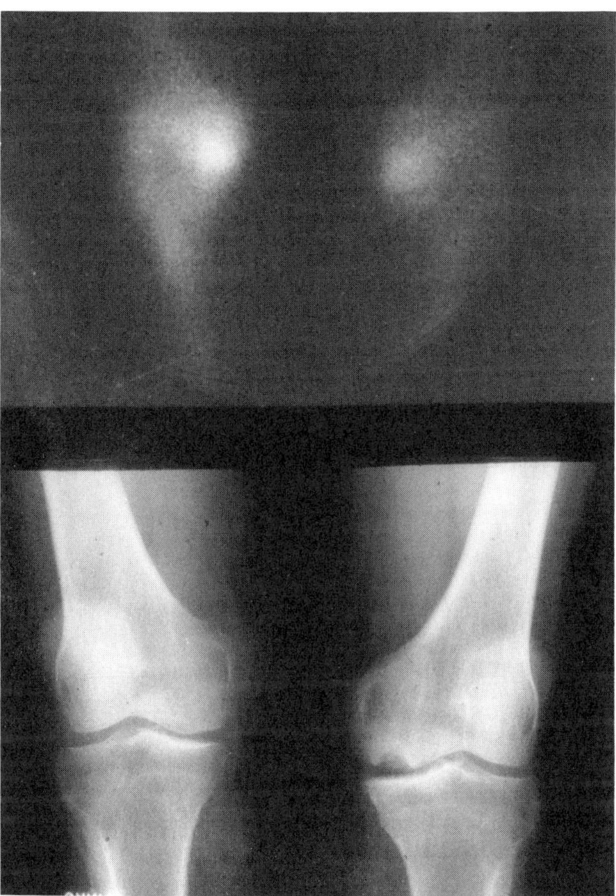

Figure 8.3 XR and scintigraphy of the knees of an 80-year-old woman complaining of pain and hydrops left knee for 1 week. She had a similar episode on the right side 2 years previously. X rays show half-moon spacing image of the medial femoral condyle and no alteration on the left side. Scintigraphy shows increased uptake of the left medial condyle and a residual increased uptake of the right femur. Scintigraphic image of recent osteonecrosis left knee.

hydrostatic pressure because of hyperhydration disrupts the collagen network (Fig. 8.4).

In the chondrocytes, the synthesis of collagen and proteoglycans is increased, as is the degradation. The disease process is aggravated by mechanical stresses and secondary inflammation. Together with cartilage degeneration, changes appear in bone including osteophytosis and eburnation. Osteophytes develop particularly at the margin of joints but may occur in other areas, for example the "peaking" of the tibial spines in OA knees. In the presence of effusion, high intraarticular pressures develop on joint movement, and when the articular surface of the bone is exposed, synovial fluid can penetrate the small crevices to produce subchondral bone cysts (Fig. 8.5).

The etiology of OA is probably multifactorial. Some regard it as a physiologic imbalance between the stress applied to the joint and the ability of the joint-supporting structures (soft tissue, cartilage, and bone) to ab-

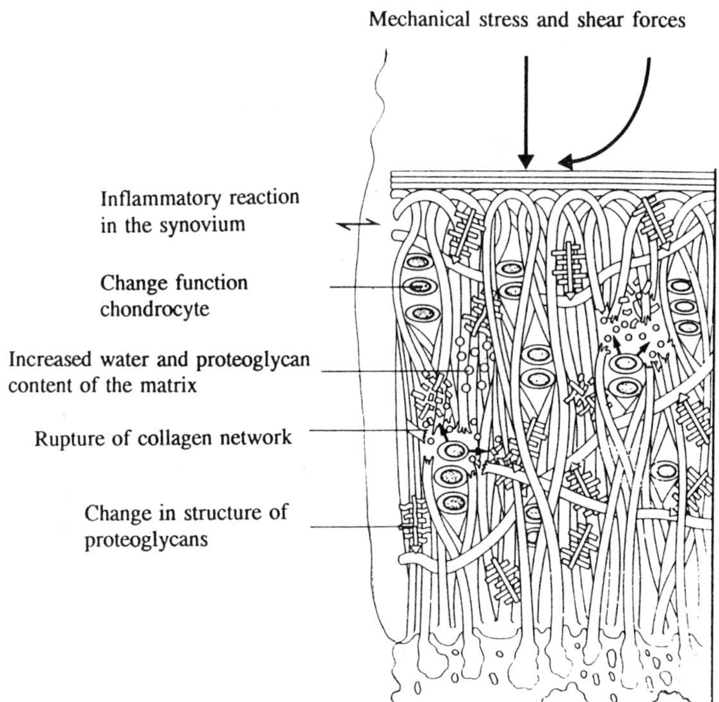

Figure 8.4 Disruption of the collagen network: Biomechanical and biochemical processes in osteoarthritis.

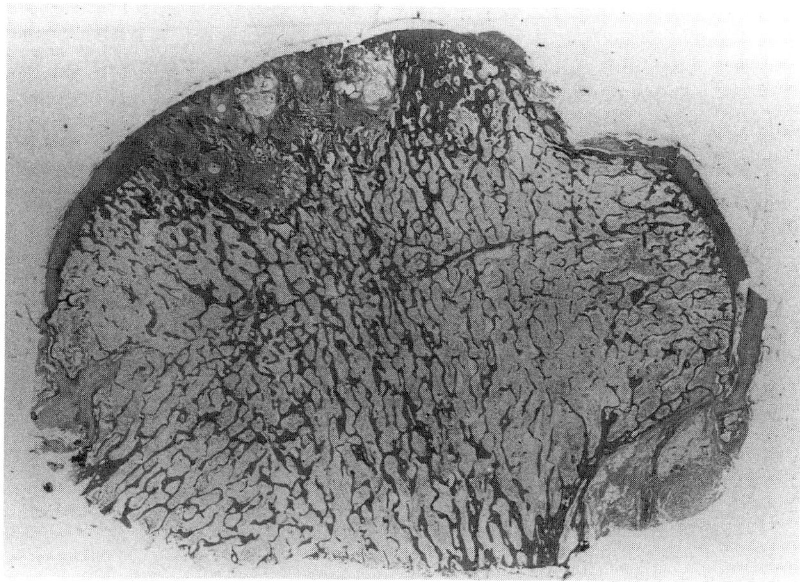

Figure 8.5 Anatomopathologic slide of an osteoarthritic femoral head with eburnation of the cartilage, subchondral cyst, and thickening of the trabeculae.

sorb and dissipate the loading stress. Age, sex, obesity, hormones, and genetic factors may play a precipitating or underlying role. There is no evidence that age per se is the cause of OA. There are biochemical differences between senescent and OA cartilage. Furthermore, not all people have OA and the severity of involvement varies widely in those affected. Multiple joint involvement is more frequent in women than in men. In generalized osteoarthritis with Heberden nodes, the inheritance is thought to be via a single autosomal gene that is dominant in females and recessive in males. Both excessive use and nonuse of joints may predispose to OA. Excessive joint movement cannot be the sole cause because the weight-bearing ankle joint is affected so uncommonly, whereas the non-weight-bearing sternoclavicular joint is frequently diseased. Preservation of the congruity of the articular surface is important, and this is particularly noticeable in the hip joint. When congruity is lost, e.g., in congenital dislocation, dysplasia, Perthes' disease, or fracture of the femur, then OA subsequently develops.

There is a link between obesity and OA in particular of the knee. It has been found that OA is more common in stout than in thin individuals and that an inverse relationship exists between OA and osteoporosis. Obesity per se does not appear to be a significant factor in the etiology or the progression of OA. Maybe hormonal factors in association with obesity play a role. Although many hormones can be shown in vitro to affect the metabolism of chondrocytes, there is at present no evidence that one hormonal factor is involved in the etiology of OA. The intricate interaction between systemic hormones and local growth factors and cytokines is at present under study. OA is seen more often in metabolic disorders as acromegaly, diabetes, alkaptonuria, and Wilson's disease.

Although OA is generally considered to be a primary disease of cartilage with chondrocyte dysfunction and secondary sclerosis, OA could conversely be a primary disorder of bone where a defect in shock absorbing capacity of the subchondral bone resulted in cartilage damage. In favor of the latter hypothesis is the finding that in patients with generalized OA bone mass and bone stiffness are increased.

1.7 Management (Table 8.4)

In early OA the patient should be encouraged to remain as physically active as possible; to reduce weight if obese; to modify lifestyle to avoid or reduce symptom-provoking activities; and to relieve pain by taking analgesics and/ or NSAIDs when necessary. NSAIDs may protect articular cartilage from degradative enzymes. On the other hand, they may inhibit glycosaminoglycan synthesis during repair.

The use of a cervical collar in cases of cervical spine involvement and walking aids, e.g., cane or Zimmer frame, should be encouraged as appropriate in addition to performing regular exercises to strengthen atrophied muscles, to reduce deformities, and to restore movement to affected joints.

In advanced OA, when pain is uncontrollable and/or function is re-

Table 8.4 Management of Osteoarthritis

Early OA:
    Remain physically active
    Reduce weight
    Modify life style
    Reduce symptom provoking activities
    Analgesics and/or NSAIDs when necessary
Advanced OA:
    Use walking aid if appropriate
    Exercise atrophied muscles
    Joint replacement when function is seriously disrupted

duced to the point where the patient's life is seriously disrupted, joint replacement surgery will considerably improve the patient's quality of life.

The so-called chondroprotective drugs as yet have no scientific basis.

1.8 Atypical Forms (Table 8.5)

A number of OA subsets have been described: primary generalized (nodal) osteoarthritis (PGOA); OA with CPPD deposition (an unusually destructive form); endemic OA. Several varieties have been described, such as Kashin–Beck disease in China and Miselini's in Africa. The precise identities of the etiopathogenetic agents are not known.

1.8.1 Diffuse Idiopathic Spine Hyperostosis

Diffuse idiopathic spine hyperostosis (DISH) (Forestier's disease, ankylosing hyperostosis) is a form of spinal disease in which new bone is laid down at the edges of the vertebral bodies, causing them to ankylose, as well as at the large joints. The result is a very rigid spine, but pain is not prominent. It occurs in elderly subjects and is associated with diabetes mellitus and acromegaly (Fig. 8.6).

1.8.2 Neuropathic Arthropathy

Neuropathic arthropathy (Charcot's joints) is an extremely destructive joint disease that occurs when the afferent sensory nerves are destroyed by disease, thereby abolishing pain and its protective function. It is seen in tabes dorsalis, syringomyelia, diabetic neuropathy, and congenital indifference to pain (Fig. 8.7).

1.8.3 Cervical Myelopathy

Occasionally severe cervical osteoarthritis due to excessive osteophytosis may compress, in addition to nerve roots, the myelon, with pain, resulting in electric shocks and loss of power in the upper limbs.

Table 8.5 Atypical Forms of Osteoarthritis

Primary generalized (nodal) osteoarthritis
OA with CPPD deposition
Endemic OA:
    Kashin–Beck disease
    Miselini's disease
Diffuse idiopathic spine hyperostosis (DISH)
Neuropathic arthropathy (Charcot's joint)

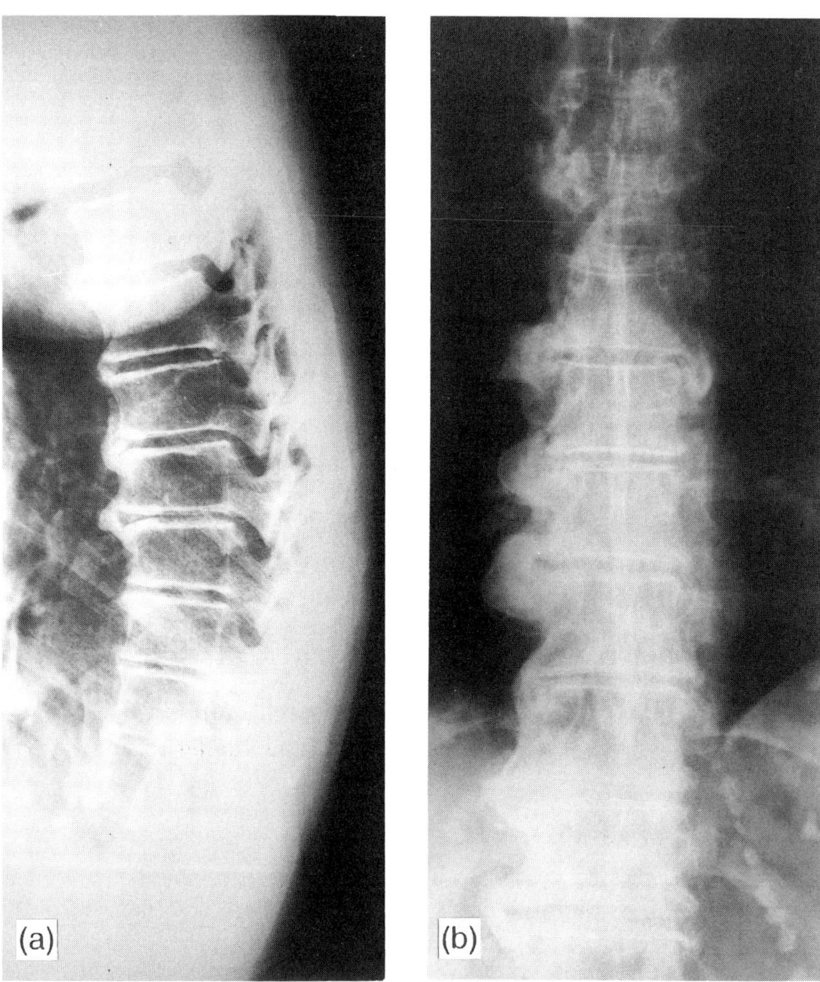

Figure 8.6 X ray showing diffuse idiopathic hyperostosis (DISH).

1.9 Impact of Disease and Prognosis

The high prevalence of OA establishes it as the single most important rheumatic disease in the community, both in terms of human suffering and in terms of economic impact — expressed as working days lost and in costs of health care. The prognosis is by no means universally gloomy. For the vast majority the disease is mild, remains mild, and progression is not inevitable.

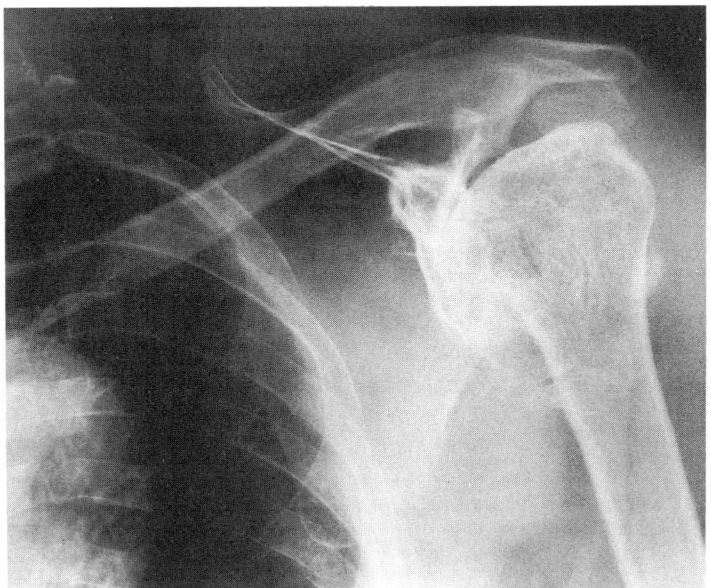

Figure 8.7 Neuropathic joint.

In some cases OA may even regress. However, in many people with OA it will advance inexorably to total joint destruction. Even then, with the development of successful joint replacement surgery, good restoration of function and gainful activity may ensue.

2 SOFT TISSUE (OVERUSE) RHEUMATISM

2.1 Definition (Table 8.6)

Soft tissue lesions comprise a group of localized affections of a traumatic nature, which affect tendons or ligaments, usually (but not exclusively) at their attachment to bone—a zone termed the enthesis. The physical loads borne by these structures are very great and their limits may be exceeded in the course of daily work or leisure activities. The term "overuse" is used to describe such chronic (often repeated) traumatic activities.

The most commonly encountered soft tissue lesions are those occurring

1. in the rotator cuff of the shoulder: supraspinatus tendonitis, bicipital tendonitis, infraspinatus tendonitis, subscapularis tendonitis, adhesive capsulitis ("frozen shoulder").

Table 8.6   Soft Tissue (Overuse) Rheumatism

Group of localized affections of tendons, bursae, or ligaments
Traumatic repetitive nature (overuse)
Shoulder-elbow: most affected
Secondary entrapment of peripheral nerve
Self-limited process
Local therapy (physiotherapy — infiltration) helpful

2. at the common extensor and flexor origins at (respectively) the lateral and medial epicondyles of the humerus: lateral epicondylitis ("tennis elbow"), medial epicondylitis ("golfer's elbow").
3. at the insertion of the plantar fascia to the undersurface of the calcaneum — termed plantar fasciitis.
4. at the sites of bursae, e.g., olecranon bursitis, bursitis trochanterium, or prepatellar and pes anserinus bursitis.
5. at the sites of entrapment of peripheral nerves, e.g., carpal tunnel syndrome (Table 8.7).

Table 8.7   Most Common Soft Tissue Lesions

Shoulder rotator cuff
    Supraspinatus tendonitis
    Bicipital tendonitis
    Infraspinatus tendonitis
    Subscapular tendonitis
    Adhesive capsulitis ("frozen shoulder")
Humerus epicondyles
    Lateral epicondylitis ("tennis elbow")
    Medial epicondylitis ("golfer's elbow")
Heel
    Achilles tendonitis
    Plantar fasciitis
Bursitis
    Olecranon
    Trochanterium
    Prepatella
    Pes anserinus
Entrapment peripheral nerve
    Carpal tunnel
    Tarsal tunnel

Table 8.8 Rotator Cuff of the Shoulder Tendonitis

Tendonitis	Painful arc	Pain on resistance	Tenderness located
Supraspinatus	Abduction	Abduction	Laterally
Bicipital	Flexion	Flexion	Anteriorly
Infraspinatus	Lat. rotation	Lat. rotation	
Subscapularis	Med. rotation	Med. rotation	

2.2 Main Clinical Features

2.2.1 Early Manifestations

The invariable presenting symptom is pain localized to the site of the lesion and occurring specifically when the damaged tendon, ligament, fascia, or capsule is used. In shoulder tendonitis the pain is reproduced during the active movement specific to that muscle/tendon ("painful arc"), and also when the same muscle is tested against resistance (Table 8.8). The range of movement is unimpaired.

Capsulitis is characterized by a concentric loss of passive movement of the shoulder in all directions. The patients experience considerable difficulty in dressing and in lifting objects above eye level.

Epicondylitis causes pain on firm gripping, so that lifting objects becomes increasingly difficult. Elbow joint movements are usually unimpaired. The characteristic findings are as follows (Table 8.9): Olecranon bursitis presents as a painful and tender prominent cystic swelling overlying the tip of the olecranon. Prepatellar bursitis ("housemaid's knee") is similar in appearance but is seen below and in front of the patella. Bursitis of trochanterium of the proximal femur presents with pain at night at the hip when the patient is lying on the affected side. On clinical examination the trochanteric area is painful on palpation and the hip movements are normal.

Carpal tunnel syndrome is an entrapment neuropathy of the median nerve in the carpal tunnel, beneath the flexor retinaculum at the wrist

Table 8.9 Epicondylitis Elbow

Lesion	Pain reproduced by	Tenderness situated
Tennis elbow	Resisted wrist extension	Lateral epicondyle
Golfer's elbow	Resisted wrist flexion	Medial epicondyle

(Fig. 8.8). The symptoms comprise pain, paresthesia, and numbness in the distribution of the median nerve, sometimes only at night. The symptoms may be provocatively reproduced by tapping over the carpal tunnel (Tinel sign) (see Chapter 1, Figure 1.8), by holding the wrist in forced flexion (Phalen sign) (Fig. 8.9), by pressure of examiner's thumb over the carpal tunnel (Table 8.10).

2.2.2 Late Manifestations

As a general rule, the soft tissue lesions referred to above, if left untreated, either resolve spontaneously or pursue a chronic course. In the latter case the severity of the symptoms may increase, but the clinical signs by and large do not change. However, in carpal tunnel syndrome severe and irreparable damage to the median nerve may result. Careful attention should be paid to the neurologic examination to detect median nerve damage (Table 8.11).

2.3 Confirming the Diagnosis—Investigations

Soft tissue lesions can all be made with confidence on clinical grounds and without recourse to investigations. X-ray and sonography of soft tissues might give additional information in complicated cases, cases of tendon rupture, etc. (Fig. 8.10).

However, both in the early and late phases of carpal tunnel, a nerve conduction test is helpful in confirming (or in refuting) the diagnosis and in

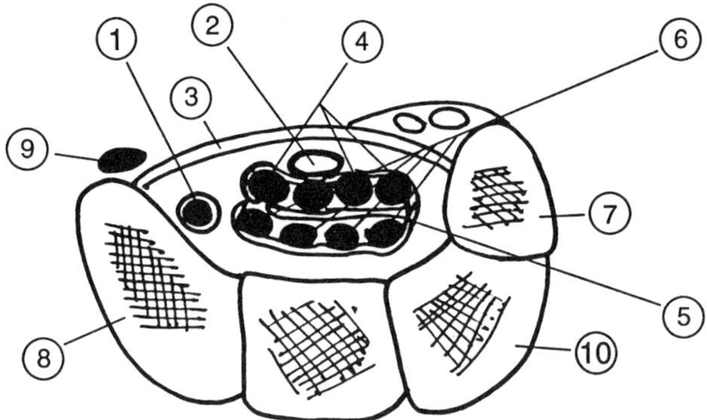

Figure 8.8 Distribution of pain in carpal tunnel syndrome. (1) Flexorpollicis longus tendon; (2) median nerve; (3) superficial flexor tendon; (4) transverse carpal ligament; (5) synovial membrane; (6) deep flexor tendon; (7) triquetrum; (8) scaphoid; (9) flexor carpi radialis tendon; (10) hamatum.

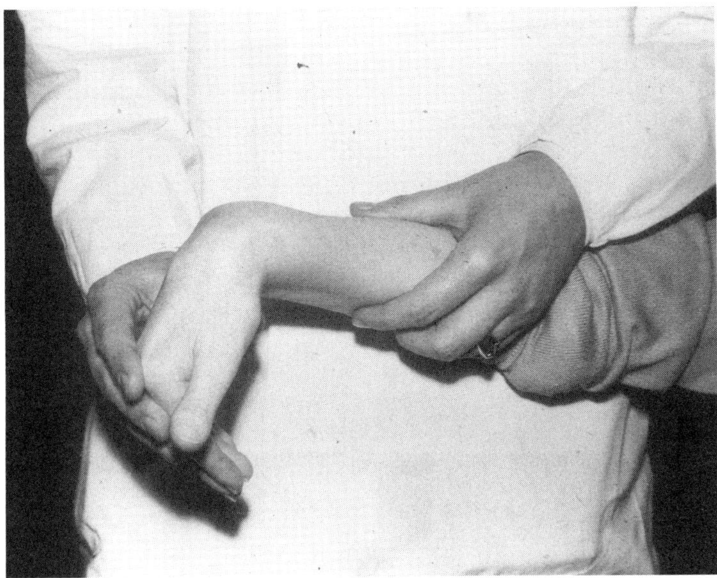

Figure 8.9 Forced flexion wrist: Phalen sign in carpal tunnel syndrome.

Table 8.10 Provocation Test Carpal Tunnel

1. Tapping over the carpal tunnel (Tinel sign)
2. Holding the wrist in forced flexion (Phalen sign)
3. Pressure of examiner's thumb over the carpal tunnel

Table 8.11 Detection Median Nerve Damage in Carpal Tunnel Syndrome

Motor function		
Wasting	Paresis	Sensory loss
Thenar mm	Abd. poll. brev. Opponens poll.	Radial 3½ fingers

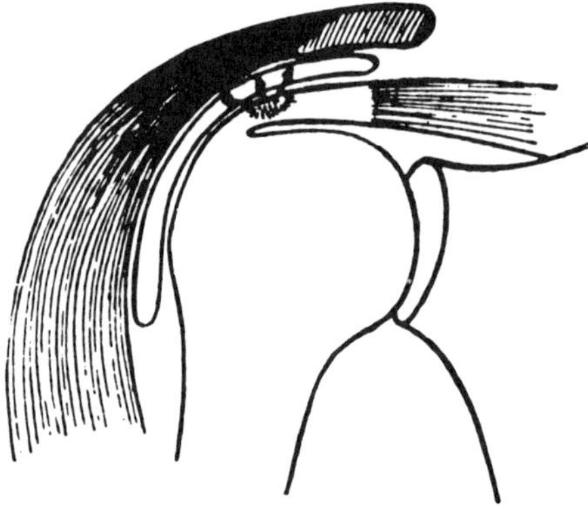

(a)

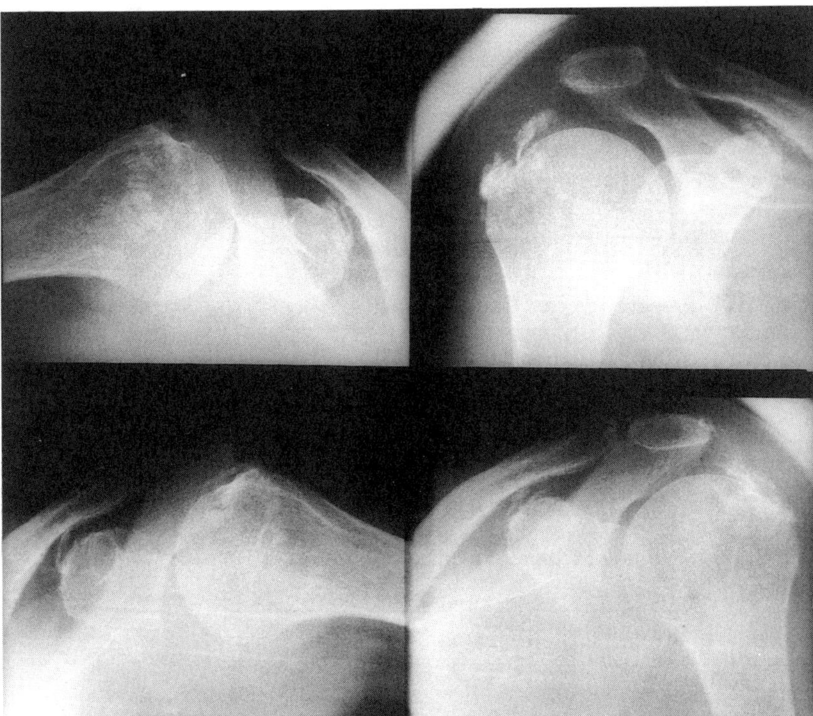

(b)

Figure 8.10 (a) Drawing showing supraspinatus tendonitis. (b) X-ray showing shoulder tendonitis. (c) Sonogram of the shoulder. (d) Sketch identifying the anatomical elements around the shoulder: a, humeral head; b, superaspinatus tendon; c, deltoid muscle; d, subcutaneous fat.

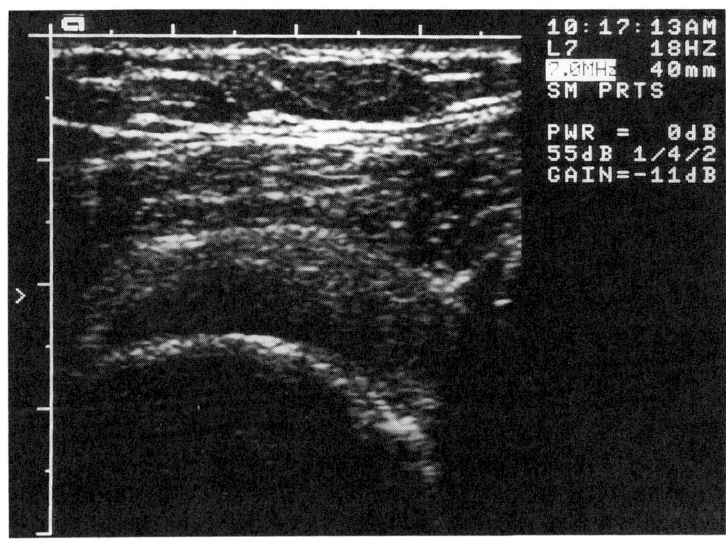

(c)

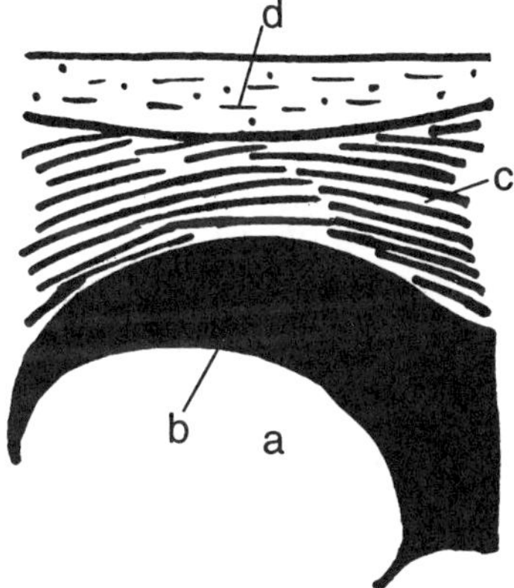

(d)

Figure 8.10   continued.

assessing prognosis, particularly in regard to potential recovery of the median nerve. A negative nerve conduction test does not, however, exclude an intermittent median nerve compression which occurs only at night.

2.4 Diagnostic Difficulties

Diagnostic difficulties are in connection with polymyalgia rheumatica (Chapter 6) and fibromyalgia (Chapter 10), both of which present with pain in soft tissues. However, the conditions considered in this chapter can usually be differentiated by the fact that they are localized lesions, which characteristically occur singly. When they apparently occur at multiple sites, one of the alternative diagnoses should be considered.

There are diagnostic difficulties in relation to carpal tunnel syndrome whereby symptoms and signs may arise from more proximal nerve lesions, e.g., cervical radiculopathy, thoracic outlet syndrome, cervical cord diseases, etc., and thenar wasting may occur in OA of the trapeziometacarpal joint as a result of disuse.

There are diagnostic difficulties in relation to cervical spine osteoarthritis. In cervical spine osteoarthritis movements of the spine are restricted and pain is relieved with a cervical collar.

2.5 Epidemiology and Historical Data

Soft tissue lesions abound in the community as a result of overuse of moving tissues in the course of daily activities. People whose employment involves heavy physical work (laborers, miners, carpenters, etc.) or who indulge in physically demanding leisure activities (jogging, aerobics, etc.) are prone. Those who are inherently hypermobile (Chapter 10) and those who lack training or who are physically unfit are particularly vulnerable.

2.6 Pathophysiology

These lesions are the result of biomechanical failure of load-bearing tissues, which have reached their breaking point. It follows that (in theory, at least) they are entirely preventable with a sensible lifestyle, on the one hand, and by the building up of tolerance with training, on the other hand. Capsulitis may occur as a result of any painful condition affecting the upper limb or shoulder girdle (particularly if as a result the arm is held immobile for any length of time). Thus it occurs after trauma (even if comparatively minor), myocardial infarction, mastectomy, etc. It may complicate a shoulder tendonitis. It is common among diabetics.

2.7 Management

A majority of these lesions will heal spontaneously, provided that the provoking physical insult is removed. Those that do not will require treatment. The most effective measure is the local infiltration of a corticosteroid preparation with or without a local anesthetic (see Chapter 11). Depot preparations can cause subcutaneous tissue atrophy and skin depigmentation. Lack of success is usually due either to incorrect anatomic diagnosis or to inaccurate placement of the injection. Recurrences are not uncommon due to the reimposition of the offending injurious activity. Alternative therapies include physiotherapy (in the form of ultrasound), local NSAID creams, and in (in resistant cases) surgical intervention.

2.8 Atypical Forms

Adhesive capsulitis may be complicated by an algodystrophy. This is a reflex sympathetic neurovascular dystrophy (see Chapter 9). The alternative name is "shoulder–hand syndrome." The hand becomes painful, diffusely tender, swollen, hyperaesthetic, hyperalgesic, and there is a progressive loss of function. Treatment is directed to a restoration of function by means of steroid infiltration of the anterior glen-humeral capsule, coupled with vigorous mobilizing physiotherapy. Stellate ganglion block is also useful in this condition.

2.9 Impact of Disease and Prognosis

Because of their high prevalence, soft tissue lesions cause much pain and economic loss in the community despite their relatively benign nature. These can be aggravated by delays in seeking skilled medical help, incorrect diagnosis, and inappropriate treatment. In a majority of cases a favorable outcome can be anticipated.

3 MECHANICAL BACK PAIN: SPONDYLOSIS

3.1 Definition (Table 8.12)

Mechanical back pain (spondylosis) is defined as mechanical pain felt between the tips of the angles of the scapulae above and the gluteal folds below. It is one of the most frequent symptoms in clinical medicine, which impinges into most areas of clinical practice.

3.2 Main Clinical Features

3.2.1 Early Manifestations

Common Back Pain (Lumbago). The vast majority of back pain episodes are short-lived and result from the injudicious use of the spine in

Table 8.12 Mechanical back pain: Spondylosis

Pain in the back: mechanical type
Common back pain: lumbago
Intervertebral disc prolapse
Facet joint pain
Trophostatic syndrome
Neurogenic claudication — spinal stenosis
Discordance X-ray images and symptoms
Conservative treatment before surgical

---

performing daily tasks such as lifting, bending, standing with a poor posture, or sitting with the back unsupported. Where a particular incident can be identified, the patient will automatically have avoided further strain and will have "rested" his back accordingly (Fig. 8.11).

In more serious injury the patient will be unable to stand and will have taken to his bed. Such pain is usually described as a severe ache and is situated in the midline at the lumbosacral junction, although it may spread to either side. On examination extremes of lumbospinal movement are painful and local midline tenderness is elicited. True reduction in lumbar spinal flexion can be measured by application of the Schober index (see chapter on physical examination). The exact source of such pain may be the muscles, ligaments, facetal joints, or the intervertebral disc.

Acute Intervertebral Disc Prolapse. This is characterized by sudden onset of severe low back pain accompanied by referred pain into the lower limb in the distribution of either the sciatic nerve (sciatica = buttock, posterior thigh, calf, and foot) or the femoral (cruralgia = anterior thigh). The pain may be aggravated by coughing or sneezing ("impulse pain"). In addition, muscle weakness may be present and paraesthesiae felt in the distribution of the relevant nerve root (Table 8.13).

Examination shows painful restriction of flexion and extension of the lumbar spine (lateral flexion remains relatively spared). Test for sciatic ("Lasègue" test) or femoral (femoral nerve stretch test) tension may be positive. Formal neurologic testing will reveal the precise root value of the compressed root. A particularly serious complication is the "cauda equina compression syndrome" in which the roots of the sacral plexus are compressed by the prolapsing disc. It presents with loss of control of the bladder and anal sphincters and impotence, which may become permanent unless the pressure is relieved rapidly.

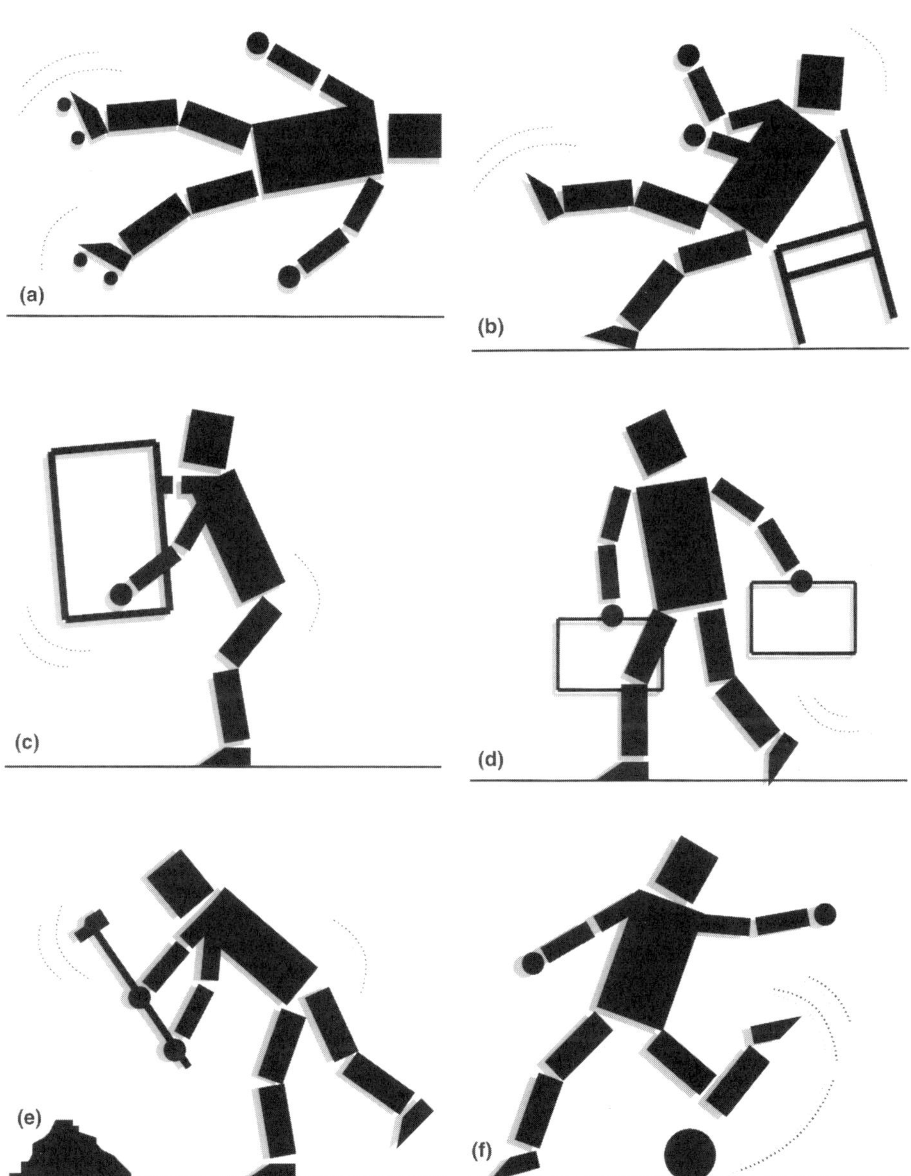

Figure 8.11 Incidents associated with mechanical back pain (a–j) and relief of back pain (k).

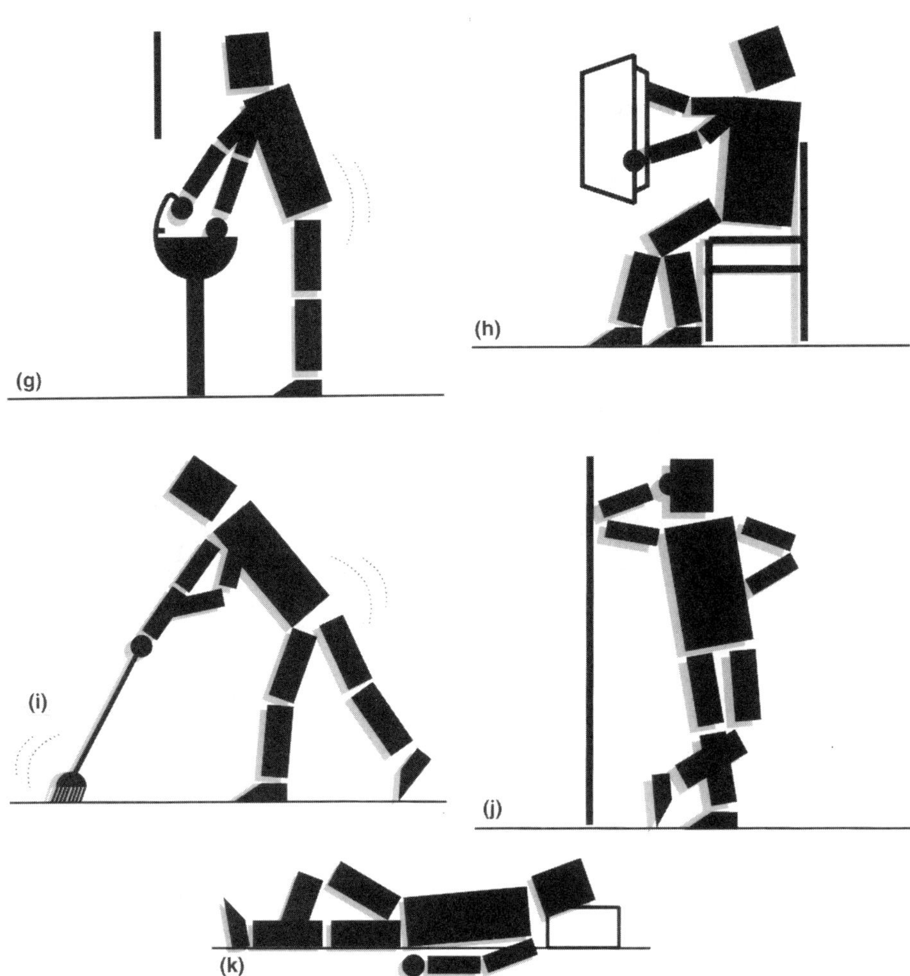

Figure 8.11 Continued.

3.2.2 Pain of Facet Joint Origin

Pain of facet joint origin is also situated in the local site of origin, but it may radiate to the posterior proximal thigh (though never below the knee). It is characteristically worst on extension and is associated with lumbar hyperlordosis, dorsal kyphosis, obesity, poor abdomen muscle strength, and neck pain.

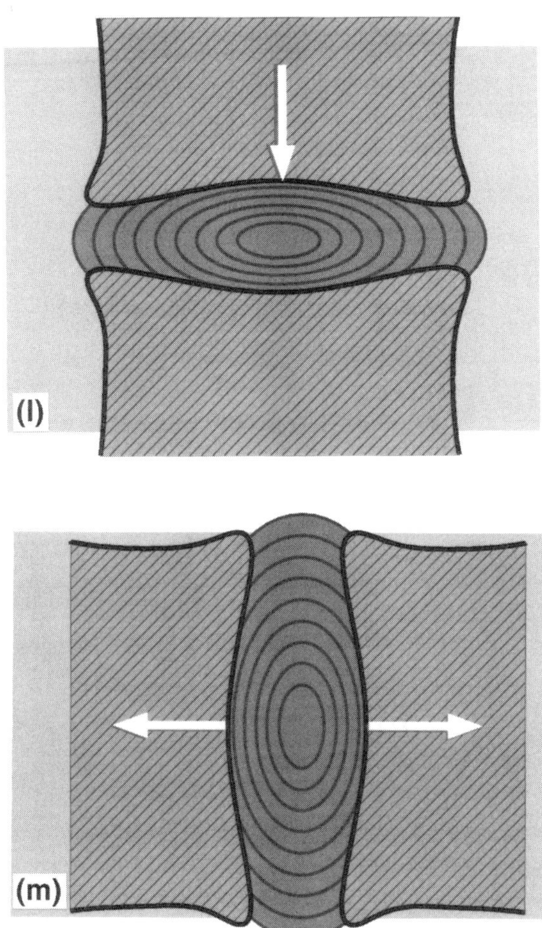

Figure 8.11 Continued.
(l, m) Effect of position, vertical or horizontal, on intervertebral disc.

In middle-aged women and men this frequent syndrome is also called the "trophostatic syndrome" (Fig. 8.12).

3.2.3 Neurogenic Claudication

The syndrome of neurogenic claudication (denoting spinal stenosis) is recognized by the occurrence of pain, paraesthesia, numbness, and/or muscle weakness after walking a certain reproducible distance. The symptoms remit within 5–10 minutes of rest but can recur after walking is resumed.

Table 8.13   Acute Intervertebral Disc Prolapse: Clinical Signs

Root	Motor weakness	Sensory loss	Reflex impaired
L4	Knee extensors Foot invertors	Medial shin	Knee jerk
L5	Foot evertors Ankle extensors Ext. hallucis long.	Lateral calf	–
S1	Ankle/toe flexors	Lateral foot	Ankle jerk
S2–4	Sphincters	Perineum	Gluteal/cremaster

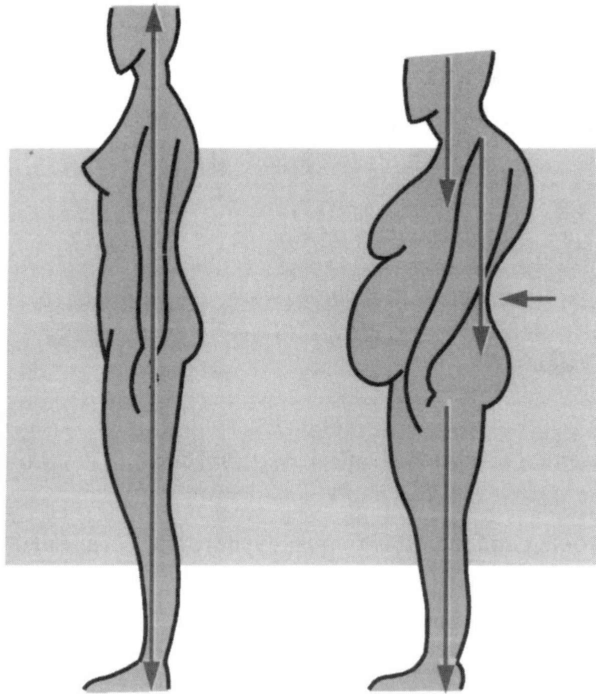

Figure 8.12   Trophostatic syndrome: lumbar hyperlordosis, dorsal hyperkyphosis, cervical hyperlordosis, poor abdomen muscles, obesity.

Table 8.14   Signals of Sinister Spinal Disease

1. Fever or night sweats
2. Weight loss
3. Severe back pain in absence of trauma history
4. Elevated sedimentation rate
5. Abnormal X ray/scintiscan

3.2.4   Late Manifestations

Chronic low back pain poses particular problems, resulting from the interaction of the chronic pain itself, disability, loss of earnings, depression, and the impact of psychosocial problems. In many cases the situation is compounded by outstanding claims for industrial or other compensation, manifesting as illness behavior.

3.3   Confirming the Diagnosis—Investigations

3.3.1   Early Phase

In common back pain the history of the precipitating injury is sufficient to satisfy the diagnosis. Under these circumstances further investigation is not required unless the pain fails to remit within a period of 3 months.

However, if "signals of sinister spinal disease" (Table 8.14) appear at any time or if otherwise unexplained back pain persists for more than 3 months, further investigation is indicated.

A preliminary back pain screen has to be done (Table 8.15). Where disc prolapse is diagnosed on clinical grounds, the back screen is required for the purpose of excluding alternative pathology. Dynamic X rays on lateral bending will disclose in the early stage which disc is involved (Fig. 8.14). Marked radiologic changes can be seen on ordinary X rays in the trophostatic syndrome, antero- and posterolisthesis T_{12}-L_1 region (L_4-L_5), and facet osteophytosis (Fig. 8.13). In the subsequent event of failure of conservative therapy definitive imaging [either by CT (Fig. 8.15) or MRI

Table 8.15   Back Pain Screen

X ray of lumbar spine + pelvis
Full blood count + ESR
Biochemical screen: calcium, phosphate, alkaline phosphatase
Protein electrophoresis, Bence–Jones protein, acid phosphatase, prostatic
  carcinoma antigen

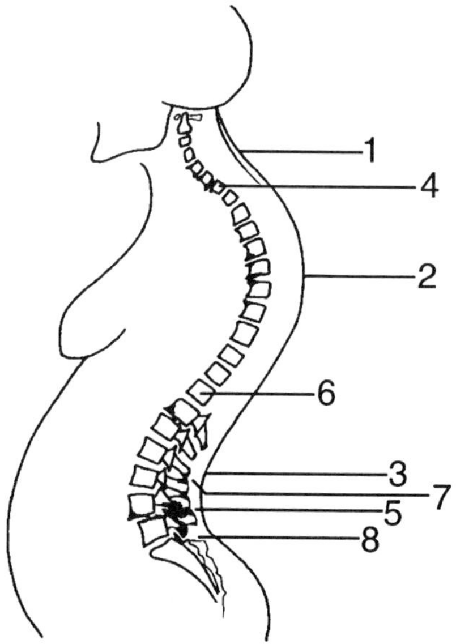

Figure 8.13 X-ray changes in trophostatic syndrome: (1) cervical hyperlordosis; (2) dorsal hyperkyphosis; (3) lumbar hyperlordosis; (4) anterior osteophytosis; (5) anterolisthesis; (6) posterolisthesis L4-L5; (7) kissing spine; (8) spinal stenosis.

(Fig. 8.16)] is indicated as a preliminary to consideration of surgical intervention in order to visualize and localize the lesion.

3.3.2 Late Phase

For reasons stated above, the full evaluation of chronic low back pain patients will include a psychological evaluation in addition to the imaging techniques referred to. Multidisciplinary back pain clinics staffed by specialists in rheumatology, pain control, orthopedics, and psychiatry provide the best environment for the investigation of such patients.

3.4 Diagnostic Difficulties

Overreliance on the X-ray appearance is a common mistake. There is a poor correlation between the occurrence of pain and degenerative changes on X ray. The latter may be asymptomatic, whereas significant disc pathology may be present despite normal X rays. Osteophytes are an X-ray sign of repair and of stability and are not in themselves painful.

Failure to take a comprehensive history may result in an important

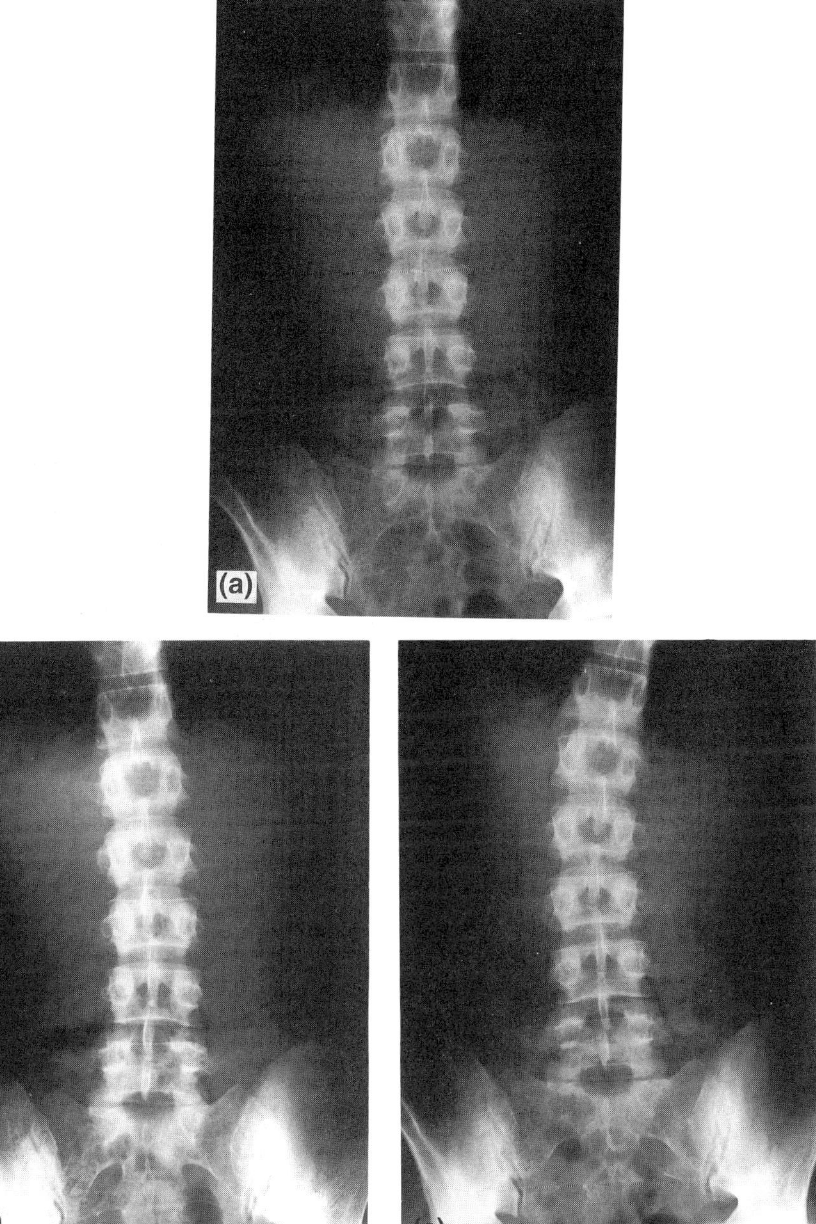

Figure 8.14   Neutral (a) and dynamic lateral bending (b, c) lumbar spine X ray: showing, when compared to the left side bending, a diminished lateroflexion to the right side with paradoxal gaping of the intervertebral disc space L4-L5 at the right side (which should become smaller than the left side in this position) as a sign of blocking caused by a right posterolateral prolapse of the intervertebral disc.

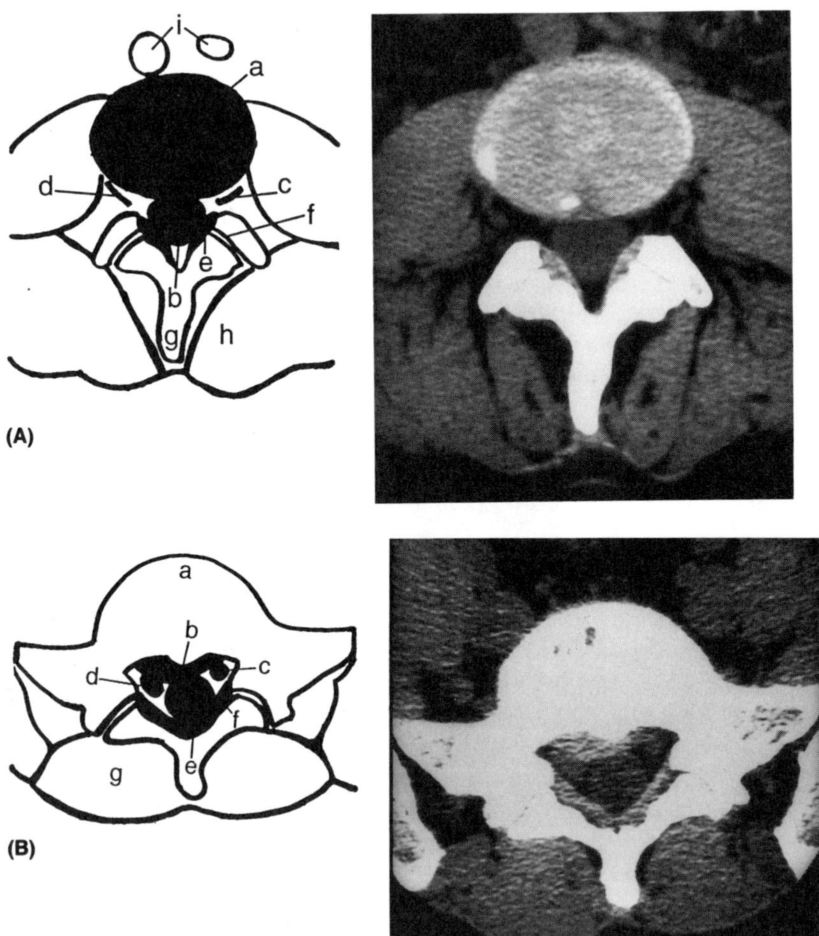

Figure 8.15 (A) Computer tomography (CT) disc bulging—transverse CT slice L3–L4 level showing loss of the normal concave posterior contour of the disc, replaced by the smooth, convex posterior contour of the bulging disc, causing some obliteration of the anterior epidural fat: (a) Intervertebral disc L3-L4; (b) dural sac; (c) left nerve root L3; (d) right nerve root L3; ligamenta flava; (f) apophyseal joint; (g) processus spinosus; (h) paraspinal muscles; (i) abdominal vessels. (B) CT nerve root compression L5–S1—transverse CT slice just below the intervertebral disc level L5–S1, showing the right side paramedical to lateral descending component of a disc hernia causing compression and posterolateral displacement of the S1 nerve root which is slightly thickened, most probably due to edema: (a) corpus vertebrae S1; (b) disc hernia; (c) left nerve root S1; (d) right nerve root S1; (e) dural sac; (f) ligamenta flava; (g) paraspinal muscles.

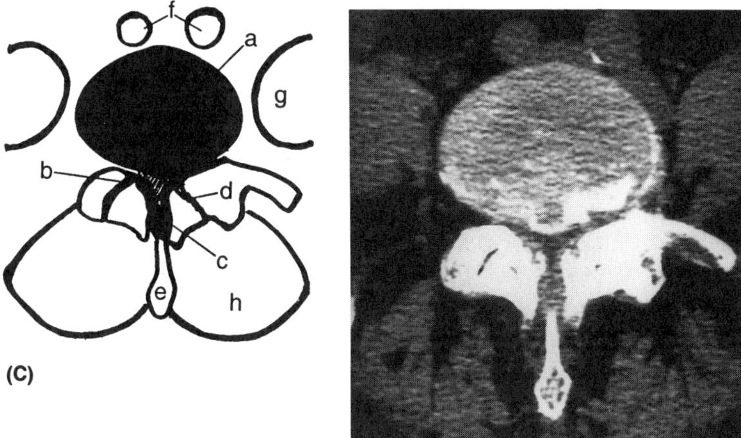

Figure 8.15 Continued
(C) CT spinal stenosis—transverse CT slice at level L4–L5, showing advanced degenerative spinal stenosis with dural sac compression caused by a combination of a bulging calcified disc, hypertrophic osteoarthritis of the facet joints, and thickening and calcification of the ligamenta flava: (a) intervertebral disc L4–L5; (b) compressed dural sac; (c) ligamenta flava; (d) degenerative apophyseal joint; (e) processus spinosus; (f) abdominal vessels; (g) psoas muscle; (h) paraspinal muscles.

diagnosis being overlooked. In particular, pain relief on exercise is suggestive of sacroileitis.

"Inappropriate" signs, such as the increase in pain when the tension in the sciatic nerve is reduced, indicates a tendency to symptom amplification consistent with illness behavior. Measurement of chest expansion may provide a clue to ankylosing spondylitis.

Osteoporosis only gives pain in the presence of a fracture.

3.5 Epidemiology and Historical Data

Back pain is the most frequent musculoskeletal symptom that presents to a general practitioner. It occurs throughout adult life and is particularly highly prevalent among workers doing heavy physical labor, e.g., porters, building laborers. Driving to work, obesity, and smoking are additional risk factors. Judging from artistic representations it was prevalent in ancient times.

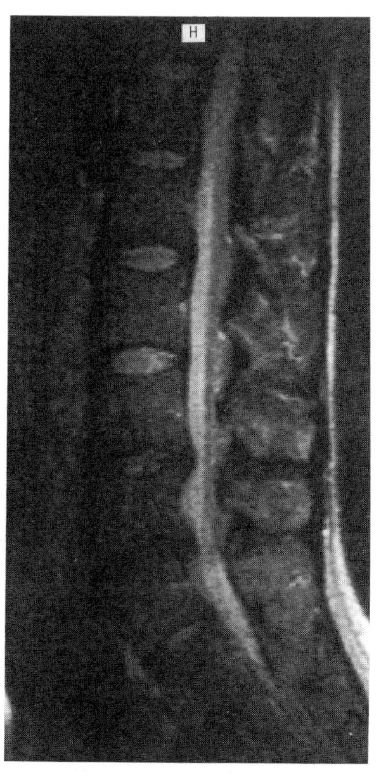

(A)

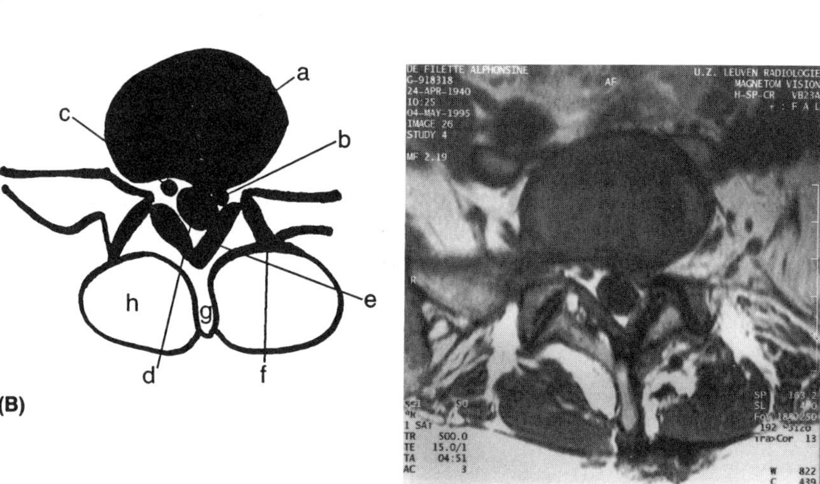

(B)

Figure 8.16 (A) Magnetic resonance image disc bulging: sagittal T2-weighted SE-image of the lumbar spine showing a marked decrease of the normal hyperin-

Table 8.16 Disease Processes Associated with Mechanical Back Pain

Site of origin	Pathologic process	Lesion
Vertebral body	Traumatic fracture	Vertebral collapse
	2rt carcinoma	
	Myeloma	
	Metabolic bone disease	
	Infection	Osteomyelitis/TB
Pars interarticularis	Fracture (if bilateral)	Spondylolysis
		Spondylolisthesis
Intervertebral disc	Degeneration	Prolapse
	Infection	Discitis
Facet joint	Osteoarthritis	Spondylosis
		Spinal stenosis
Sacroiliac joint	Inflammation	
Ligament/muscle injury		Tear

3.6 Pathophysiology

Localized pain can arise from any of the various musculoskeletal structures of the lumbosacral region and as the result of a variety of disease processes (Table 8.16).

3.7 Management

Common back pain is treated in many different ways according to whether the training and beliefs of the practitioner concerned is more toward rest and immobilization in surgical corset or toward mobilization. These days

---

tense disc signal (compared to the other levels) at L3–L4 and L4–L5, typical sight of disc degeneration. At both levels the posterior longitudinal ligament is displaced, with some slight impression on the dural sac, due to disc bulging. (B) Magnetic resonance image root compression — axial T1-weighted SE-image through the intervertebral disc L5–S1, showing the hypointense intervertebral disc with loss of the normal straight posterior contour caused by a left paramedian disc hernia with posterior displacement of the nerve root S1. This root is thickened and has an increased signal intensity as a sign of inflammatory edema: (a) intervertebral disc L5-S1; (b) left nerve root S1; (c) right nerve root S1; (d) dural sac; (e) ligamenta flava; (f) apophyseal joint; (g) processus spinosus; (h) paraspinal muscles.

more and more back pain patients self-refer themselves to physiotherapists, osteopath, and chiropractors, who may adopt manipulative treatment without a clinical examination and appropriate investigations. Fortunately, most such patients recover irrespective of treatment (and in spite of it!). Disc prolapse with nerve root entrapment can be treated by epidural steroid injection or intermittent spinal traction. Failure of conservative treatment is an indication for surgical discectomy.

Spinal stenosis (if epidural steroid injection fails) or cauda equina syndrome require decompressive surgery. Severe spondylolisthesis with instability may require spinal fusion, an operation that is also undertaken for disc prolapse without radiculopathy.

Care of the back is an important area of preventive medicine. Avoidance (or treatment) of obesity will help to minimize hyperlordosis with its attendant facet joint overloading, as will muscle-strengthening exercises directed to the anterior abdominal muscles (Fig. 8.17).

3.8 Impact of Disease and Prognosis

Low back pain is the single most highly prevalent musculoskeletal disorder. The national cost both in terms of loss of productive income and in terms of social benefits and health care cost is enormous. In human terms the cost is incalculable. Nevertheless, 70% of all back pain incidents recover within 1 month and 90% within 3 months. Thus only a small proportion of back pain patients (out of a large total) require specialist care and investigation. A small core will remain permanently disabled despite all efforts.

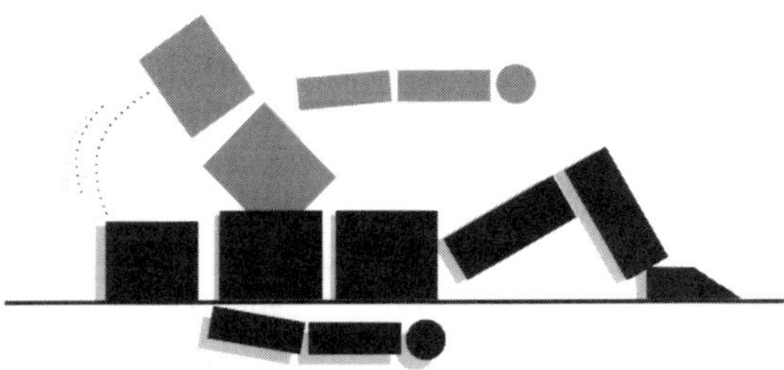

Figure 8.17 Simple exercises for strengthening internal abdominal muscles without straining the lower back. Patients lay down with knees bended (in order to straighten out lumbar lordosis), then bend forward with shoulders lifted and hands touching the knees. Tap the knees 10 times —relax—repeat 10 times, two times a day (morning and evening).

4 HYPERTROPHIC OSTEOARTHROPATHY

4.1 Definition (Table 8.17)

Hypertrophic osteoarthropathy (HOA) or achropachy is a syndrome characterized by excessive proliferation of skin and bones at the distal parts of the extremities. Its most conspicuous clinical feature is a unique bulbous deformity of the tips of the digits, conventionally known as clubbing. In advanced stages, periosteal proliferation of the tubular bones and synovial effusion become evident.

The classification of HOA is outlined in Table 8.18. The degree of association of clubbing with the diverse illnesses varies from it being a constant finding, as in cases with cyanotic heart diseases, to being a rare manifestation, as in patients with cancer of the lung, liver cirrhosis, or Graves disease.

Synonyms for the deformity, besides clubbing, include drumstick, pendulum, and hippocratic fingers. Primary HOA is also known as pachydermoperiostosis.

A patient should be classified as having the primary form of the syndrome only after a careful scrutiny fails to reveal an underlying illness.

The importance of recognizing HOA cannot be overstated. If in a previously healthy individual any of the manifestations of the syndrome becomes evident, a thorough search for an underlying illness should be undertaken. Special attention must be directed to the chest because nowadays the most frequent cause of and "acute" onset of HOA in adults is malignant lung tumors, either primary or metastatic. On the other hand, if a patient previously diagnosed with any of the chronic illnesses outlined in Table 8.18 develops clubbing, this by itself is a bad prognostic sign indicating that the disease has reached an advanced stage.

4.2 Management

Apart from the unsightliness, clubbing is usually asymptomatic and does not require therapy. Patients with painful osteoarthropathy generally respond best to nonsteroidal antiinflammatory drugs. Correction of a heart

Table 8.17 Hypertrophic Osteoarthropathy

Clubbing
Periostitis
Bone pain, extremities
May be association with pulmonary tumor

Table 8.18 Classification of Digital Clubbing and Hypertrophic Osteoarthropathy

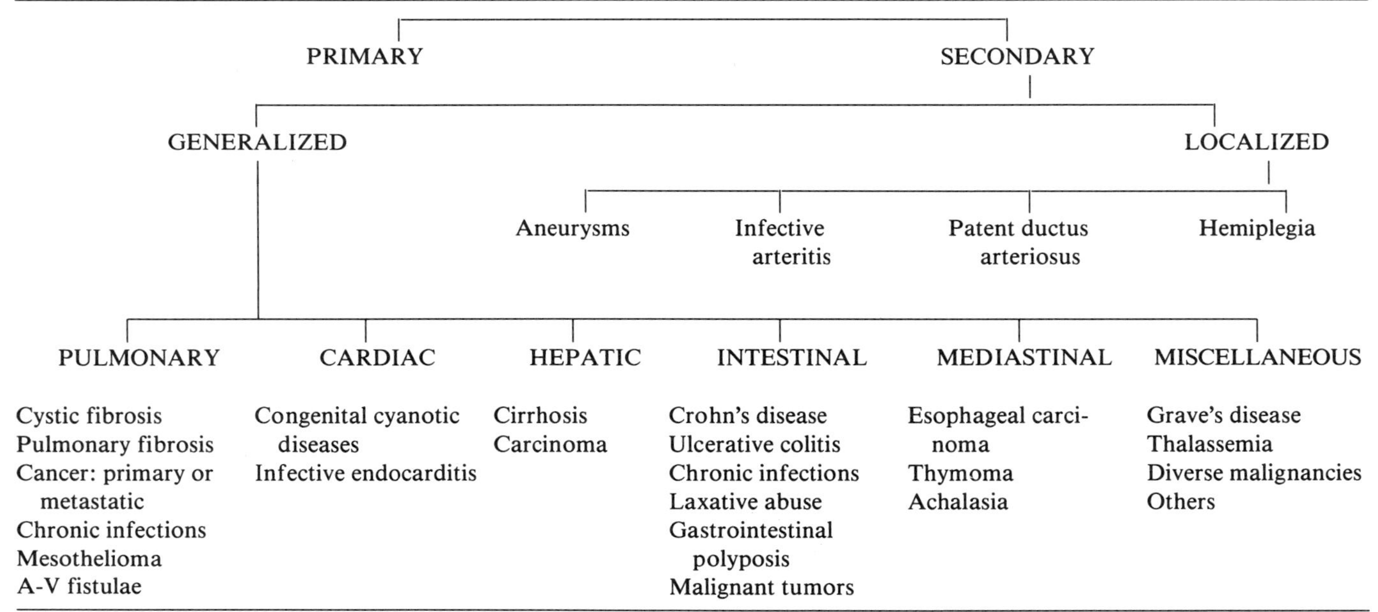

malformation, removal of a lung tumor, and successful treatment of endo-carditis can produce a rapid regression of all symptoms.

5 FIBROMYALGIA

5.1 Definition (Table 8.19)

Fibromyalgia, also known as fibrositis, is characterized by diffuse nonin-flammatory musculoskeletal pain which is quite common, affecting about 3–5% of women in Western Europe and the United States. Fibromyalgia may occur in the absence of any other musculoskeletal condition or may be present with any other musculoskeletal condition. Most patients are women aged 30–60 years.

5.2 Main Clinical Features

The primary clinical feature of fibromyalgia is diffuse musculoskeletal pain. Patients frequently have tender points, the most common of which involve the shoulders, but also seen in the lower back, arms, and legs. Joints may be tender but the tenderness is not limited to joints. A definition proposed by the American College of Rheumatology (ACR) involves at least 11 tender points documented by examination (Fig. 8.18).

A major clinical feature of fibromyalgia involves poor sleep (reported by more than 90% of patients). Most patients report that they do not feel rested upon arising in the morning, and many comment, "I feel like I need a good night's sleep." Patients generally are deconditioned, with little or no regular exercise, and sometimes comment that they have too much pain for regular exercise.

Fibromyalgia is often seen in individuals who report somatization problems (Table 8.20), defined as reporting of symptoms in the absence of structural abnormalities of organs. Thus it is common for patients with fibromyalgia to report a history of conditions such as irritable bowel syn-drome, hyperventilation syndrome, headaches of unknown etiology, and to

Table 8.19 Fibromyalgia

Diffuse musculoskeletal pain
Middle-aged women
Tender points positive
Sleep disturbance
Somatization problems
Management difficult

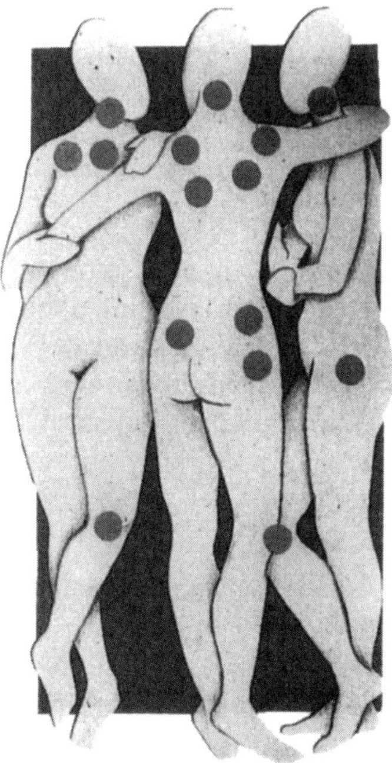

Figure 8.18   Multiple tender points.

have undergone extensive evaluations for potential severe and life-threatening somatic diseases of the cardiovascular, pulmonary, gastrointestinal, and nervous systems, with negative findings. Therefore, patients with fibromyalgia are often among the most difficult to treat because of the severity of their symptoms and the absence of abnormalities on investigation.

Fibromyalgia is also frequently accompanied by severe fatigue and presents similarly to the chronic fatigue syndrome, which is sometimes difficult to distinguish from fibromyalgia. Patients may have substantial

Table 8.20   Fibromyalgia — History

Widespread pain not limited to joints — may be "all over"
Frequent report of other somatization problems: headaches, GI distress, chest pain, dyspnea
Dysfunctional sleep
In some premorbid hyperactivity

anxiety and/or depression, which contribute to fatigue and somatic symptoms.

5.3 Confirming the Diagnosis and Investigations (Table 8.21)

In principle, the diagnosis of fibromyalgia depends on extensive diffuse musculoskeletal pain in the absence of structural disease defined by radiographs or inflammatory disease defined by laboratory tests. Therefore, patients often receive extensive evaluations of radiographic and laboratory studies.

Two important problems are associated with this approach. In the first place, the majority of patients, who are females aged 30–60, will show some abnormalities on radiographs, which typically would involve early osteoarthritis of the cervical spine. Thus, the widespread musculoskeletal pain is interpreted to be secondary to osteoarthritis. Furthermore, serologic tests are positive in 1–5% of normal individuals, most notably the antinuclear antibody (ANA) test, RAF, and the test for Lyme disease (*Borrelia burgdorferi*). These tests therefore are positive in up to 5% of individuals with fibromyalgia. More people who receive a "label" of systemic lupus erythematosus (SLE) or Lyme disease have fibromyalgia than actually have lupus or Lyme. These considerations render it undesirable to base the diagnosis of fibromyalgia strictly on the basis of negative radiographs or laboratory tests.

The second problem with this approach is that there are individuals who have rheumatoid arthritis (RA), SLE, ankylosing spondylitis, or other disease whose primary clinical manifestations may resemble fibromyalgia. This is an important matter because these patients are often approached with the suggestion of more aggressive antiinflammatory therapy, which is not as helpful as measures directed to fibromyalgia.

These considerations would render it desirable to approach a diagnosis of fibromyalgia on the basis of positive findings, i.e., an individual with

Table 8.21 Fibromyalgia — Investigations

Physical Exam:
    Muscle spasm
    Tender points
    No joint swelling or limited motion
Radiographs:
    Osteoarthritis seen, but nonexplanatory, especially cervical spine
Laboratory Tests:
    Generally normal, but 5% may have positive ANA, elevated uric acid

widespread musculoskeletal pain, with a somewhat characteristic history involving poor sleep. Analyses using patient self-report questionnaires indicate that patients with fibromyalgia tend to have high pain scores relative to their difficulty in performing activities of daily living, in contrast to individuals with conditions such as rheumatoid arthritis, whose pain scores and scores for difficulty in activities of daily living are more correlated. This information is not yet used in routine clinical care, but clinicians may suspect fibromyalgia in patients who report unusually significant pain relative to limitations in functional capacity.

5.4 Diagnostic Difficulties

Fibromyalgia is a difficult diagnosis in part because it can mimic any condition associated with widespread pain. Thus, a major possibility that must be considered includes early rheumatoid arthritis. The absence of specific signs of RA can usually be used to exclude this diagnosis.

Osteoarthritis should be noted in the differential diagnosis, but usually it is very easily distinguished from fibromyalgia in that osteoarthritis involves specific joints and is associated with definite radiographic changes. Soft tissue rheumatism, such as tendonitis and bursitis, can be associated with fibromyalgia and confused with fibromyalgia but, in general again, is related to a specific group with anatomic definition on physical examination. The pain associated with neoplasia is often an unarticulated but important concern for patients who require reassurance that widespread pain does not indicate malignant disease.

5.4.1 Stress-Related Conversion

Pain is the most frequent conversion reaction and the location in the musculoskeletal system calls more attention of the public. Conversion is often associated with a stressed personality and theatrical behavior. Conversion reaction is the consequence of psychological stress in relation to setback, conflict, unsatisfactory relationships, or loss of important personality.

5.5 Epidemiology and Historical Data

Fibromyalgia has been recognized for many years as psychogenic rheumatism, or fibrositis, but has not received prominent attention until the last decade. It is not clear as to whether the actual prevalence of disease is increasing or whether it is being recognized more commonly. Fibromyalgia diagnoses may be increasing in part as a result of the modern technologically oriented approach to musculoskeletal symptoms. For example, 20 years ago a patient seen because of shoulder and neck pain might have been reassured that there was no evidence of serious progressive disease, without further tests. However, today this patient will often have several laboratory tests, radiographs, and, in the United States, some type of MRI scan. An evaluation involving considerable cost leaves a patient concerned about serious disease, and it is often difficult to provide reassurance that such serious disease is not present.

Fibromyalgia is one of the most common rheumatic conditions in the population, thought to effect 3–7% of women in studies in the United States and the United Kingdom. Indeed, in the age group under 60, fibromyalgia is probably more common than osteoarthritis, and many patients labeled as having osteoarthritis in the population are individuals who have fibromyalgia. This distinction is not simply of academic interest, as the approach to management of the patient depends on recognizing whether symptoms result from a structural process such as osteoarthritis versus a more functional process such as fibromyalgia.

5.6 Pathophysiology

The pathophysiology of fibromyalgia is very poorly understood and there is at present no organic explanation for fibromyalgia. Many new biochemical or structural lesions have been described in fibromyalgia, but no long-term confirmable lesions have been identified other than repeated documentation of poor sleep. Indeed, the reader (and any person) can mimic the type of problems experienced by patients with fibromyalgia in recognizing the type of musculoskeletal symptomatology found after a poor night's sleep or a need to be awake through the night or a work-related problem or an airplane flight. There is aching of the shoulders and legs, but a physician would not identify the presence of a disease. Most of the patients with fibromyalgia syndrome have a generalized lower pain threshold probably induced by psychogenic mechanisms secondary to surmenage, difficulty in coping with life stress, personality problems such as "pain proneness" and/ or frustrated bodily narcissism, and premorbid hyperactivity (see section on atypical forms).

5.7 Management

The management of fibromyalgia is directed to correcting the poor sleep and deconditioning the patients, which generally are the most powerful measures to improve the symptomatology.

The first principle of management (Table 8.22) is to reassure the patient that the problem of fibromyalgia is quite common and is probably found in at least 1 in 20 (5%) women. The second principle is to reassure the patient that the pain experienced by people with fibromyalgia is quite "real," as pain is not ascertained by any radiograph or laboratory test but

Table 8.22 Fibromyalgia—Treatment

Treatment:
    Frank discussion
    Pain is real
    Exercise program
    Better sleep
Drugs:
    Tricyclic antidepressants
    Nonsteroidal antiinflammatory drugs
    Avoid narcotics

---

rather is experienced by an individual. A third major point to emphasize is that the improvement in fibromyalgia is generally more in the hands of the patient than in the hands of a physician or health professional. That is, if the patient does not follow through on an exercise program, the likelihood of improvement is greatly reduced, and this is obviously in the hands of the patient. A good doctor–patient relationship is essential for successful psychotherapy.

The two major therapeutic goals are to improve sleep and improve physical conditioning through an exercise program, which often results in better sleep. Patients are often resistant to this suggestion, indicating that exercise exacerbates generalized musculoskeletal pain. Reassurance is needed that exercise will not result in any permanent long-term damage or be harmful to the patient. Emphasis must be made that a small amount of physical activity on a regular basis is much more desirable than a large amount of sporadic activity.

The goal of improved sleep is often advanced through use of drugs, primarily tricyclic antidepressant drugs, which may be used in low doses. Indeed, 10-mg preparations of amitriptyline and doxepin were developed initially to treat patients with fibromyalgia. The practice of the doctor is generally to suggest that the patient begin with 10-mg 3 hr before bedtime (not at bedtime because the effect will not begin for a while) and to continue this for a week. If there is no effect, the patient can advance to two pills for another week, and continue to advance until he or she experiences a good night's sleep. At some point, the good night's sleep may be accompanied by a "hangover," with the patient feeling sleepy in the morning, in which case it is necessary to lower the dose. Most patients find a satisfactory level in the range of 20–30 mg/day, 3 hr prior to bedtime.

Nonsteroidal antiinflammatory drugs (NSAIDs) are often valuable as an adjunct to antidepressant drugs in the management of fibromyalgia. However, it should be emphasized that NSAIDs alone are rarely helpful to patients. Indeed, the absence of any response to NSAIDs may be, in fact, a helpful point in establishing a diagnosis of fibromyalgia. In addition, fibromyalgia does not respond to corticosteroids, which should *not* be used in the management of this condition, although a short-term trial over 30 days of prednisone 5 mg is sometimes useful in attempting to differentiate fibromyalgia from early mild inflammatory arthritis.

5.8 Atypical Forms

Fibromyalgia is atypical, but it is seen in males—about 5–10% of patients. Patients may experience limited musculoskeletal pain similar to fibromyalgia not due to structural disease in any part of the body, which may be regarded as atypical fibromyalgia. Some clinicians are beginning to regard many forms of somatization, including chronic fatigue syndrome, irritable bowel syndrome, and floppy mitral valve syndrome, as forms of fibromyalgia, using the term to connote somatization. There are also occasional patients who are quite physically fit but nonetheless suffer from fibromyalgia (but who lead productive lives or have stopped doing so because of fibromyalgia). These patients should be encouraged to ignore their symptoms and maintain their productive lifestyle.

5.8.1 Premorbid Hyperactivity (Bulldozer Syndrome; It-Is-Now-My-Turn Syndrome)

One of the possible mechanisms behind fibromyalgia syndrome in men and women is a premorbid life and workstyle characterized by an excessive hyperactivity. From their youth onward, because of a well-built body and physical fitness, they have been engaged in hard physical labor, sports, free time exercises, and double-day working hours. Around the age of 35–40 they experience a simple musculoskeletal injury as lumbago or tendonitis, at which point they discover that their body is no longer the best, the strongest. This induces a "trauma to their narcissism" and creates a frustrated passivity–activity behavior expressed in a chronic musculoskeletal pain syndrome. Despite an above-average well-built musculoskeletal system, they state: "Before I could do everything and now I can do nothing." Allegorically these syndromes can be called "bulldozer syndrome" and "it-is-now-my-turn syndrome." Bulldozer syndrome is seen more in males, whereas it-is-now-my-turn syndrome is seen more in females. In the latter syndrome the premorbid hyperactivity was most manifest in the household activities (first up—last in bed), in the care for everyone in the neighborhood including grandparents, and a high level of engagement in all parish or local social and cultural work. When an underlying psychogenic mechanism can be disclosed, the therapy will be easier and the patient can better understand the syndrome.

5.9   Impact of the Disease and Prognosis

The impact of fibromyalgia on society is substantial and greatly underrecognized. Many individuals suffer the symptomatology of fibromyalgia briefly and generally transiently without long-term consequences. However, many individuals under the age of 60 are receiving disability pensions, including quite a few under 50, who have no physical basis for incapacity to work. Indeed, not working rarely improves symptoms and may exacerbate them on the basis of lost self-esteem. The problem of disability in fibromyalgia is quite costly to individuals and the society at large.

Overall, results in management of fibromyalgia are comparable to those in management of other rheumatic diseases. About one third of patients appear to improve, about one third stay the same, and one third do poorly. It is important to recognize that patients with fibromyalgia often consult many different physicians prior to diagnosis and after diagnosis, although with insight and sympathy many patients may be managed effectively. Early recognition and diagnosis of fibromyalgia together with a good management may reduce considerably medical costs and invalidity.

9

Bone Diseases

1 OSTEOPOROSIS

1.1 Definition (Table 9.1)

Osteoporosis is an age-dependent bone disease characterized by a decreased bone mass and increased susceptibility for fractures with minimal trauma. Osteoporosis without fractures is commonly distinguished from osteoporosis with fracture by the term *osteopenia*, whereas the term *osteoporosis* is reserved for those who have a fragility fracture. In this way, the relation between osteopenia and osteoporosis is comparable with the relation between hypertension and cerebrovascular accident. An additional important aspect of the definition of osteoporosis is that the decrease in bone mass is not associated with a change in bone composition, i.e., the ratio of mineral to matrix. In this way, osteoporosis can be distinguished from osteomalacia, which is characterized by an inadequate mineralization of the bone matrix due to an alteration of the vitamin D metabolism (Fig. 9.1).

1.2 Main Clinical Features

1.2.1 Early Manifestations

Osteopenia, or the gradual loss of bone over decades until the bone becomes so weak that it cannot sustain minimal trauma, is a silent process. Therefore osteoporosis is often called the silent thief or the silent epidemic.

Table 9.1   Osteoporosis

Age-dependent disease characterized by fragility fractures (wrist, spine, proximal femur).
Frequent in postmenopausal women and elderly men.
Osteoporosis can be secondary to immobilization and corticosteroid treatment and sex hormone deficiency.
Low bone mass (osteopenia) predisposes to osteoporosis.
No characteristic biochemical abnormalities in urine and serum.
Patients at risk can be identified by bone densitometry.
Preventive and curative therapy are possible but diverse.
Calcium at bedtime and good vitamin D status are a preventive and first therapeutic measure.

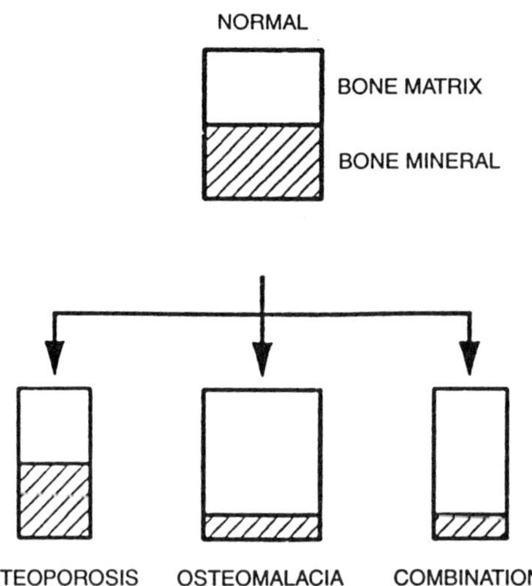

Figure 9.1   Schematic illustration of the difference between osteomalacia and osteoporosis. In osteoporosis the ratio of organic bone matrix to bone mineral is normal, whereas in osteomalacia the amount of bone mineral is decreased due to a deficit in the mineralization of bone matrix. The two disorders may coexist particularly in the elderly.

The first symptom of osteoporosis is an acute episode of pain in the spinal column, either at the midthoracic or at the thoracolumbar region, experienced during an activity of daily living such as standing up, bending, or lifting. The pain is sudden and may irradiate girdle-like to the front of the chest or to the loin. The patient can usually indicate the level where the pain started. The mobility of the spine is much reduced in particular when turning in bed. The pain increases when sitting or standing and is relieved on lying down. Coughing, sneezing, or pressing can induce an exacerbation of the pain. Paravertebral muscle spasms are often visible and palpable. Pain on tapping the spine is limited to the affected region. Some subjects with wedging of the midthoracic vertebrae experience few symptoms, except for discomfort along the ribs, loss in height, and mild thoracic kyphosis. Spinal cord compression is extremely rare in osteoporotic deformation of the spine. The clinical picture of a peripheral fracture (Colles fracture at the forearm or proximal femur fracture) is quite evident (Fig. 9.2).

A fracture of the distal parts of the radius occurring during a fall on the outstretched wrist shows a typical bayonet-like deformity. This fracture can be the first sign of an underlying osteopenia.

A fracture of the proximal femur at the femoral neck or at the trochanteric area is usually very evident. The affected leg is shortened and externally rotated. The patient, often a frail elderly person, is lying on the floor after a trivial slip and is unable to move his or her leg because of pain.

Femoral neck (intracapsular) fractures of the femur occur most com-

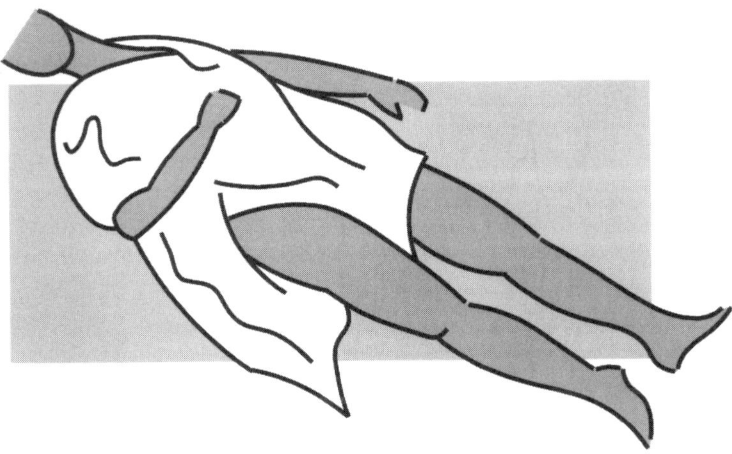

Figure 9.2 Clinical pictures of fragility fractures at the proximal femur. Note typical external rotation and shortening right leg.

monly between the ages of 65 and 75, whereas the incidence of intertrochanteric fractures peaks nearly 10 years later between the ages of 75 and 85.

1.2.2 Late Manifestations

With time, multiple vertebral fractures can occur. The body height will become reduced, thoracic kyphosis will become more prominent, whereas the lumbar lordosis becomes less. A discrepancy between body height and arm span length is now evident. Each vertebral collapse can reduce height by 2–4 cm. A marked thoracic kyphosis in osteoporosis is called "dowager's hump."

The change in stature leads to a reduced abdominal space with abdominal protrusion; the ribs may reach to the pelvic rim. In this stage, the patient may experience difficulty in breathing and eating. The cosmetic effect of the statural changes often causes psychological problems (Fig. 9.3).

In between the episodes of vertebral collapse, the patient is pain-free. The change in stature, however, can be associated with permanent vague back pain complaints. Before fracture, the osteoporotic patient has no pain. Back pain and bone pain without fracture should not be diagnosed as osteoporosis. Other diseases have to be looked for. In postmenopausal women, back pain is most often due to degenerative back lesions associated with hyperlordosis and osteoarthritis of the facet joints in the lumbar re-

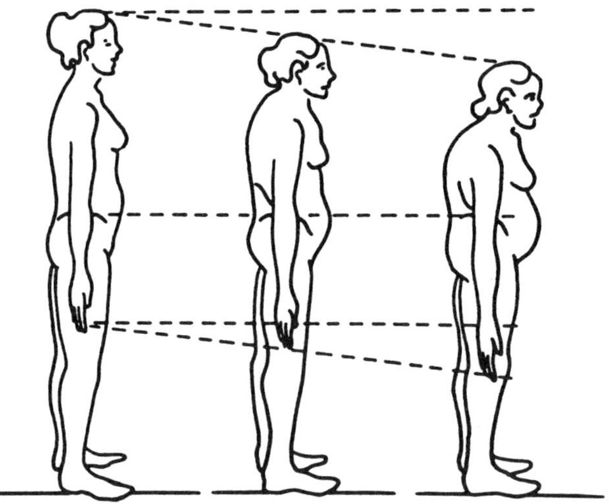

Figure 9.3   Stature changes in osteoporosis.

gion. However, other possible diagnoses should not be overlooked, e.g., bone metastasis and multiple myeloma.

1.3 Confirming the Diagnosis—Investigations

1.3.1 Early Phase

Imaging. The diagnosis of a fragility fracture, such as vertebral collapse, Colles fracture, or fracture of the proximal femur, has to be objectified by an X ray of the appropriate region in several directions. As a rule, this does not create any problem because of the typical X-ray picture. Figure 9.4 shows the typical fracture outlines for the forearm, spine, and hip.

Bone scintigraphy will give high-uptake pictures at the fracture sites (vertebrae, ribs, and pelvis). This investigation can be useful for the differential diagnosis with other diseases affecting the skeleton, e.g., bone metastasis and osteomalacia.

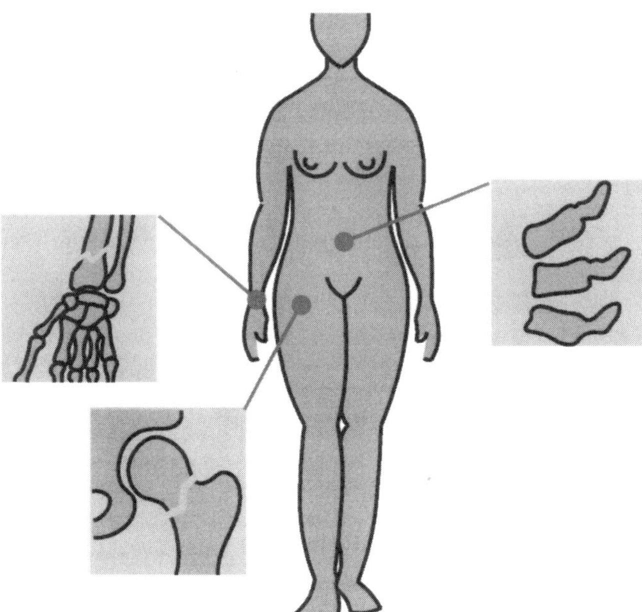

Figure 9.4 The most common types of osteoporotic fractures are those of the wrist, the spine, and the hip, but osteoporotic women fracture any bone more easily than healthy women.

Biochemistry. There are no characteristic or pathognomonic biochemical tests for osteoporosis in contrast with other metabolic bone diseases such as osteomalacia, hyperparathyroidism, and Paget's disease. After a recent fracture, serum alkaline phosphatase activity can be temporarily increased. The use of biochemical tests such as serum calcium, phosphorus, alkaline phosphatase, parathyroid hormone, and vitamin D levels only makes sense in connection with the exclusion of other diseases. Often a fasting 2-hr morning urine calcium/creatinine ratio, hydroxyproline/creatinine ratio, or D-pyridinolinium/creatinine ratio is requested in osteoporosis cases in order to determine if the patient at the time of diagnosis is at a high- or low-turnover bone status.

The fasting morning urine is collected after a voiding of the bladder in the morning. The patient should be fasting and not have had calcium the night before. The Ca/Cr ratio > 0.15 is an indication of calcium loss during the night and of high turnover. A 24-hr calcium excretion is a measure of calcium absorption, normally > 100 mg/24 hr. Excretion of > 250 mg/24 hr is indicative of hypercalciuria. A 24-hr hydroxyproline excretion, and even better the collagen crosslink pyridinolinium, is a measure of bone resorption. Hydroxyproline excretion is normally < 50 mg/24 hr if the diet is not rich in gelatin, fish, or ice cream.

Osteocalcin is a protein that is specific for the osteoblast. It is a better measure of bone formation than alkaline phosphatase activity, although the latter, in the absence of liver disturbances, is also reliable. Increased levels of osteocalcin and alkaline phosphatase activity are seen in high-bone-turnover states.

These calcium metabolism parameters can be of help for therapeutic decision making. Table 9.2 summarizes the usefulness of the calcium metabolism parameters.

1.3.2 Late Phase
Primary and Secondary Osteoporosis. When an osteoporotic fracture is diagnosed clinically and by X ray, then one has to determine if the fracture is the consequence of primary or secondary osteoporosis. In order to do this correctly, a complete medical history, clinical examination, and extra blood and urine tests have to be done. Table 9.3 summarizes the main causes of secondary osteoporosis.

When secondary osteoporosis is excluded, then one can be sure about the diagnosis of primary osteoporosis. In the diagnostic group "primary osteoporosis," two types can be distinguished (Table 9.4): postmenopausal osteoporosis, with mainly trabecular bone loss and its associated fractures at the forearm and the spine; and senile osteoporosis, with trabecular as well as cortical bone loss leading to hip fracture.

Table 9.2 Calcium Metabolism Parameters in Metabolic Bone Diseases

	Osteoporosis	Osteomalacia	Hyperpara-thyroidism	Renal bone dystrophy	Multiple myeloma
Serum Ca	Normal	↓	↑	↓-Normal	Normal — sometimes ↑
Serum P	Normal	↓	↓	↑	Normal — sometimes ↑
BUN	Normal	Normal	Normal	↑	Normal — sometimes ↑
A1-P	Normal	↑	↑-Normal	↑-Normal	Normal — sometimes ↑
M Protein	(−)	(−)	(−)	(−)	(+)
PTH	Normal ↑ ↓	Slightly ↑	↑	↑	Normal
1,25(OH)$_2$D$_3$	↓-Normal	↓	↑	↓	Normal

BUN, blood ureum; A1-P, alkaline phosphatase; M protein, monoclonal protein (electrophoresis); PTH, parathyroid hormone.

Table 9.3 Causes of Secondary Osteoporosis

Endocrine diseases
    Hypogammagonadism
    Cushing's syndrome
    Hyperthyroidism
    Hyperparathyroidism
Gastrointestinal diseases
    Gastrectomy
    Malnutrition
    Anorexia nervosa
Bone marrow diseases
    Multiple myeloma
    Bone metastasis
Connective tissue diseases
    Osteogenesis imperfecta
Others
    Immobilization
    Alcohol abusus
    Chronic heparin treatment

Table 9.4 Types of Primary Osteoporosis

Factor	Postmenopausal	Senile
Age	51–70	>70
Ratio women/men	6 : 1	2 : 1
Type of bone loss	Mostly trabecular	Trabecular and cortical
Fracture places	Vertebrae, distal radius	Vertebrae, hips
Causes	Menopause	Aging

Noninvasive Methods to Measure Bone Mass and Bone Density (Fig. 9.5).

X-ray. Simple X-ray of the spine is not useful to estimate the amount of bone and bone density. Osteopenia cannot be precisely diagnosed on plain X-ray films because of many artifacts. Of bone loss, 20–30% has to have occurred before it can be detected in this way.

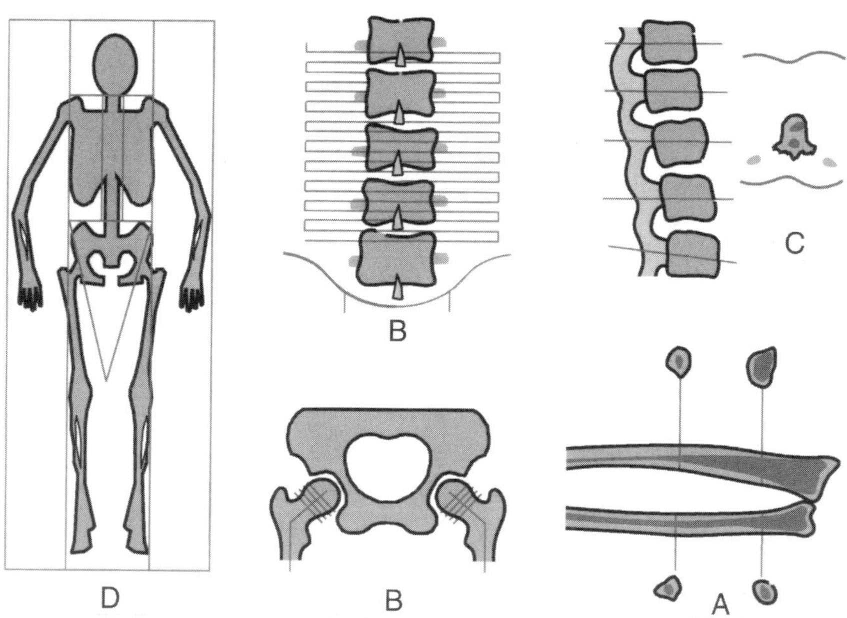

Figure 9.5 Noninvasive methods to measure bone density: (A) single- and (B) dual-energy absorptiometry (DXA), (C) quantitative computed tomography (QCT), (D) total body DXA densitometry.

When a fracture occurs, the diagnosis of osteoporosis can be made with routine radiographic evaluation of the skeleton without resorting to sophisticated new methods.

Radiologic vertebral osteoporosis index. The vertebral collapses are graded according to a radiologic vertebral index. This index grades the morphologic changes from thoracic IV to lumbar V (Fig. 9.6).

Radiogrammetry. Measurement of cortical thickness on X rays of the hand can, in experienced hands, be a good measure for cortical bone mass.

Quantitative computed tomography can be used for evaluation of pure trabecular bone density of the spine and of the distal radius, but this measurement has to be done in specialized centers by experienced personnel.

Photon absorptiometry. Bone densitometry can now be done with specialized equipment, using single- or dual-energy photon absorptiometry at the forearm, at the spine, at the proximal femur, or on the total skeleton. These measurements are simple, precise, and accurate. They give information on bone capital at the cortical and trabecular sites. They are particularly useful for screening purposes in order to detect patients at risk for osteoporosis and thus those

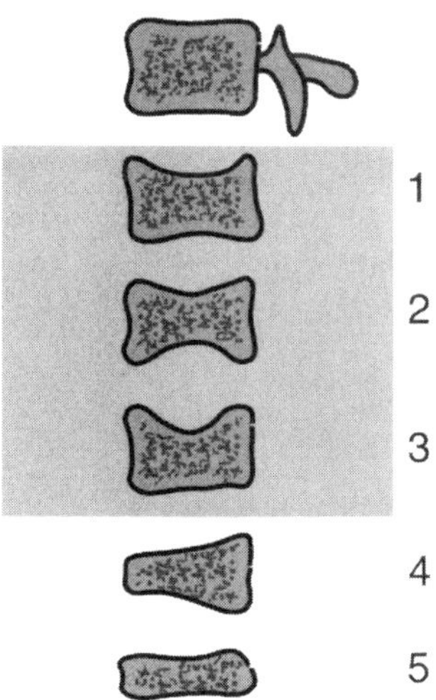

Figure 9.6 Radiographic vertebral osteoporosis index. (1) Monoconcave vertebra. (2) Biconcave vertebra. (3) Fracture of one vertebral plate. (4) Fracture of two vertebral plates or wedge compression. (5) Full compression. The minimum score is 0 and the maximum score 70.

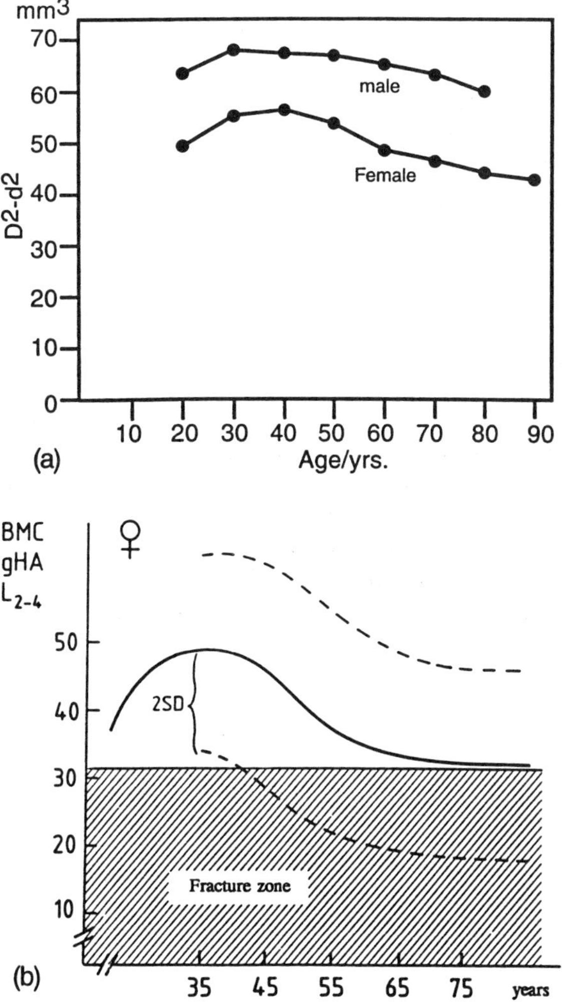

Figure 9.7 (a–c)   Bone density changes over life span in men and women.

with osteopenia. The measurement can be used for follow-up but only after a 2- or 3-year interval because the measurement error has the same magnitude as the yearly loss of bone.

Figure 9.7a shows the typical profile of bone mass changes over the life span in men and women. Women have less bone than men; they lose

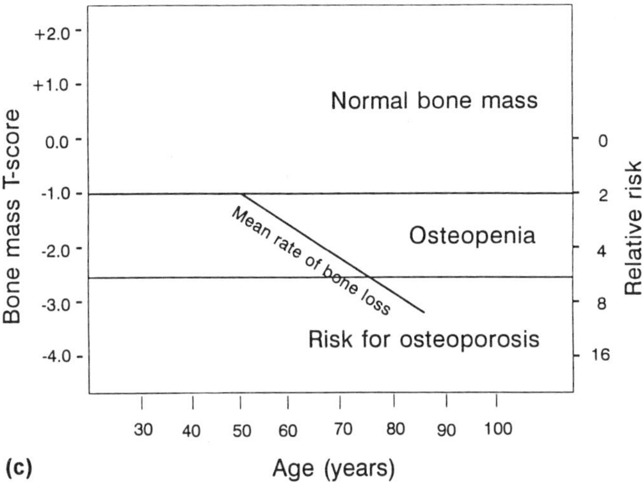

Figure 9.7 Continued

bone more rapidly with aging, in particular just after the menopause. For each sex–age group there is a considerable variability in bone densities (±30%), so some have ±30% more or less bone than the others for the same age and sex.

Most patients with osteoporotic fracture have a bone value below 2.5 standard deviations of peak bone mass (T score). Therefore this limit is called the fracture threshold and indicates the zone where the risk of fracture increases considerably (Fig. 9.7b). The lower the value, the greater the risk for fracture. Because bone loss can be prevented (see below), it is important to detect in time, before loss has occurred, those who are at risk. A risk score for osteoporosis is not a diagnosis for symptomatic osteoporosis but it serves as a sound clinical guideline for decision making, to consider serious preventive measures, to inhibit bone loss or improve bone density.

Invasive Method to Measure Bone: Biopsy. At present, bone biopsy for the diagnosis or differential diagnosis of osteoporosis is not often practiced. The above described methods and biochemical tests are in most of the cases of bone failure sufficient to confirm the diagnosis. In unusual cases, bone biopsy can give more information on bone turnover, or can help to exclude osteomalacia.

1.4 Diagnostic Difficulties

1.4.1 Osteomalacia
Definition (Table 9.5).
Osteomalacia (rickets) is a curable bone disease characterized by weak bone due to inadequate mineralization of bone matrix because of a disturbance in the vitamin D metabolism, caused by deficiency (lack of sunshine, diet), malabsorption, or liver or kidney disease.
Clinical Manifestations.
EARLY STAGE. Osteomalacia can have as presenting symptoms bone fracture, bone pain, and muscle weakness. The symptoms are not acute and become worse gradually. The muscle weakness may lead to a waddling gait (duck's gait).
LATE STAGE. Weight bearing produces a bowing deformity of the long bones. Prominences of the costochondral junction, the so-called rachitic rosary, can also be seen in particular in children.
Confirming the Diagnosis — Investigations.
EARLY STAGE. The calcium biochemical tests are manifestly altered with low serum calcium and phosphorus, high alkaline phosphatase, low urinary calcium excretion, low 25–vitamin D levels, and, in particular, high parathyroid hormone levels in the serum.
LATE STAGE. The late stage is characterized by the same biochemical parameters as in the early stage but more marked X-ray changes. Osteomalacia has a typical X-ray picture in its late stage with enlargement of the metaphyses in children, and pseudofracture, Milkman–Looser lines at the pelvis, hip, and ribs seen on X ray and bone scintigraphy in adults (Fig. 9.8).
Differential Diagnosis
PAGET'S DISEASE. The bowing of the bones, particularly the femur and tibia, may be confused with osteomalacia. In Paget's disease, however, bowing is asymmetric and biochemical parameters show no deficiency of calcium metabolism, except for a high alkaline phosphatase.

Table 9.5 Osteomalacia

Rickets
Weakness
Stress fractures
Mineralization defect
Vitamin D deficiency
Curable
Subclinical form in the elderly

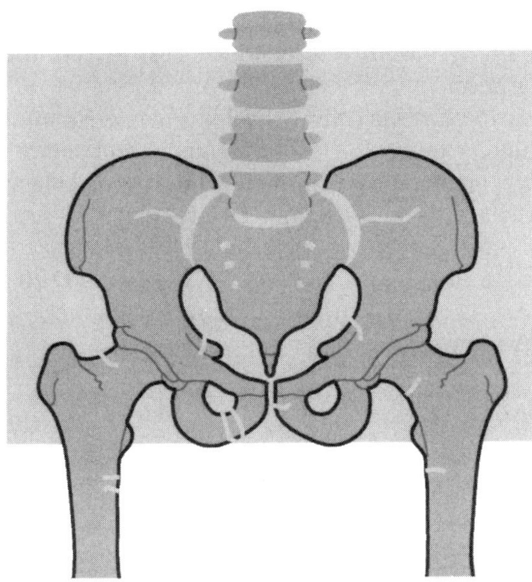

Figure 9.8 X-ray features of osteomalacia: Milkman–Looser lines.

STRESS FRACTURE. Stress fractures, or fatigue fractures, resemble fractures seen in osteomalacia. They occur most often at the metatarsal bones after prolonged unusual physical exercise. No abnormalities in bone parameters will be found.

Epidemiology and Historical Data. Osteomalacia was a very frequent disease in the 19th century in industrialized urban Europe, particularly in children. Adult osteomalacia was endemic in India, in China in 1900, and in Europe in the Second World War.

Even in modern times osteomalacia is frequently seen in Asian populations, particularly when they come to live in northwestern Europe where sunshine is less abundant. In the present economic climate of western Europe, nutritional osteomalacia and rickets are very rare. Sporadic osteomalacia is mostly due to gastrointestinal diseases with malabsorption of vitamin D. The main cause is glutenenteropathy and, more rarely, gastrectomy. In the latter, osteomalacia often occurs 10 years postgastrectomy, more frequently in women (0.4%) than in men (0.1%).

Pathophysiology. Vitamin D deficiency through lack of adequate sunlight, lack of dietary vitamin D in fish oil and milk products, malabsorption of vitamin D, poor hydroxylation in the liver and/or kidney of vitamin D results in osteomalacia or rickets. Rickets is a disorder of mineralization of the bone matrix or osteoid. Because of hypocalcemia and hypophosphatemia, secondary hyperparathyroidism results which also affects the bones by increasing bone resorption.

Management. The basic mechanism behind the deficiency of vitamin D has to be treated. In addition, vitamin D (1500–3000 units) replacement daily should be given orally or parenterally when there is no liver or kidney disease. In those with liver disease (lack 25-vitamin D) or kidney disease, or resistant to vitamin D, the most active form of $1,25(OH)_2$ (0.15–0.5 μg/day)(calcitriol) should be given. In case of liver disease, 25-OH vitamin D 20–30 μg/day should be given. A brusque rise in serum phosphate within 2–3 weeks will be observed and muscle weakness will disappear soon.

Atypical Forms. Phosphate diabetes or hypophosphatemic vitamin D–resistant rickets-osteomalacia is seen in a number of hereditary syndromes: Fanconi's syndrome, renal tubular acidosis, and in association with mesenchymal tumors. These cases need for their management large amounts of phosphate salts and supraphysiologic doses of 1,25-vitamin D. In tumor-associated cases the tumor has to be removed.

Impact of the Disease and Prognosis. The prognosis is excellent in most cases when vitamin D deficiency is corrected in time. The addition of vitamin D to the nutrition of children has almost eradicated rachitis in the countries where this is the rule. Systematic addition of vitamin D and calcium in the nutrition of the very elderly may result in a considerable reduction of femoral neck fracture cases.

1.4.2 Bone Metastasis

The first symptom of cancer and metastatic spread from cancer can be a fracture of, for example, the hip or vertebral collapse. Breast, kidney, thyroid, and prostate cancer in particular are known to reveal themselves sometimes by bone metastasis. Careful clinical examination should be done. Scintigraphy can be helpful to detect symptomless invasion of other parts of the skeleton (Fig. 9.9).

1.4.3 Multiple Myeloma

Kahler's disease (multiple myeloma) can have as the first presenting symptom demineralization of the skeleton locally, e.g., in the pelvis, or generalized with vertebral collapse. This diagnosis should be thought of if the patient has, in addition to fracture, a high erythrocyte sedimentation rate (ESR) or a changed electrophoretic protein pattern with a monoclonal peak (Fig. 9.10). In rare cases of myeloma light chains are produced that are quickly filtrated in the kidney and the ESR in these cases is normal as is the electrophoretic protein pattern. Bone marrow examination, however, will confirm the diagnosis. Typical X-ray lesions are shown in Fig. 9.11.

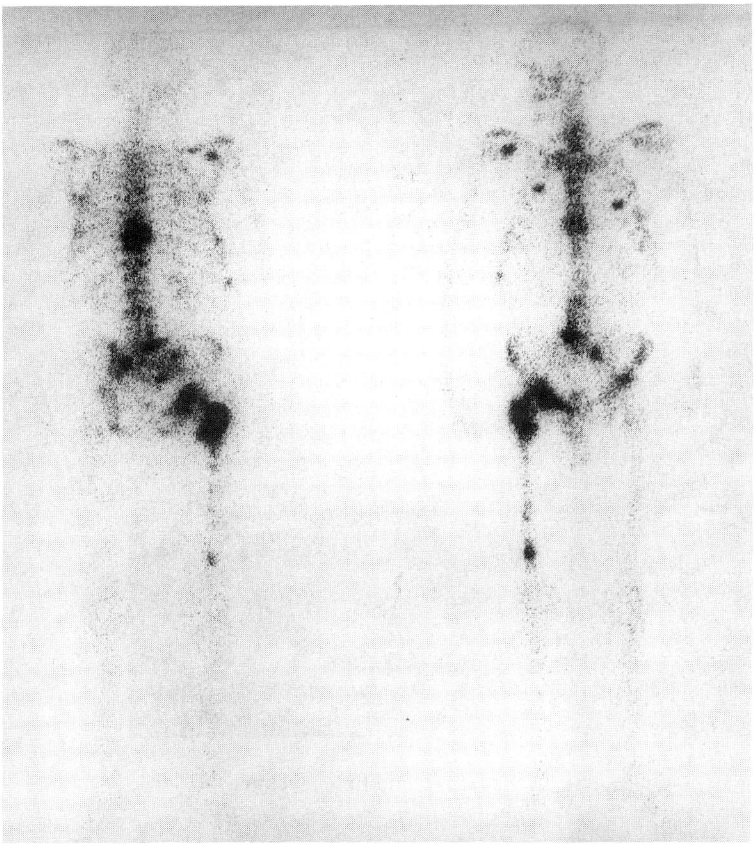

Figure 9.9   Bone scintigraphy and bone metastasis.

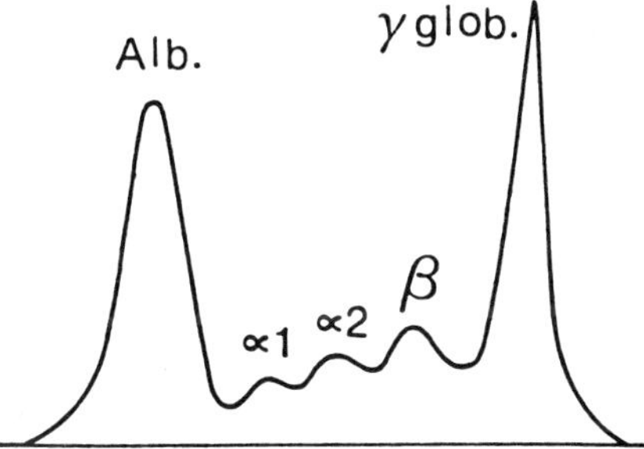

Figure 9.10   Typical protein electrophoresis in a case with multiple myeloma.

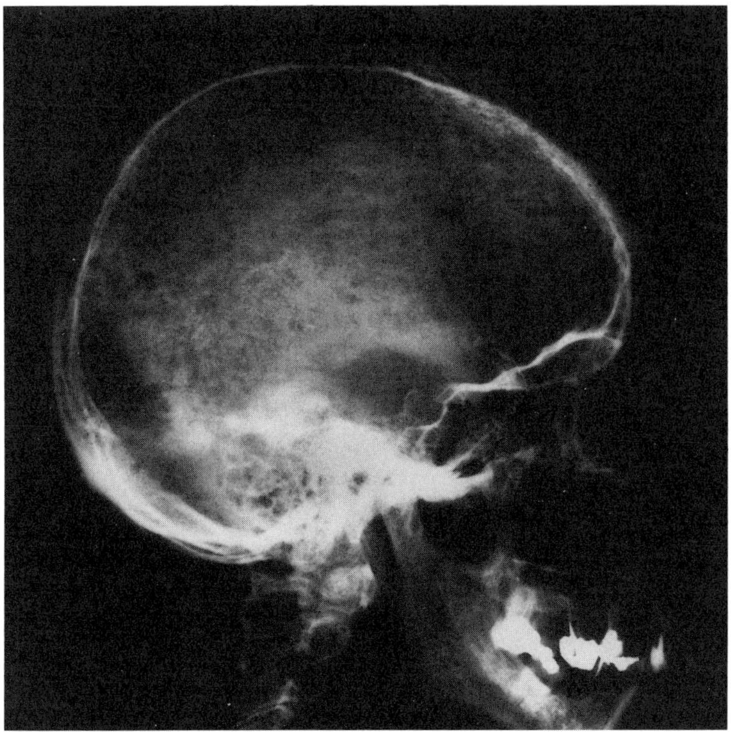

Figure 9.11   X-ray changes at the skull in multiple myeloma.

1.4.4   Hyperthyroidism and Hyperparathyroidism

Hyperthyroidism and hyperparathyroidism are two metabolic bone diseases that have a profound effect on bone, in particular in the elderly, and may disclose themselves by bone failure as the main symptom. The diagnosis is in general easily excluded by biochemical tests: hypercalcemia or direct hormonal estimation in the serum.

1.4.5   Degenerative Kyphosis: Osteoarthritis, Scoliosis, Scheuer–Manns Disease

THORACIC OSTEOARTHRITIS.   Kyphosis of the thoracic spine with wedging and reduction in body height also occurs in patients suffering from osteoarthritis of the spine. The typical osteophytes and disc narrowing visible on lateral X ray of the spine makes the differential diagnosis easy (Fig. 9.12).

Structural scoliosis is accompanied by asymmetric development of

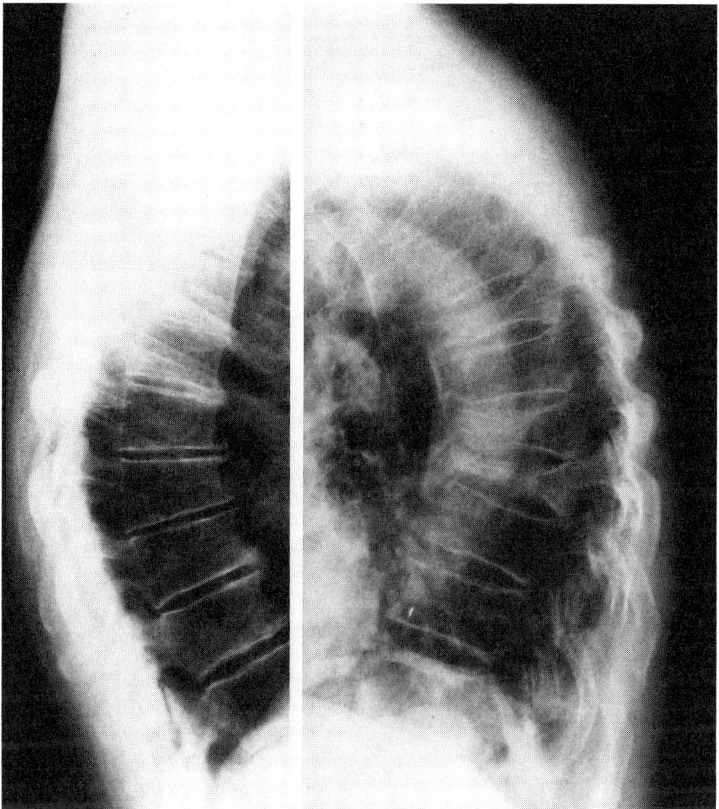

Figure 9.12 X-ray of the thoracic spine in a case with osteoarthritis of the thoracic spine (left), compared to a case with vertebral collapse (right).

vertebral bodies and this should not be confounded with vertebral collapse.

Scheuermann's disease of the thoracic spine is characterized by thoracic wedging and irregular deckplates. This also should be differentiated from osteoporosis (Fig. 9.13).

Epidemiology and Historical Data. Bone loss as a syndrome was first recognized by Pommer in 1855. The credit for its introduction as a disorder of clinical interest (osteoporosis), however, goes to Fuller Allbright and Edward Reifenstein (1948). Pommer differentiated osteoporosis from rickets and osteomalacia, pointing out that the distinguishing characteristic of osteoporosis is a poverty of bone tissue. It is noteworthy that Allbright delineated postmenopausal osteoporosis from "senile" and acute juvenile osteoporosis and from other bone diseases. The antiquity of osteoporosis

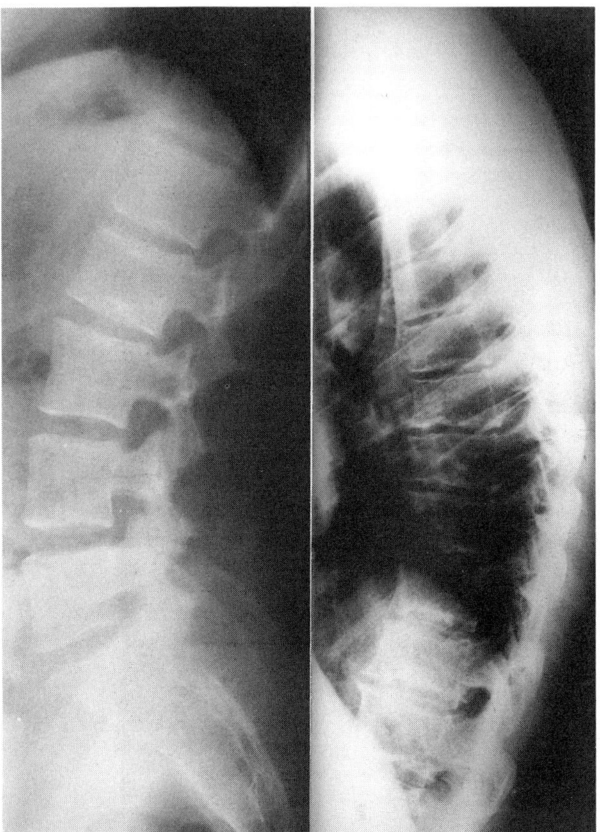

Figure 9.13 Radiologic features of Scheuermann's disease, which may be confused with vertebral collapse: wedged vertebra, Schmorl nodules, free epiphyseal growth center, and irregular endplates.

has been documented in paleopathologic population studies in ancient Nubia (350 B.C.–1400 A.D.) and in American Indians (2500–2600 B.C.).

Studies of contemporary populations support the paleopathologic findings that women have less bone than men, that women still lose more bone than men, and that this bone loss is noticeable earlier in life in females.

The older accounts of osteoporosis were minute accurate descriptions of advanced clinical manifestations of vertebral fractures with low back pain, kyphosis, and loss of stature. At later dates, the diagnosis of osteoporosis was made at an earlier stage by X-ray evidence of vertebral deformity and not necessarily accompanied by kyphosis, pain, or pronounced loss of height.

Despite these striking observations, it was only after 1960 that technical tools became available for the quantitative evaluation of bone in vivo. Since then, several noninvasive tools for quantifying bone mass at the appendicular and axial skeleton have been developed.

Osteoporosis is the most common of the diseases that affect bone. Osteoporosis is more common in women than in men in Europe and Northern America, but the problem in men is by no means insignificant, in particular in Asian and developing countries. Osteoporosis is less prevalent in blacks than in whites. One third of white women over 65 will have vertebral fracture; the lifetime risk of hip fracture in white women is 16% and in men 5% (Fig. 9.14).

With more and more people reaching a higher age and in particular

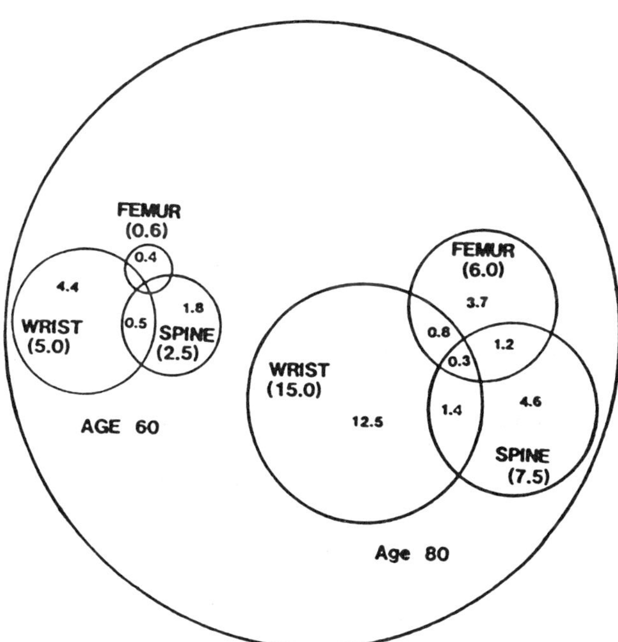

Figure 9.14 Fracture prevalence (%) in women age 60 and age 80. The outer circle represents the whole population; the inner circles represent the fracture populations drawn to scale. The overlapping areas represent cases with more than one fracture. The number denotes the percentages of the total population who have sustained the different fractures. (Ref. 1.)

with more and more women reaching the age beyond the menopause, the incidence and prevalence of osteoporosis is increasing. Osteoporosis is now becoming a worldwide health problem. In Europe, the raise of hip fractures is more than just a consequence of demographic changes. Osteoporosis is associated with a high morbidity and increase mortality (20 times higher than expected in the case of hip fracture). Osteoporosis is of considerable socioeconomic importance because of the high prevalence of fracture and the enormous costs in health care funds required to deal with the consequences of these fractures.

Pathophysiology.   A low bone mass is the main risk factor for osteoporotic fracture. The quality of bone and falls, however, are important cofactors in particular in the older age group. When osteoclasts resorb more bone than the osteoblasts can fill in, then bone loss occurs and a negative bone balance becomes evident.

In order to understand the pathophysiology of osteoporosis, it is important to have a basic knowledge of the physiologic mechanisms of bone modeling and remodeling.

MACROANATOMY.   Bone has unique physical and chemical attributes that mirror the diversity of its functions. The most obvious function of course is its supportive one: strong, hard bones make useful limbs. A second function is that of protecting vital soft tissues such as the brain, spinal cord, heart, and bone marrow. Third, bone is involved in calcium homeostasis.

Bone is an ideal supporting material by virtue of its remarkable strength. It is a two-phase material, consisting of two contrasting substances: fibrous protein collagen (which is strong in tension) and the mineral apatite (which is strong in compression). The crystallites of apatite (or calcium phosphate) are exceedingly small and are aligned along the collagen fibrils.

Bone tissue consists of two major types: compact or cortical bone and trabecular or cancellous bone (Fig. 9.15). Cortical bone forms the shell of the bones and trabecular bone forms an intricate spongy three-dimensional scaffolding with cortical shells. The proportion of cortical to trabecular bone differs from one bone to another. Trabecular bone is mainly present in the distal radius, vertebral bodies, and in the femur, in the intertrochanteric area. Cortical bone is seen in the diaphysis of lone bones, as well as in the proximal femur and in the femoral neck. Because of the greater proportion of free surface to bone volume, trabecular bone is more sensitive to metabolic alterations.

REMODELING.   Peak bone mass is reached for cortical bone between 35 and 40 years and for trabecular bone sooner. The bone becomes more porous, resulting in the condition known as osteoporosis. It is less able to

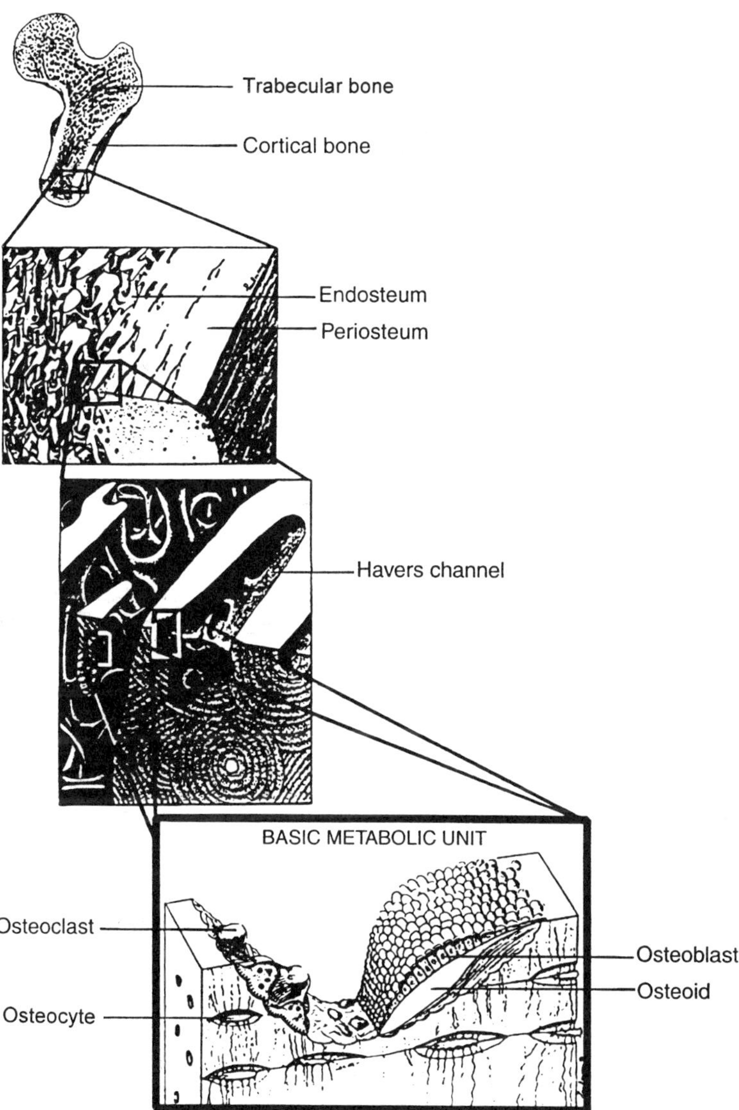

Figure 9.15 Anatomic and histologic reminder of bone tissue.

withstand the strains normally placed on it and becomes more liable to fracture.

During adult life, in the adult skeleton, a continuous remodeling goes on at the microscopic level. Osteoclasts resorb bone and osteoblasts fill up the hole (basic metabolic unit). In adulthood there is a delicate equilibrium between these two processes, which only begins to break down in old age, when the rate of resorption is greater than the rate of redeposition.

Osteoclasts and osteoblasts are coupled in time, space, and intensity (bone turnover). The speed of bone turnover can be measured by blood and urine parameters (Fig. 9.16).

MEDIATORS OF BONE REMODELING. Many stimulators and inhibitors of osteoclast function are known (Fig. 9.17). The mechanism of bone turnover is complicated, entailing communication between several cell types, which respond to systemic hormones and locally released factors. The coupling of the catabolic and anabolic phases of bone remodeling is conserved under many pathologic conditions. This explains why the ability of the major bone-resorbing hormones, as parathyroid hormone (PTH) and 1,25-vitamin D, stimulate bone formation.

RISK FACTORS FOR OSTEOPOROSIS. Factors that influence peak bone mass and factors that increase bone turnover are considered to be risk factors for osteoporosis. The bone-depleting effect of estrogen deficiency is well documented. Patients at high risk for osteopenia are women with premature estrogen deficiency, whether of surgical or natural origin. Other causes of estrogen deficiency associated with bone loss are anorexia nervosa, excessive playing of sports, and history of smoking. Smoking not only reduces serum estrogen levels but also induces an earlier menopause.

There seems to be general agreement about the risk factors for osteoporosis as summarized in Table 9.6. Women are more at risk than men. In particular, western European women have a greater risk than women originating from the Mediterranean area. In the black population osteoporosis is rarely seen. Such anthropometric descriptors as slenderness, small stature, fair, thin, pale skin are associated with osteoporosis. Low-calcium diet, no children, alcohol, and smoking increase the risk for osteoporosis. A family history of osteoporosis is an important risk factor, indicating a genetic predisposition. A sedentary life, intercurrent diseases, and use of glucocorticosteroids accelerate the age-related bone loss.

There is an inverse relationship between osteoporosis and osteoarthritis. Patients with osteoporosis have no or few signs of osteoarthritis and osteoarthritis patients rarely develop fragility fractures (Fig. 9.18). Since the first clinical signs of generalized osteoarthritis (Heberden and Bouchard nodes) are readily observable around the menopause, it is of particular interest to look for these negative risk factors on screening. Osteoarthritic

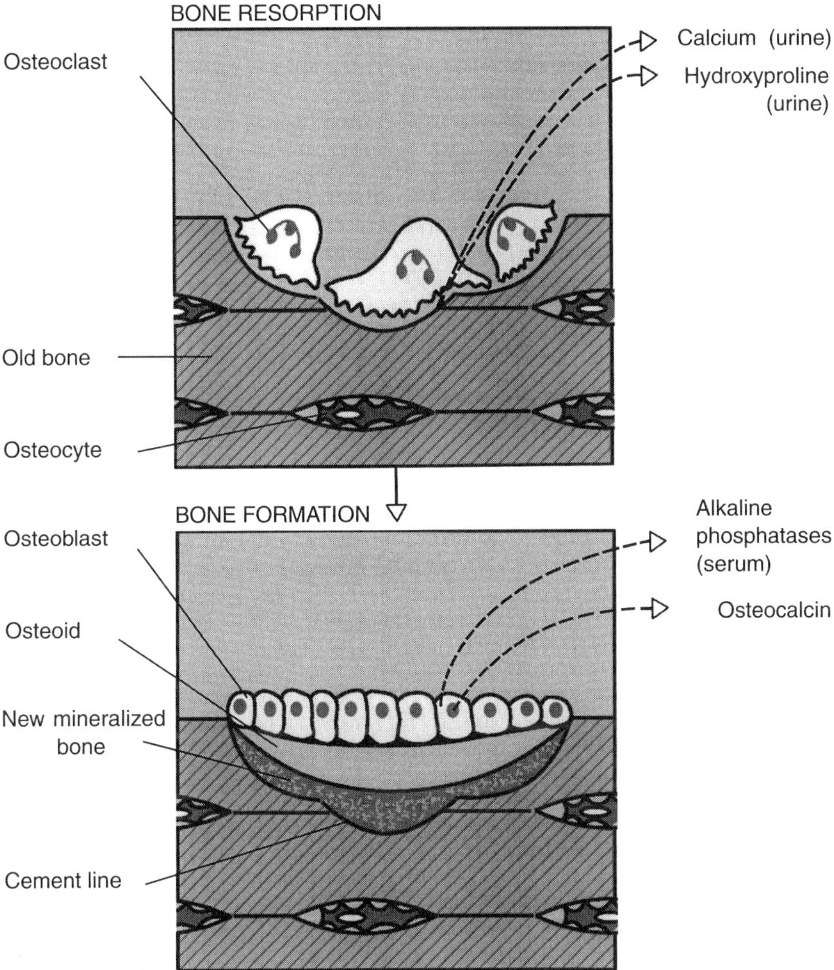

Figure 9.16 Bone resorption by osteoclasts is followed by bone formation by osteoblasts, with production of biochemical parameters.

patients have an excess of body weight, skinfold thickness, and muscle girth and strength. Obese patients have a better estrogen production after the menopause because of peripheral aromatization of androstenedione to estrone.

Bone Loss — Pathophysiology. The key problem in the pathophysiology of osteoporosis, apart from the amount of peak bone mass attained at adult life, is increased resorption and/or decreased bone formation.

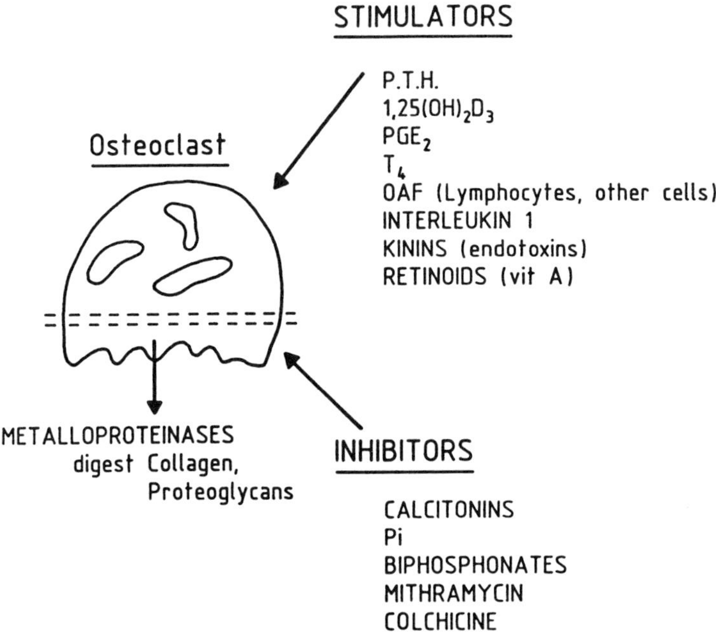

Figure 9.17 Activators and inhibitors of osteoclasts function assessed by calcium mobilization and matrix degradation. PTH, parathyroid hormone; 1,25-$(OH)_2D_3$, 1,25-dihydroxyvitamin D_3; PGE, prostaglandin E; T_4, thyroxine; OAF, osteoblast-activating factor; P_i, inorganic phosphate.

There is evidence that the parathyroid hormone (PTH) plays a major role in this enhanced bone resorption. In order to summarize the various pathologic processes that may produce bone resorption with PTH as a mediator, a possible sequence of events in the development of increased bone resorption and the rationale of pharmacologic interventions is traced in Fig. 9.19.

In most instances the role of PTH is probably indirect by a change in end-organ sensitivity due to hormonal changes, estrogens/androgens, and immobilization.

Calcium deficiency due to a lack of input (diet, malabsorption) or a change in output (hypercalciuria) certainly plays a role by reducing serum ionized calcium levels and stimulating parathyroid activity. Even the small decrease of ionized calcium during the night because of fasting might be sufficient to induce a negative calcium balance in postmenopausal women, which is responsible for the silent bone loss. This is reflected in the increased calcium/creatinine and hydroxyproline/creatine ratio found in the fasting morning urine in women after the menopause.

Table 9.6 Risk Factors for Osteoporosis

Genetic
    Females more than males
    Whites more than blacks
    Family history of osteoporotic fracture
    Absence of generalized osteoarthritis
Anthropometric
    Small stature
    Fair, thin, pale-skinned
    Slenderness
Hormonal
    Premature menopause: natural, iatrogenic
    Nullipara
    Anorexia nervosa
Dietary
    Low calcium diet: adolescence, menopause
    Excess proteins?
Lifestyle
    Sedentary
    Alcohol abuse
    Smoking
Concurrent illness and medication
    Gastrectomy, hyperparathyroidism
    Hyperthyroidism, rheumatoid arthritis
    Corticosteroids
    Neurologic disease: cerebrovascular accident, Parkinson's disease, etc.

The possible deficiency of calcitonin reserve, 1,25-vitamin D hydroxylase or coupling factor, is not fully elucidated and needs further research.

In the absence of estrogens, PTH will take out more calcium from the bone than necessary for homeostasis of serum ionized calcium. Calcium will be preferentially mobilized from the trabecular bone. The efficacy of calcium absorption from the gut is 50% less in postmenopausal women and these women very often have a low-calcium diet. The combination of a low calcium intake and a low estrogen level explains the increase of the incidence of fracture after the menopause. That not all women develop clinical osteoporosis can be explained by a difference in peak bone mass, a better calcium intake, and/or a smaller estrogen deficiency because of peripheral production.

Management.

PREVENTION. The best prevention is to ensure that the peak bone mass is as high as possible and to achieve this bone growth should be

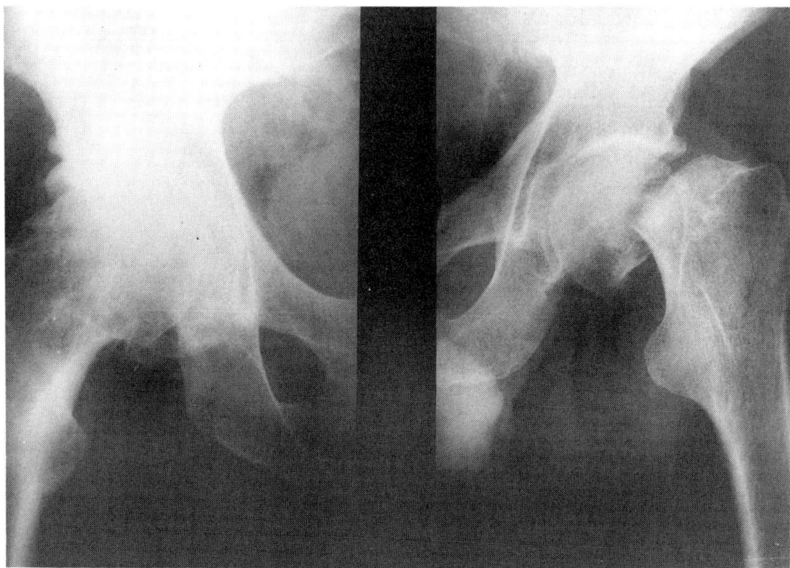

Figure 9.18 Inverse relationship osteoarthritis-osteoporosis: X-ray picture of hip osteoarthritis (loss of cartilage, sclerotic subchondral bone) compared to X-ray picture of femoral neck fracture (well-preserved cartilage, low bone density).

optimal during childhood. Therefore, sufficient calcium intake, vitamin D, and physical activity are necessary. Calcium remains an important mean to reduce bone loss during the peri- and postmenopause. Calcium should preferentially be taken at bedtime in the form of one or two glasses of milk or yogurt. Yogurt is better tolerated in persons with lactase deficiency. The need for calcium increases after the menopause is up to 1500 mg/day instead of 750 mg before the menopause. One should not forget that the menopause is not an abrupt phenomenon, except iatrogenically induced. Long before menstruation ceases, calcium supplementation should be started. When milk products are not well tolerated, calcium carbonate 1000 mg/day as a supplement to the diet is advised. Calcium carbonate contains more calcium per weight unit than calcium lactate or calcium gluconate. Calcium supplementation of 1 g and vitamin D 800 units have been shown to reduce femoral neck fracture incidence by 25% in institutionalized elderly.

As prevention, oral contraception can also be prescribed for a longer period because it has been shown that women who used oral contraceptives conserved better bone mass. Substitution therapy with estrogens for preven-

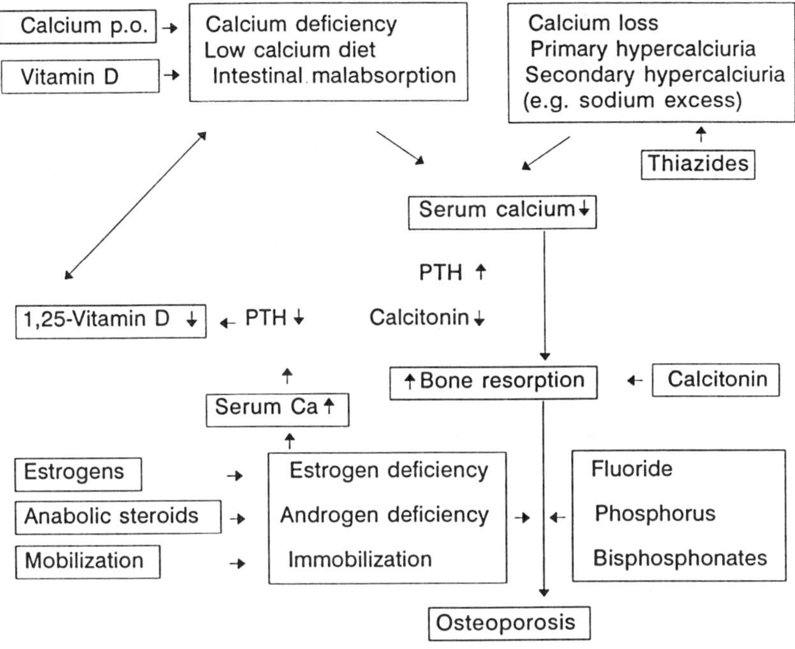

Figure 9.19 Pathophysiology of osteoporosis (PTH, parathyroid hormone; CT, calcitonin). Rationale and place of pathophysiologic interactions of various pharmacologic agents used in the treatment of osteoporosis.

given for climacteric symptoms. Patients with an intact uterus need a dosage equivalent to 0.625 mg conjugated estrogens or 2 mg estradiol-valerate, to be taken 21 days a month. From the 10th until the 21st day, progestogen is added to prevent endometrium hyperplasia. An elegant way to administer estrogens is percutaneously. The minimal duration of a preventive hormone replacement therapy (HRT) is 10 years. This has to be discussed openly with the patient. When HRT is stopped, bone loss will recur. It is the intention of preventive therapy to keep the patients at risk out of the fracture risk zone until a late age. An absolute contraindication for estrogen use is a personal or family history of estrogen-dependent mammary carcinoma. Long-term (>5 years) estrogen therapy in elderly persons over 60 has been shown to increase breast cancer in a large-population study. Ideally, hormonal therapy for prevention of osteoporotic fractures should be given for at least 5 years and preferably for 10–15 years. Some even advocate giving it indefinitely, but in reality compliance with hormonal therapy is low.

There are several reasons for this low compliance: withdrawal bleed-

There are several reasons for this low compliance: withdrawal bleeding and fear of breast cancer are the two most important. The risk of endometrial cancer, considered the greatest risk of estrogen replacement therapy, is now much reduced by the concomitant use of progestogen. However, the introduction of progestogen in itself may reduce considerably the reported benefits of estrogens for cardiovascular disease. The risk for breast cancer is probably the most important reason for refusal of starting HRT and for the low compliance in a large proportion of the postmenopausal population.

The chance of any women having breast cancer during her lifetime is about 1 in 12, and thus, even a slight increase in risk will yield a substantial increase in the number of cancers. HRT should be more optimally targeted to individuals with a high risk of cardiovascular disease and avoided in individuals with a risk of breast cancer.

One of the alternatives for HRT, particularly in post- and perimenopausal women, is the estrogen analog (raloxifene, tibolone, etc.).

CURATIVE TREATMENT. Before starting treatment for osteoporosis, it is necessary to search for the cause of osteoporosis and to alleviate the causative factors as much as possible. Osteoporosis is a heterogeneous syndrome because mechanisms of bone failure are diverse. Insufficient bone resistance to load can be due to a low buildup of bone during adolescent growth; an increased breakdown during mature life, e.g., immobilization, corticosteroid treatment; accelerated loss of bone at the menopause and old age; or a combination of several factors. At the time of failure (fracture), the bone metabolism can be in a high or low turnover state or bone reserves can be low at the trabecular site and normal at the cortical site or vice versa, or low at both sites.

At present, it is well established that some drugs have preferential effects on cortical or trabecular bone and that some drugs work through antiresorbing activity while others have a bone formation–stimulating activity.

A decision tree for determining treatment based on physiopathology is shown in Fig. 9.20. A treatment program should be based on the biochemical disturbances underlying the osteoporotic state at the time of fracture. For example, when a low 24-hr calcium excretion is found, calcium and vitamin D should be prescribed to increase calcium absorption in the gut. When a high fasting urinary calcium/creatinine ratio is observed, indicating high-turnover bone loss, then antiresorbing drugs as calcitonin, estrogens, bisphosphonates, and anabolic steroid treatments are more appropriate. If there is a high 24-hr calcium excretion, thiazides can be prescribed in order to reduce urinary calcium excretion. In the case of an important pain syndrome, calcitonin can temporarily be given subcutaneously in com-

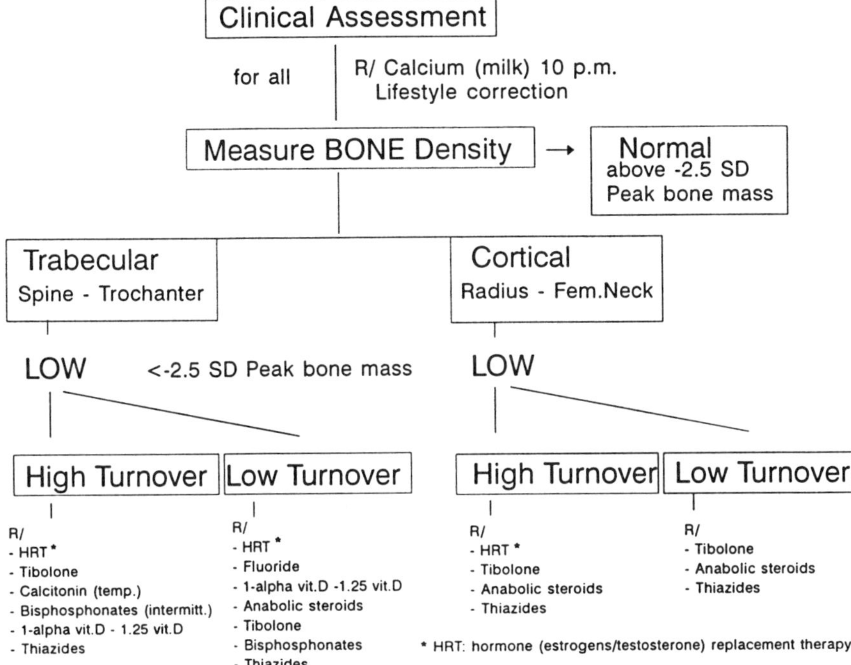

Figure 9.20 Decision tree for determining treatment choice.

bination with bedrest. Vitamin D metabolites and fluoride are more active on the trabecular bone and are currently underinvestigated. They might be useful in corticosteroid induced osteoporosis.

REHABILITATION AND EXERCISES. The prevention of further fractures is not only a question of arresting bone loss, increasing bone mass, and enhancing bone quality but of improving the quality of life by endeavoring to eliminate the risk of falls. Improving the quality of life and living conditions calls for a positive rather than a negative (nihilistic) approach to the patient. General rehabilitation measures should be available as soon after fracture as possible, involving the services of a multidisciplinary team of committed nurses, physiotherapists, social workers, and occupational therapists working in close cooperation with physicians. Exercises shaped according to the stage of the patient can be found useful and are outlined in Fig. 9.21.

In Fig. 9.21a are shown the main exercises for stage I patients who are still bedridden because of back pain. They do the following exercises in consecutive sequence: (1) flex and extend the right and left leg; (2) elevate

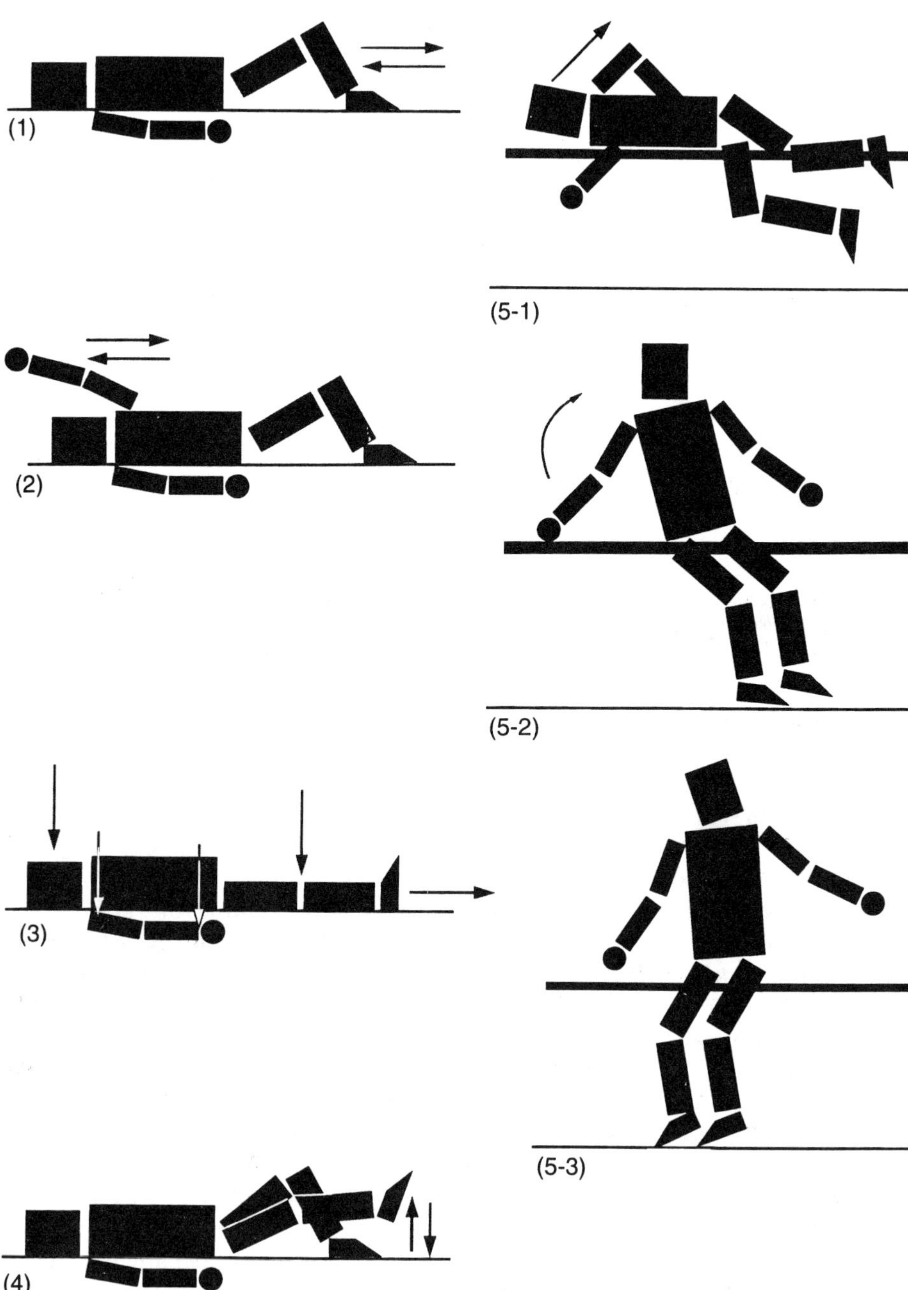

Figure 9.21a Stage I exercises for osteoporotic patients (1–5).

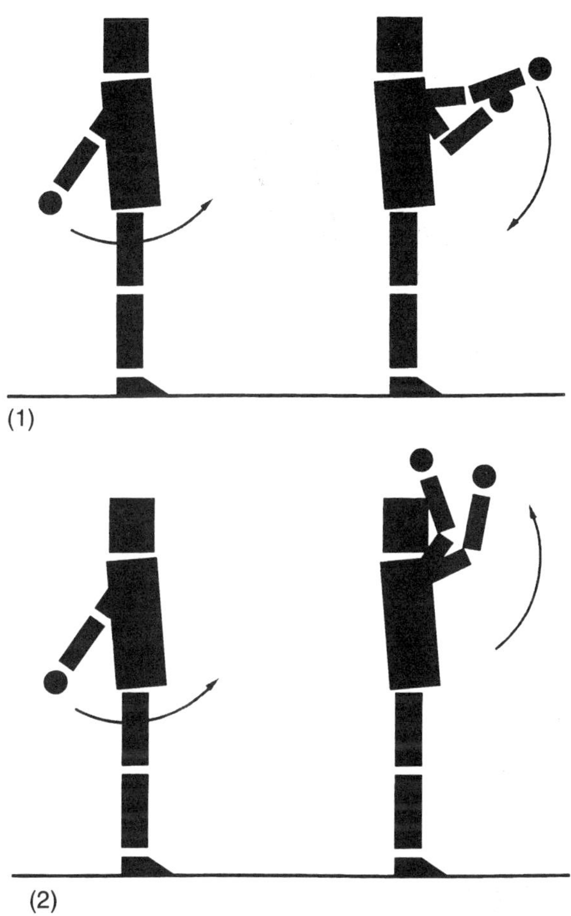

Figure 9.21b Stage II exercises for osteoporotic patients (1–6).

the left and right arm; (3) stretch isometrically the back muscles, triceps, and quadriceps while pushing into the mattress; (4) with knees in moderate flexion and the heels on the bed, extend right and left knee alternatively; (5) in order to learn how to come out of the bed without pain, the patient turns from lateral decubitus with a straight back in bloc in a sitting position at the border of the bed.

As soon as the patient can sit and stand without too much pain, the exercise of stage II (Fig. 9.21b) can be started: (1) arms balanced forward and backward; (2) arms elevated to the maximum; (3) marching on the spot; (4) sitting with the back against the wall, standing exercises and auto-lengthening while pushing head and arms backward; (5) with the hands on

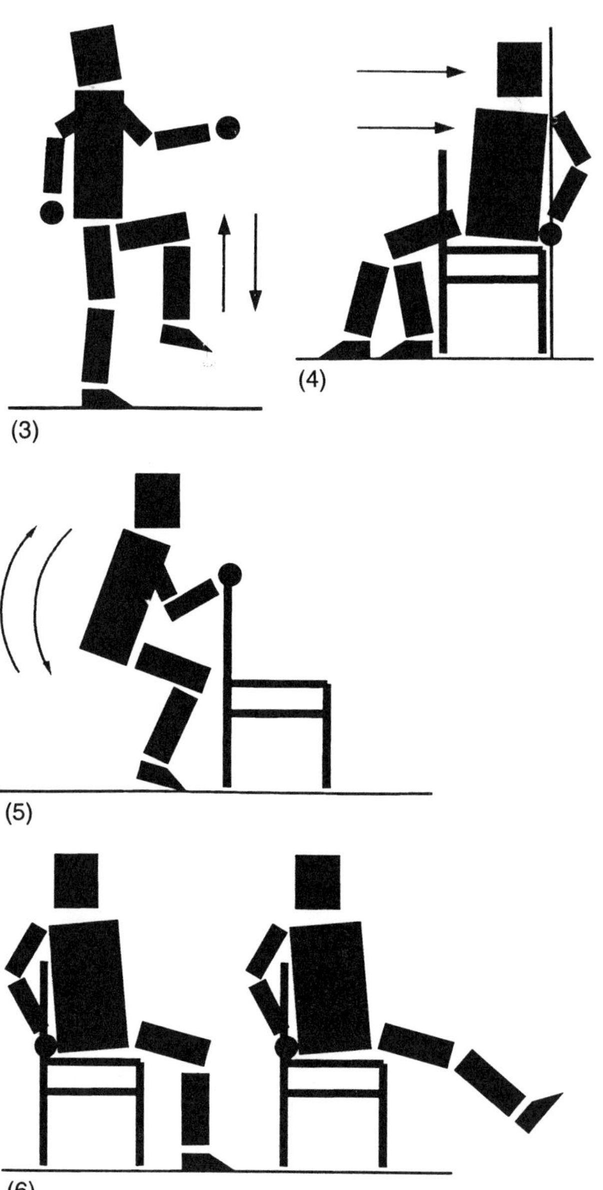

(3)

(4)

(5)

(6)

Figure 9.21b Continued.

a table or on the back of a chair, flexing knees up to 90°; (6) flexing-extending the knees in a sitting position.

Furthermore, patients learn what to avoid during activities of daily living, in particular avoiding lifting objects with a flexed position. Situp exercises for abdominal muscle training are not indicated in osteoporotic patients with back pain.

Patients who continue to have back pain after periods of activity may benefit from long-term use of a canvas corset or a more rigid hyperextension orthosis. Too early use of rigid corsets should be discouraged because they are in general not well tolerated due to a progressive change in profile of the patient. Short periods of intermittent bedrest, 15–20 min several times each day, may also help to relieve discomfort.

1.5 Atypical Forms

1.5.1 Osteogenesis Imperfecta

Osteogenesis imperfecta, "brittle bone disease," is a heritable disorder of connective tissue in which the pathogenesis of nearly all clinical types appears to involve an abnormality in the synthesis or structure of type I collagen. The hallmarks of osteogenesis imperfecta are osteopenia with fracture diathesis, blue sclerae, and deafness due to osteosclerosis. Patients with osteogenesis imperfecta have the peak incidence of fractures during childhood and adolescence, experience fewer fractures after puberty, and again become prone to fracture after the menopause.

1.5.2 Glucocorticoid-Induced Osteoporosis

Cushing's disease or chronic treatment with pharmacologic doses of glucocorticoids frequently produces a severe osteoporosis that clinically resembles age-related osteoporosis. On occasion, typical cushingoid features may not be apparent, and the osteoporosis can be the major presenting problem. The disorder can be the result of (1) direct glucocorticoid suppression of osteoblastic bone forming activity and (2) increased osteoclastic bone resorbing activity caused by increased PTH secretion. Bone loss is more severe in those regions of the skeleton with a high content of trabecular bone. Thus fractures are especially common in the ribs, vertebrae, and ends of long bones. Chronic glucocorticoid therapy is by far the most common iatrogenic cause of osteoporosis and is a major risk factor for bone loss. The reported incidence of bone fracture in steroid-treated patients ranges from 8% to 18% and is two- to threefold greater than in similar patients treated with other agents.

Age, menopausal status, and activity level are important determinants of fracture risk. The incidence of clinically significant osteoporosis is highest in children, postmenopausal women, patients of both sexes over the age of 50, and relatively immobilized individuals.

X rays of the spine of corticosteroid-induced osteoporosis may demonstrate not only multiple vertebral wedge fractures but also characteristic marginal condensations due to exuberant callus of compressed vertebra endplates (Fig. 9.22).

1.5.3 Osteoporomalacia

A certain degree of hypovitamin D is often encountered in the elderly and may play a role in the pathogenesis of fractures of the proximal femur. The interaction of aging, malabsorption, and decrease in renal function is illustrated in Fig. 9.23.

About 10% of femoral neck fracture cases have histologic evidence of osteomalacia. 25-Hydroxy vitamin D serum levels are low in these cases (<10 mg/ml). 25-Hydroxy vitamin D serum levels show marked seasonal

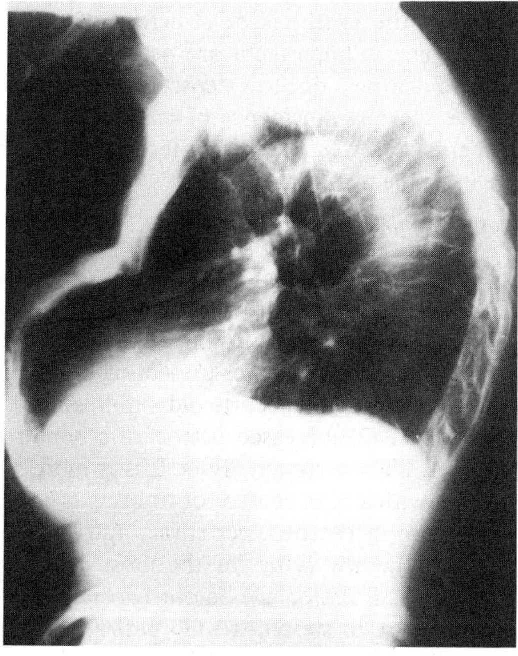

Figure 9.22 Corticosteroid-induced osteoporosis in a 60-year-old woman. This lateral X ray of the thoracic spine demonstrates multiple vertebral wedge fractures and fracture of the sternal bone.

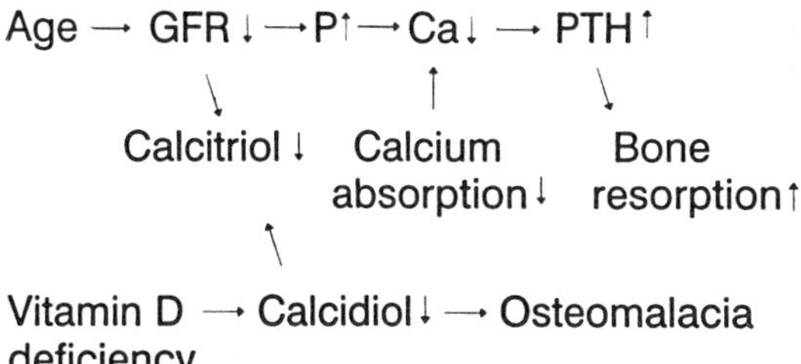

Figure 9.23 Pathophysiology of osteoporomalacia in the elderly.

variation. In Europe the maximum level is ±20–25 ng/ml in September and the minimum level is ±10 ng/ml in March. Levels below 5 ng/ml are associated with deficiency disease.

1.6 Impact of Disease and Prognosis

Osteoporotic fractures heal well but deformities may remain. During the intervals (often years) between compression fractures, most patients are totally pain-free. However, some continue to be plagued with chronic, dull, aching, postural pain in the midthoracic and upper lumbar region that responds symptomatically to frequent, intermittent horizontal rest.

With each episode of segmental vertebral collapse and progressive kyphosis, the patient's height may decrease by 2–4 cm. Women may notice a change in the way clothes fit and may have to raise the hemline of their dresses. This may upset them psychologically.

In 95% of postmenopausal patients with symptomatic osteoporosis, more than six radiographically evident vertebral fractures occur over a period of approximately 10 years. Seventy-five percent of patients lose at least 10 cm in height. The progression of the dowager's hump and the decrease in height provide reliable clinical signs of the early progress of the disease. Once the spine has collapsed to the point where the lower rib comes to rest on the iliac crest, further significant loss in height is not likely, although loss of bone mass may continue.

Two of the clinically disturbing, long-term side effects of progressive vertebral compression fractures occur as a result of the decrease in size of the thoracic and abdominal cavities. The patient becomes aware of diminished exercise tolerance as a result of disease-related postural changes. Early satiety is noted, with abdominal protrusion secondary to severe lumbar vertebral collapse. The patient feels bloated after ingesting small amounts of food. Circumferential pachydermal skin folds develop at the rib and pelvic margins as the disease progresses.

The fracture of the distal radius after a correct reposition as a rule does not give adverse effects, but sometimes a carpal tunnel syndrome or a reflex sympathetic algodystrophy may appear.

Progression of hip fracture is clearly less favorable. The mortality is 12–20% higher the first 3 months after fracture, compared to age- and sex-matched populations. Possibly part of this increased mortality is due to underlying or concomitant diseases rather than to the fracture itself. Of the patients who were independent at home before the fracture, 15–25% had to be admitted to a nursing home and this for longer than 1 year after the fracture. In addition to this, 25–35% became dependent on others or on walking aids or wheelchairs. Usually the disease does not involve only one fracture. The chance of developing new fractures after an initial collapse is very high and this also applies to peripheral fractures.

2 PAGET'S DISEASE

2.1 Definition (Table 9.7)

Paget's disease of bone (osteitis deformans) is a localized disorder of bone remodeling of unknown origin, leading to bones expanded in size, less compact, more vascular, and more susceptible to deformity or fracture than normal bone.

2.2 Main Clinical Features

Clinical signs and symptoms will vary from one patient to the next, depending on the number and location of affected skeletal sites as well as the rapidity of the abnormal bone turnover. It is believed that most patients are asymptomatic, but a substantial minority may experience a variety of symptoms, including bone pain, secondary osetoarthritic problems, bone deformity, excessive warmth over bone from hypervascularity, and a vari-

Table 9.7 Paget's Disease

A localized disorder of bone remodeling of unknown origin.
The bones affected are expanded in size, have a chaotic structure, and are susceptible to deformity and fracture.
Secondary osteoarthritis, nerve compression, and cardiac failure may occur.
Disease is often unnoted except from the finding of an elevated serum alkaline phosphatase activity.
Affects mainly elderly.
Management is medical (anti-bone-resorbing drugs) and/or surgical.

ety of neurologic complications due in most instances to compression of nerves adjacent to Pagetic bone.

2.3   Confirming the Diagnosis—Investigations

2.3.1   Early Phase

Paget's disease is often detected on routine blood screening where the elevation of alkaline phosphatase attracts attention. If this is an isolated finding (no other biological signs of liver disease), the next step is to request a bone scan.

Bone scintigraphy is more sensitive than radiography in the detection of early disease and of particular value in assessing the extent of the disease activity (Fig. 9.24).

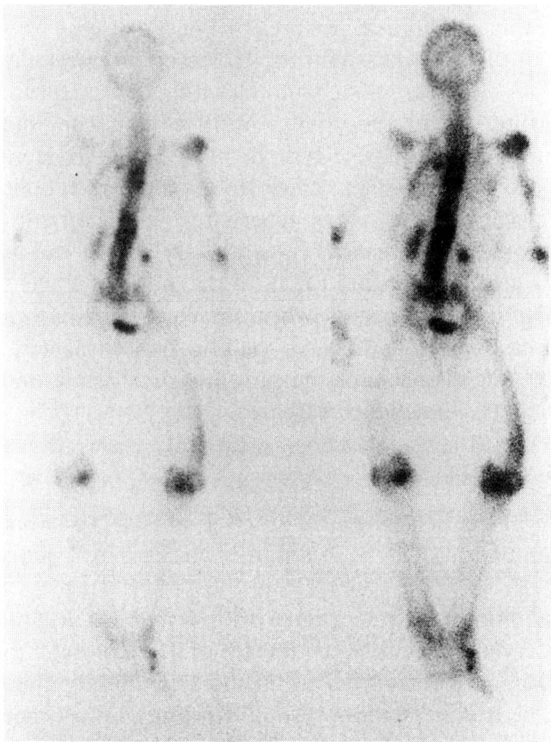

Figure 9.24   Scintigraphic evidence of Pagetic lesions affecting parts of the dorsal and lumbar spine, both femora and right proximal humerus.

Disease activity is assessed by measuring alkaline phosphatase activity in the serum and hydroxyproline excretion in the urine.

Paget's disease gives typical X ray features: the bone is enlarged, the cortical thickening is associated with an increased intracortical porosity, while the adjacent trabecular bone has thickened trabeculae (Fig. 9.25).

2.3.2 Late Phase

Paget's deformities may be crippling, particularly in the limbs (bowing of the legs; Fig. 9.26), may induce osteoarthritis in particular of the hip and knee, and may be aesthetically unfavorable, e.g., facial bones (leonthiasis ossea). When the skull is affected, this may lead to deafness, cranial nerve involvement, platybasia, basilar invagination, hydrocephalus, and verte-brobasilar insufficiency. If vertebrae are involved, spinal cord compression may occur.

2.4 Diagnostic Difficulties

The characteristic radiographic and clinical features of Paget's disease usu-ally eliminate problems with differential diagnosis. However, occasionally an older patient may present with severe bone pain, elevations of the serum alkaline phosphatase and urinary hydroxyproline, a positive bone scan, and less than characteristic radiographic areas of lytic or blastic change. Here the question of metastatic disease to bone or some other form of metabolic bone disease (e.g., osteomalacia with secondary hyperparathyroidism) must be considered. Old radiographs and laboratory tests are very helpful in this setting, as normal studies a year earlier would make a diagnosis of Paget's disease less likely. A similar dilemma occurs when someone with known and established Paget's disease develops multiple painful new sites; here, too, the likelihood of metastatic disease must be carefully considered, and bone biopsy for a tissue diagnosis may be indicated.

2.5 Epidemiology and Historical Data

Sir James Paget is credited for the first magistral description (1877) of what he felt was a chronic inflammation of bone and named the disease osteitis deformans.

Paget's disease affects both men and women with a slight male pre-ponderance. It is rarely observed to occur below the age of 25, is thought to develop after the age of 40 in most instances, and is most commonly diag-nosed in persons in their 50s. It may be monostotic, affecting only a single bone or portion of a bone, or may be polyostotic involving two or more bones. The most common sites of involvement include the pelvis, femur, spine, skull, and tibia. The anatomic prevalence is between 3% and 7%.

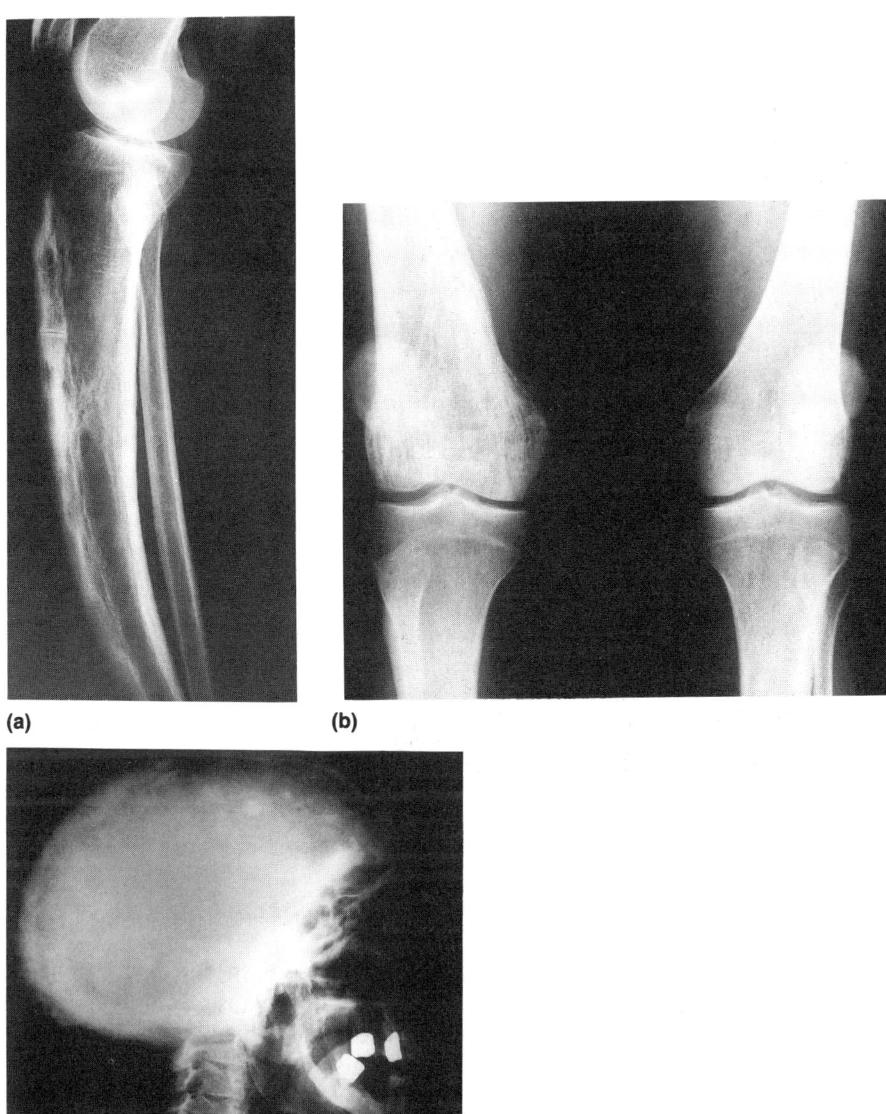

Figure 9.25 Radiographic features of Paget's disease: (a) Tibia: hypertrophy and increased anterior curvature of the tibia (1), fibrillar and disorganized appearance of the bone trabeculae (2), fissure fractures anteriorly (3), lower third of tibia normal with V-shaped demarcation (4). (b) Femur: coarse-grained bone structure with translucent areas and widening of the femoral metaphysis. (c) Skull: coarse-grained structure with sclerotic areas and platybasia.

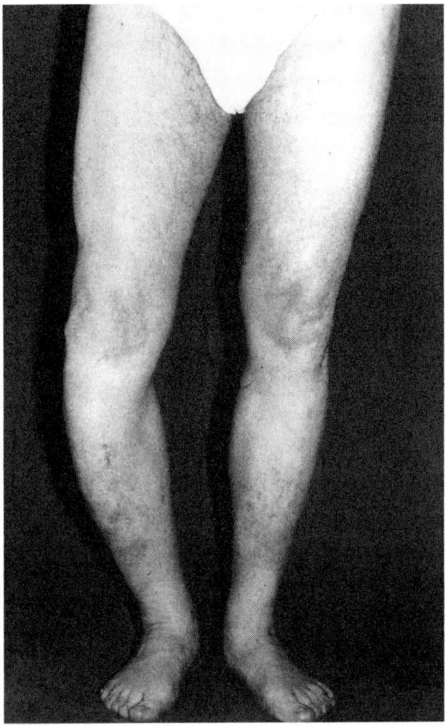

Figure 9.26   Bowing of the leg due to Paget's disease.

The clinical prevalence is much lower and very often detected by chance because of an unexplained elevated alkaline phosphatase. In only one third of the patients is the diagnosis made before death. The disease is sometimes seen in families and more often in individuals of Anglo-Saxon descendence.

2.6 Pathophysiology

The process is initiated by increases in huge multinucleated osteoclast-mediated bone resorption, with subsequent compensatory increases in new bone formation, resulting in a disorganized mosaic of woven and lamellar bone at affected skeletal sites. This structural change produces bone that is expanded in size, less compact, more vascular, and more susceptible to deformity or fracture than normal bone.

The initiation of the Paget's process could be a slow virus (canine distemper virus?), but this remains a hypothesis.

2.7 Management

Therapy consists of calcitonin or bisphosphonates. Both drugs will reduce disease activity (alkaline phosphatase) by 70%. Indication for therapy is pain, bowing of the bones, progressive neurologic syndromes, fissure fractures, immobilization, hypercalcemia, heart failure, osteolytic lesions in weight-bearing bones, strong elevation of alkaline phosphatase activity in the serum, and/or hydroxyprolinuria.

When Paget's disease is an accidental finding, then often no treatment is required.

2.8 Impact of Disease and Prognosis

As the late manifestations of the disease can be disfiguring and give rise to important deformities, Paget's disease will induce psychological stresses, in particular when the face and skull are involved.

Treatment usually can control the pain syndrome. When nearby joints are affected with osteoarthritis, joint reconstruction has to be advised, in particular at the hip and the knee. Only rare cases come to the development of intracranial problems such as hydrocephalus or basilar invagination.

When Paget's disease affects more than 35% of the skeleton, it may cause high cardiac output failure, precisely because of the increased bone blood flow. Pagetic bones are brittle and may fracture spontaneously, in particular the femur, the tibia, the humerus, and the forearm. In about 0.2% of the cases malignant degeneration may occur.

3 REFLEX SYMPATHETIC ALGODYSTROPHY SYNDROME

3.1 Definition (Table 9.8)

Reflex sympathetic algodystrophy syndrome (RSD) is a symptom complex characterized by severe pain, swelling, autonomic dysfunction, and impaired mobility of an extremity, which may occur without a precipitating cause.

Table 9.8 Reflex Sympathetic Algodystrophy Syndrome

Symptom complex of severe pain, swelling, autonomic dysfunction, and impaired mobility of an extremity.
Many precipitating situations including psychological stress.
When occurring after trauma: this condition is called Südeck's syndrome.
Bone scintigraphy gives typical images and the vascular scan can stage the disease.
Management is difficult.

The variable presentations of the syndrome have resulted in its having several names, including algodystrophy (the preferred European term), Sudeck's atrophy, reflex neurovascular dystrophy, shoulder–hand syndrome, traumatic angiospasm, migratory osteoporosis, and transient osteoporosis.

3.2 Main Clinical Features

3.2.1 Early Manifestations

Typical signs and symptoms include pain and swelling of an extremity, usually unilateral, which may become bilateral in 30% of patients. The pain is usually burning, aching, or even "bursting" and can be sufficiently intense to prevent movement of an affected digit or joint. Blowing on the skin may produce discomfort. Affected lower limbs may become more painful during weight bearing. Signs of autonomic instability are usually present, including tight, shining, warm, and ruddy skin. Pallor, cyanosis, coldness, nonpitting edema, and hyperhidrosis may also be present (Fig. 9.27).

The involved area is not limited to a dermatome, myotome, or peripheral nerve distribution, but may involve a foot, hand, knee, or shoulder. Partial or incomplete forms may exist involving a portion of the hand or foot, or one only of the femoral condyles at the knee may be involved with

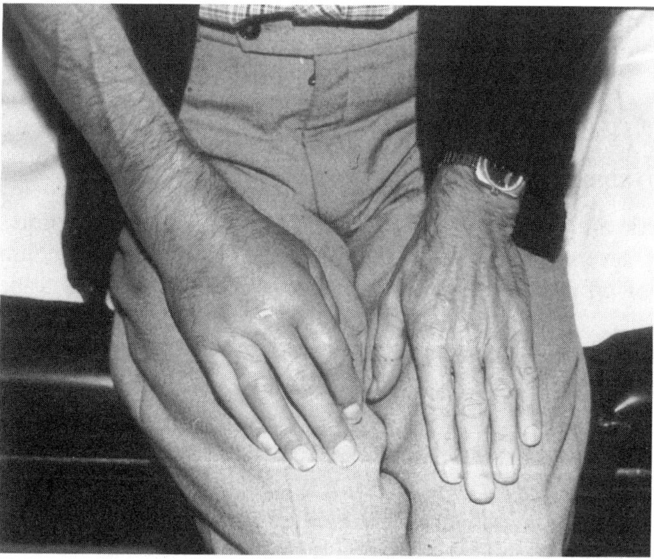

Figure 9.27   Clinical signs of algodystrophy.

symptoms and signs localized to that side of the joint. Affected joints occasionally develop small noninflammatory effusions.

3.2.2 Late Manifestations

Three distinct clinical stages of the syndrome have been described. While most patients pass through these distinct phases in a predictable pattern, overlap may be noted or one stage may be completely bypassed.

Stage I may have a dramatic onset and last from 1 to 6 months. The main symptom is persistent deep burning pain aggravated by movement, contact, or emotional disturbance. The skin is warm, dry, or moist; hyperaesthetic; tender to minor pressure; and accompanied by nonpitting edema. Usually, all digits are painful in the interarticular as well as the articular sites and are sensitive to palpation.

Stage II may last 3–6 months with partial resolution of some of the symptoms of stage I followed by a tendency for atrophy of the subcutaneous tissue, wasting of the interstitial muscles, thickening of joint capsules, stiffness with flexion deformity of the fingers, induration of the skin, and features reminiscent of scleroderma. At this juncture there is usually a marked degree of osteopenia.

Stage III is characterized by trophic changes and contracture of the skin and joints with X-ray evidence of severe demineralization.

While single episodes are most common, symptoms may follow a migratory pattern. Individual episodes may last 6–9 months followed by spontaneous or assisted resolutions. A patient may experience six or more episodes.

3.3 Confirming the Diagnosis

There are usually no characteristic biochemical abnormalities. The urinary hydroxyproline excretion may be elevated in the early phase of the disease. Radiologic changes may occur rapidly during the first 3 or 4 weeks. The majority of patients have patchy demineralization in the affected area, involving either a whole region (hand, foot) or a portion of the limb (Fig. 9.28).

Bilateral X rays are suggested because the earliest changes may be subtle. The most marked changes occur in the articular surfaces of subchondral bone where the support trabeculae may rapidly diminish in size and number. Trabecular bone loss exaggerates the definition of the subchondral plate, which appears as a pencil line between the joint space cavity and remaining trabeculae, and may give a picture resembling erosions (pseudoerosions). The pattern of bone loss is often patchy in the early phases of hip and knee involvement, with only a segment of the end of the bone affected.

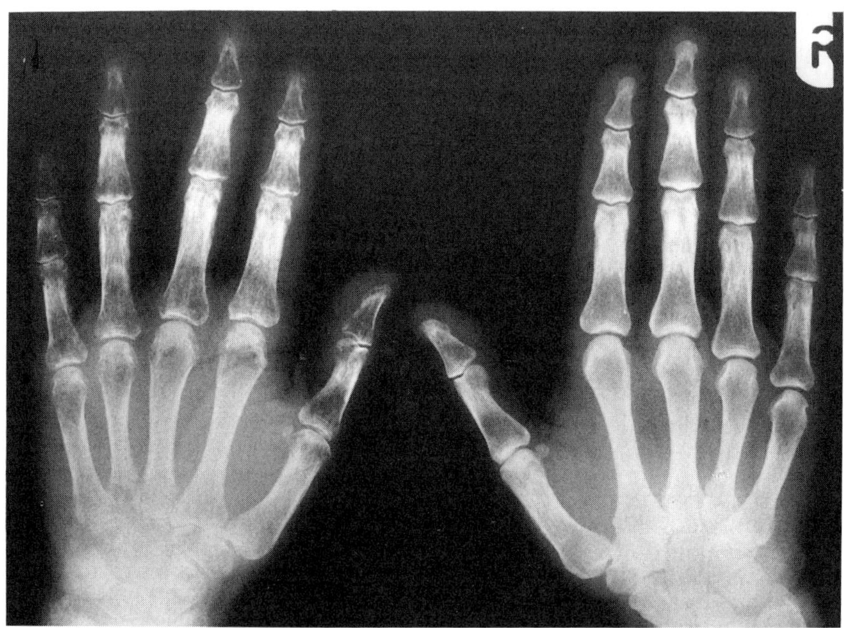

Figure 9.28   Radiologic features of algodystrophy, left hand.

3.3.1 Scintigraphy

A positive bone scan with technetium pertechnitate may develop before X-ray changes are evident and may identify early involvement of the opposite limb. In children, however, a negative scintigraphy is often seen (Fig. 9.29).

Vascular scintigraphy with albumen-marked technetium, comparing the affected (pathologic) to the nonaffected (normal) side, shows hemodynamic flow patterns (0'–20') that are strikingly different in stage I than in stage II and III algodystrophy. The ratio of the counts in the early and plateau phase P/N (pathologic/normal) is high in stage I and low in stage II and III.

This hemodynamic pattern corresponds to a phase of increased blood flow and blood volume, representing vasodilatation, whereas in stage II there is a low blood flow and blood volume (representing vasoconstriction).

Precipitating events that have been associated with reflex sympathetic dystrophy include trauma, surgical operation, acute cerebrovascular injuries, stroke, myocardial infarction, intrathoracic disease, primary diseases of the joints, drug therapy (barbiturates, antiepileptic agents and antituber-

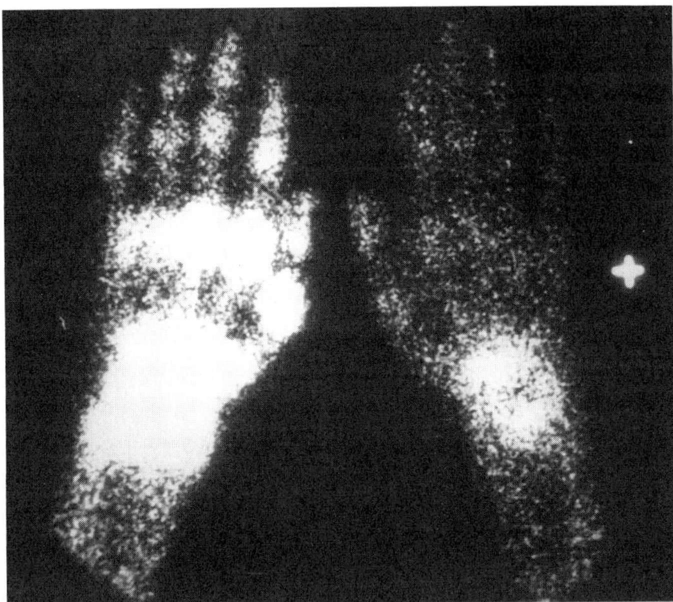

Figure 9.29 Scintigraphic features of algodystrophy. Note hypercaptation of left hand.

culous agents), malignancy, and pregnancy. Many cases of reflex sympathetic dystrophy syndrome have no precipitating event. Although typical forms involving a single site may be readily diagnosed, many partial forms are overlooked.

3.4 Epidemiology and Historical Data

Men and women are affected with equal frequency, and reflex sympathetic dystrophy syndrome has been reported in both children and young adults. In the latter, reflex sympathetic dystrophy syndrome is often associated with a peculiar psychological background, characterized by emotional lability or hyperreactivity and tendency to anxiety and depression.

The development of an acute painful, swollen extremity following trauma, infection, or burn has been recognized for many centuries. Weir Mitchell in 1864 gave the classical description of the syndrome he called causalgia which followed gunshot injury to a major nerve of the limb. Reflex sympathetic dystrophy syndrome is the term applied to a similar set of symptoms and signs when the peripheral nerve has not been injured.

3.5 Pathophysiology

The pathogenesis of these syndromes is not clear. In order to explain the diverse features and associated conditions of reflex sympathetic dystrophy syndrome, there must be a regulation disturbance of the autonomic nervous system. Normally there is a dynamic balance in the central nervous system that is influenced by cognitive and perceptual processes, as well as by impulse of the sympathetic nervous system. Stimulation of the efferent sympathetic nerves by ascending pain elements (trauma), descendent cognitive or perceptive mechanisms (CVA, medication, psychological effects), or direct irritation of the receptor centra (CVA, medication, spine myelolesions) may produce a reflex sympathetic dystrophy syndrome.

Table 9.9 shows the conditions often associated with reflex sympathetic dystrophy.

3.6 Management

Early therapeutic intervention is important. Pain control with NSAIDs is the initial choice but stronger analgesics may be necessary. Protective and assisted mobilization of the affected limb is essential to prevent disuse and to control peripheral edema. Vigorous physical therapy is essential and treatment of any underlying condition imperative.

Psychosocial counseling is often necessary as well as supportive psychiatric therapy.

Oral glucocorticoids (30–40 mg prednisone) in the first 4–6 weeks for 2 weeks may be useful to reduce the high-turnover metabolic state. This therapy was often used in the past. At present, preference is given to calcito-

Table 9.9 Conditions Often Associated with Reflex Sympathetic Dystrophy

Trauma
Heart infarction
Spinal cord lesion
Hemiplegia
Epilepsy
Herpes zoster
Lesion of the shoulder capsule
Tuberculosis
Tuberculostatics
Barbiturates
Cervical osteoarthritis
Hysterical personality?

nin treatment in the early phase of reflex sympathetic dystrophy (100 IU daily for 4 weeks) with tapering off the doses and frequency after that. Sympathetic blockade with local anaesthetic (lidocaine) have been useful. Beta-blocking agents such as propranalol have been used and require monitoring of the peripheral pulse. Guanethidine can be injected into vessels proximal to the occlusion. None of these therapeutic programs has been tested by double-blind trials. The use of antidepressants, splints, psychotherapy, acupuncture, and electric simulation (transcutaneous nerve stimulation) have also been used with other therapeutic regimens, with inconclusive results.

3.7 Atypical Forms

Focal and migratory regional osteoporosis are often missed. The scintigraphic picture of a localized hyperactive zone is often helpful.

3.8 Impact of Disease and Prognosis

Although single episodes are most common, symptoms may follow a migratory pattern. Individual episodes may last 6–9 months, followed by spontaneous or assisted resolutions. A patient may experience six or more episodes.

The course of the disease can be prolonged over years and end up manifested in a painless contracted functionless appendage with cool shiny skin. In most cases, the symptoms of the disease cease gradually without important sequelae within 2 years. The impact of the disease on the patient and family is not negligible, in particular because it may affect young adults in the most productive time of life. Because of its chronicity, patients often seek help in the alternative medical circuit or change from doctor to doctor with unnecessary financial consequences. Therefore it is of primary importance for the physician to assist these patients comprehensively, including psychosocial counseling of both the patient and the family, and explain to them that this is a temporary syndrome that resolves spontaneously, usually with very few sequelae.

REFERENCE

1. Nordin BEC. Osteoporosis with particular reference to the menopause. In: Avioli LV (ed.), The Osteoporotic Syndrome, New York: Grune and Stratton, 13–43.

10

Hereditary Connective Tissue Disorders

The molecular composition and organization of connective tissue are extraordinary complex. Much remains unknown about the genes—their number, structure, chromosomal location, and regulation—that control synthesis, organization, and metabolism of this tissue.

Figure 10.1 shows the physiopathology of collagen metabolism and the different points where alterations may occur. This section will briefly consider heritable disorders of connective tissue not including genetic bone disorders or mucopolysaccharidose.

1 BENIGN JOINT HYPERMOBILITY SYNDROME

1.1 Definition (Table 10.1)

Hypermobility is a common, benign, heritable disorder of connective tissue (HDCT), characterized by joint laxity, tissue fragility, and a predisposition to the effects of trauma, overuse, and mechanical failure. It is an overlap syndrome, which encompasses many of the features encountered in the "classical" heritable disorders of connective tissue such as the Marfan and Ehlers-Danlos syndromes and osteogenesis imperfecta, but in a much more benign form. There are no life-threatening complications. It is therefore generally referred to as the benign joint hypermobility syndrome (BJHS).

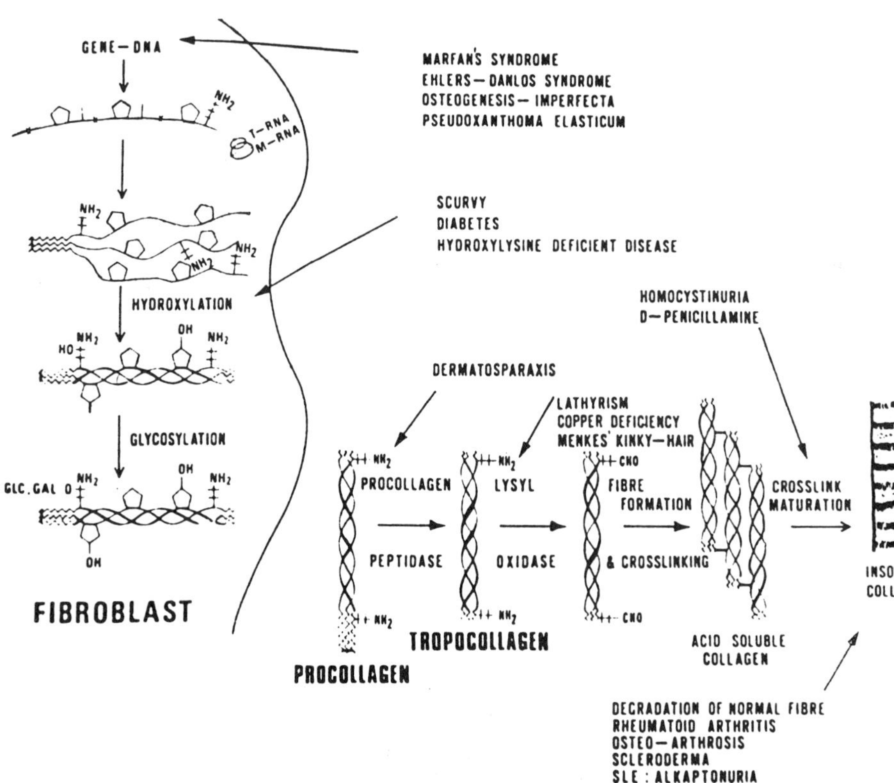

Figure 10.1 Pathophysiology of collagen diseases.

Table 10.1 Benign Joint Hypermobility Syndrome (BJHS)

Heritable disorder of connective tissue characterized by joint laxity, tissue
    fragility, and mechanical failure.
Arthralgias due to tendonitis, capsulitis, recurrent dislocations.
Active teenagers and young adults.
Benign prognosis—adaptation of life style.

1.2 Main Clinical Features

1.2.1 Early Manifestations

Joint laxity manifest as hypermobility being inherent is present from birth and persists throughout life, although it diminishes progressively from infancy. For many (perhaps the majority) hypermobility is an asset, assisting their indulgence in sport and in the performing arts; for most it causes no symptoms and they may be unaware of it; for the unfortunate few it may, depending on their lifestyle, be the source of frequent and varied musculoskeletal problems that may include the whole range of traumatic and overuse lesions described in Chapter 8. The term hypermobility syndrome is reserved for hypermobile subjects with such symptoms. Although symptoms not infrequently commence in childhood, the more athletically active teenage years are when problems are most likely to arise. The common modes of presentation are summarized in Table 10.2.

1.2.2 Late Manifestations

As the years go by the patient is likely to be continued to be troubled by the various conditions in the list. It should be emphasized that these afflictions occur in all people but are more frequent and more varied in hypermobile subjects. With advancing age the progressive loss of hypermobility may be accompanied by

1. Fewer overuse/traumatic lesions
2. The onset of symptoms of osteoarthritis
3. Visceral problems resulting from weakness of connective tissues including supporting structures.

Table 10.2 Common Modes of Presentation BJHS

Muscle/ligament tear
Epicondylitis
Tendonitis/capsulitis
Carpal tunnel syndrome
Plantar fasciitis
Traumatic arthritis
Chondromalacia patellae
Soft tissue back pain
Spondylolysis/spondylolisthesis
Disc prolapse
Stress fracture
Recurrent dislocation
Nonspecific arthralgia/myalgia

Table 10.3 Late Features in BJHS

Nonspecific arthralgia/myalgia
Osteoarthritis (esp. hip/knee)
Disc prolapse/spondylosis/spinal stenosis
Uterine/rectal prolapse
Hernia/varicose veins
Mitral valve prolapse (mild)
Depression

1.3   Confirming the Diagnosis—Investigations

1.3.1   Early Phase

Benign joint hypermobility syndrome is often overlooked for the simple reason that hypermobility is not tested for in the clinical examination. The time-honored 9-point Beighton system is simple to perform and takes seconds. It involves the ability to perform four paired passive and one active maneuvers. A score of >2 usually denotes widespread laxity (Fig. 10.2).

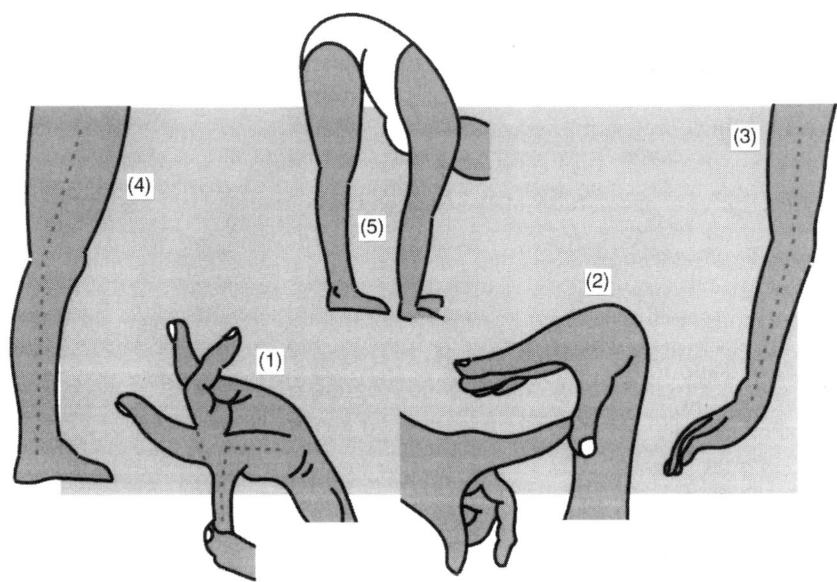

Figure 10.2   Nine-point Beighton score.

1.3.2 Late Phase

For reasons stated above, it will be appreciated that the actual Beighton score diminishes with age to the extent that it may reach zero. Many subjects will, however, recall their earlier ability to perform several of the maneuvers, especially no. 5, to create a "historical" score.

1.4 Diagnostic Difficulties

The principal bar to diagnosis is (1) lack of awareness of the condition and (2) failure to look for evidence of hypermobility as part of the examination of the musculoskeletal system. This results in

1. Misdiagnosis—usually in favor of rheumatoid/juvenile chronic arthritis or of psychoneurosis
2. The inappropriate use of useless and potentially harmful drug therapy
3. Unnecessary suffering, frustration, and loss of faith in orthodox medicine

Specialist expert advice may be needed in distinguishing benign joint hypermobility syndrome from other heritable disorders of connective tissue (see next section).

Benign joint hypermobility syndrome should not be confused with Marfans or Ehlers–Danlos syndrome (see next section).

1.5 Epidemiology and Historical Data

Hypermobility has been identified in population surveys in all parts of the world, with the prevalence varying from 5% to 20% depending on age, gender, and ethnic background. There is general agreement that it is most prevalent in people of Indian origin, followed by those of African origin, followed by Europeans. Women are more hypermobile than men. There are few data on the epidemiology of the hypermobility syndrome (as opposed to hypermobility itself). Clinical data suggest that (if recognized) it is an important source of morbidity.

Hypermobility has been recognized since the days of Hippocrates.

1.6 Pathophysiology

The basis for many of the features of benign joint hypermobility syndrome is mechanical failure on the part of connective tissue, which is genetically imperfect (or at least different) and as a result ill equipped to meet the physical demands of daily life. Thus, traumatic and "overuse" lesions of soft tissues are prominent. However, all collagen-bearing tissues (skin, muscle, bone, cartilage, tendon, ligament, heart valve, etc.) are at risk and may be affected in one way or another. The molecular genetic defect in benign joint hypermobility syndrome has yet to be identified.

1.7 Management

The principles of management are as follows:

1. Establish the correct (and disabuse incorrect) diagnosis.
2. Inform and educate the patient about her or his condition.
3. Treat identifiable lesions along conventional lines.
4. Modify lifestyle to avoid provoking factors where possible.
5. Symptomatic treatment for nonspecific complaints.

1.8 Atypical Forms

It should be noted that hypermobility may occur solely in one joint or in a few joints (mono- or pauciarticular hypermobility). Yet it may nevertheless explain the symptoms in that/those joint(s).

1.9 Impact of the Disease and Prognosis

Benign joint hypermobility syndrome is a much neglected and underrecognized condition. Patients who experience difficulty in having the source and nature of their condition explained derive considerable satisfaction in the knowledge that their symptoms are not imagined and are capable of logical explanation and relief (even if not cure!). Benign joint hypermobility syndrome does not diminish life expectancy. Most patients who understand the limitations imposed on them by their condition are able to adapt their lifestyle accordingly and enjoy a reasonably full life. There is a core of less fortunate individuals who remain invalid despite all efforts to the contrary.

2　MARFAN'S SYNDROME

2.1　Definition (Table 10.4)

Marfan's syndrome is a heritable disorder of connective tissue characterized by long slender extremities, dislocation of the ocular lens (ectopia lentis), and aortic dilatation and/or aneurysm formation.

2.2　Main Clinical Features

2.2.1　Early Manifestations

Tall stature, long slender arms and legs, spidery fingers (arachnodactily), scoliosis, joint laxity, pes planus, hallux valgus, ectopic lentis may be apparent in infancy or early childhood.

Table 10.4   Marfan's Syndrome

Hereditary connective tissue disorders
Tall stature
Ectopia lentis
Arachnodactily
Aortic aneurysm (adulthood)
Collagen

2.2.2   Late Manifestations

During the adolescent growth spurt the abnormalities in body shape (marfanoid habitus) become more pronounced, especially tall height, scoliosis, and thoracic cage deformities (pectus excavatum and carinatum). Aortic aneurysm may occur in adult life, which may result in fatal rupture. Mitral valve prolapse can also occur.

2.3   Confirming the Diagnosis—Investigations

Diagnosis remains based solely on clinical features and the autosomal dominant inheritance pattern.

The marfanoid habitus is confirmed by

1.   Span:height ratio > 1.03
2.   Upper segment:lower segment ratio < 0.09
3.   Hand:height ratio $> 11\%$
4.   Foot:height ratio $> 15\%$
5.   Arachnodactily
6.   Scoliosis
7.   Pectum excavatum/carinatum
8.   Ectopia lentis

Aortic root dilatation can be recognized by serial echocardiography.

2.4   Diagnostic Difficulties

Marfanoid habitus is seen (without aortic dilatation or ectopia lentis) in the benign joint hypermobility syndrome (see previous section) and in contractual arachnoidactily. The unsuspecting, undiagnosed Marfan's syndrome may be at great risk of fatal aortic aneurysmal rupture, either because a diagnosis of Marfan's syndrome has been overlooked or because dilatation is asymptomatic in the early stages.

2.5 Epidemiology and Historical Data

Marfan's syndrome is seen in all ethnic groups. The prevalence is approximately 1 in 10,000. Antoine Marfan described the skeletal features in 1895. The hereditary, ocular, and cardiac features were reported in the first half of the 20th century. The link with the fibrillin gene was discovered in 1990.

2.6 Pathophysiology

The disease is transmitted as autosomal dominant, but mutations are common. The skeletal, ocular, and cardiac manifestations result from an intrinsic weakness of connective tissues in the organs concerned due to a deficiency of fibrillin, a glycoprotein in which they are normally rich. Both the gene for Marfan's syndrome and that for fibrillin have been located on the 15th chromosome.

2.7 Management

Regular echocardiographic examinations are undertaken to detect early and/or increasing aortic root dilatation. Patients are maintained on β-blocker drugs, which lower blood pressure and thereby slow down the rate of dilatation. Contact sports are avoided. Aortic graft operations are undertaken when dilatation is established in order to forestall aneurysm formation. Operations may also be required to treat the scoliosis and/or pectus deformities.

2.8 Atypical Forms

An incomplete clinical picture may be acceptable for diagnosis if unequivocal first-degree relatives are known to have the disease. Homocystinuria is an autosomal recessive disorder that resembles Marfan's syndrome. It is caused by a deficiency of the enzyme cystathionine β-synthetase. It is believed that hyperhomocystinemia may influence fibrillin adversely. The clinical features comprise ectopia lentis/myopia, osteoporosis/scoliosis, increased length of long bones, joint hypomobility, vascular occlusions, mental retardation, and seizures (Table 10.5).

Management includes methionine restriction (to decrease homocystine load); cystine to avoid cysteine deficiency; pyridoxine to increase residual activity of the enzyme and to prevent/correct folate deficiency; betaine to increase remethylation of homocysteine to methionine; and antithrombotic agents to inhibit platelet function.

Table 10.5 Clinical Features of Homocystinuria

Ectopia lentis/myopia
Osteoporosis/scoliosis
Increased length of long bones
Joint hypomobility
Vascular occlusions
Mental retardation/seizures

2.9 Impact of the Disease and Prognosis

Sudden death of a family member is always a catastrophe, so that people suspected of having Marfan's syndrome or who are family members of known cases *must* be screened. Self-help groups provide information, comfort, and support.

3 OSTEOGENESIS IMPERFECTA

3.1 Definition (Table 10.6)

Osteogenesis imperfecta is a common disorder of bone fragility associated with blue sclerae.

3.2 Main Clinical Features

3.2.1 Early Manifestations

In severe cases death may occur in utero from multiple fractures. In less severe cases fractures are less frequent, but severe deformities may result in short stature.

3.2.2 Late Manifestations

Other features may include blue sclerae and deafness.

Table 10.6 Osteogenesis Imperfecta

Hereditary connective tissue disorder
Blue sclerae
Bone fragility in the youth period

3.3 Confirming the Diagnosis

3.3.1 Early Phase

The finding of a positive family history, blue sclerae, and recurrent fractures will point to the correct diagnosis.

3.3.2 Late Phase

In some cases the disease becomes clinically apparent with the onset of osteoporosis in middle age.

3.4 Diagnostic Difficulties

The differential diagnosis is between osteogenesis imperfecta and nonaccidental injury, with which it can be confused.

3.5 Epidemiology and Historical Data

Osteogenesis imperfecta is seen in all ethnic groups. Evidence suggests that it dates back to antiquity.

3.6 Pathophysiology

The disease has a mainly dominant role of inheritance. Recessive forms are rare. It is in effect a congenital form of osteoporosis, due in most cases to a mutation(s) in collagen I genes (COL1A1; COL1A2).

3.7 Management

Fractures are treated by conventional orthopedic measures using lightweight casts. There is no known way of strengthening the weakened bone matrix.

3.8 Atypical Forms

Minor phenotypically distinct forms of osteogenesis imperfecta are seen sporadically.

3.9 Impact of the Disease and Prognosis

The fetal form may lead to stillbirth. Late milder forms may be compatible with a normal life span.

4 EHLERS–DANLOS SYNDROME

4.1 Definition (Table 10.7)

Ehlers-Danlos syndrome is a heritable disorder of connective tissue (HDCT) characterized by a triad of articular hypermobility, skin hyperextensibility, and cutaneous scarring. It is a heterogeneous condition.

Table 10.7 Ehlers–Danlos Syndrome

Hereditary connective tissue disorder
Articular hypermobility
Skin hyperextensibility
Ruptured arteries

4.2 Main Clinical Features

4.2.1 Early Manifestations

The skin is thin and splits easily leaving ugly gaping pigmented, papyraceous scars, especially over the knees and scalp. Joint laxity can lead to recurrent dislocations and instability, commonly with effusions.

4.2.2 Late Manifestations

Rupture of major arteries occurs (only) in Ehlers–Danlos syndrome type IV. A tendency to bleeding is seen. Osteoarthritis occurs frequently in unstable joints.

4.3 Confirming the Diagnosis—Investigations

4.3.1 Early Phase

This is based on the positive family history and the clinical features.

4.3.2 Late Phase

In Ehlers–Danlos syndrome type IV there is a deficiency of collagen type III.

4.4 Diagnostic Difficulties

Difficulties may arise in distinguishing Ehlers–Danlos syndrome from other heritable disorders of connective tissue that share common features, e.g., benign joint hypermobility syndrome, osteogenesis imperfecta, Marfan's syndrome.

4.5 Epidemiology and Historical Data

Types I (gravis), II (mitis), and III (hypermobile) are relatively common, whereas the remaining seven types (including the serious type IV) are comparatively rare.

4.6 Pathophysiology

The primary defect of types I-III are not known. In type VI there is deficiency of lysyl hydroxylase; in type IX a reduction in lysyl oxidase; and in type X a probable defect in fibronectin.

4.7 Management

Physiotherapy with exercises to promote muscle strengthening and the use of casts to support unstable joints are helpful. Skin protection is essential. Violent sports and unsuitable occupations should be avoided. Surgery is difficult and requires additional suturing. Genetic counseling is advisable, because there is 50% chance of progeny being affected.

4.8 Impact of the Disease and Prognosis

Since many family members may be affected, the disease can cause great anxiety. Information, support, and advice is now available through self-help groups.

11

Current Intra- and Periarticular Injection Techniques in Rheumatology

The local intra- and periarticular administration of corticosteroids is an attractive treatment of rheumatic diseases. A quick and maximal effectiveness is to be expected with a minimum of systemic effects. The side effects remain limited on the conditions that the indication for administration was correct and that the technique and aseptic conditions are perfect, and that the number of injections is kept to a minimum.

This therapeutic approach, developed by Hollander in the early 1950s, remains a half century later an important adjunctive treatment for rheumatic diseases. Rheumatoid arthritis and related conditions, osteoarthritis in an active phase, and periarticular rheumatic diseases are the most prominent indications for this kind of management.

The corticosteroid preparations used are suspensions of methylprednisolone, triamcinolone, or paramethasone. Rarely the combination suspensions and solutions are indicated. This is also true for the association of corticosteroids and anesthetics. The local tolerance of the products is excellent. In very rare cases, a microcrystal arthropathy and pain can immediately follow injection.

Joint destruction has been reported after local injection because hypoalgesia induced by infiltration could predispose to articular overloading and therefore accelerate the process of chondrolysis and osteolysis.

Table 11.1 Guidelines for the Local Administration
of Corticosteroids

Correct indication
Perfect injection technique
Strict asepsis
Injection of moderate dosages
Maximal spreading of injections

All joints can be infiltrated. In daily practice, knees, shoulders, and
wrists pose no problems. Somewhat more complicated are the infiltrations
of the elbows, ankles, hand, and feet. However, when using precise techniques, as shown on the pictures and schemes of the next pages, one should
not encounter major problems.

The basic rules are as follows:

1. Local asepsis should be assured. The patient's skin should be
    cleaned with iodine alcohol 1% or Isobetadine, and the doctor's
    hands must be washed profusely before injection.
2. The use of appropriate material is essential: a syringe of 2 ml to
    be used only once; disposable needles (20G × 2″ 0.90 × 50 −
    21G × 1½″ 0.80 × 40 − 24G × 1″ 0.55 × 25 − 25G × 5/
    8″ 0.50 × 16).
3. For maximal efficacy, 24-hr functional rest after injection is ad-
    vised.
4. When not experienced, only inject joints when you can palpate
    intraarticular fluid. This will facilitate this procedure consider-
    ably.

1 UPPER LIMBS

1.1 The Shoulder

Infiltration in the shoulder can be given intra- or periarticularly based on
the pathologic finding.

1.1.1 Intraarticular Shoulder

Scapulohumeral Joint (Fig. 11.1). The anterior approach is more
easy than the posterior one and therefore should be preferred.

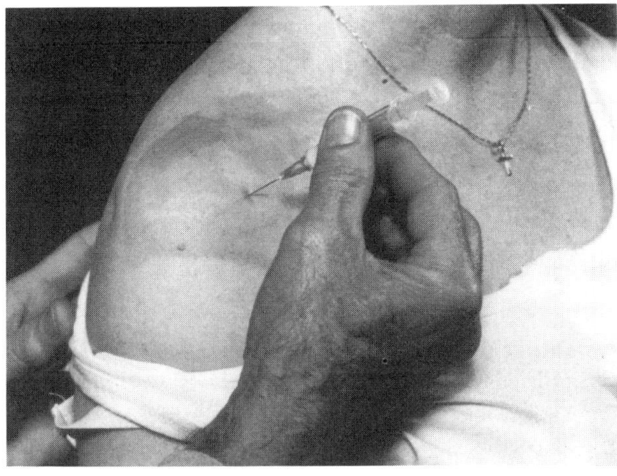

(a)

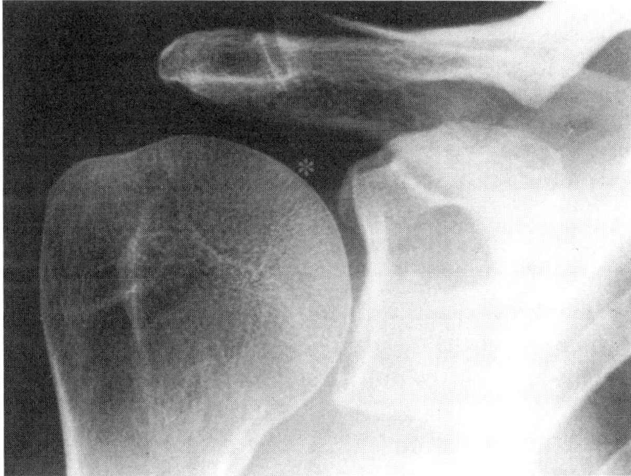

(b)

Figure 11.1 (a) Intraarticular injection scapulohumeral joint; (b) corresponding injection location on X-ray.

Technique: The patient sits with the shoulder in external rotation. The punction site is located on the crossing of the line which runs a finger width under the clavicula and a finger width medial of the external board of the acromion. The needle should be brought into the joint space perpendicularly.
Material: Needle 0.55 × 25 mm or 0.80 × 40 mm.
For punction: 0.90 × 50″.
Local anesthesia is not necessary.
Product: Methylprednisolone, triamcinolone, paramethasone.
Amount: 1 ml.

Acromioclavicular Joint (Fig. 11.2).

Technique: This joint is easy of access. The patient sits with the shoulder in external rotation. One marks with the finger the prominence at the external end of the clavicula. The needle is inserted perpendicularly just beside this prominence.
Material: Needle 0.55 × 25 mm.
Sometimes local anesthesia is necessary because the injection of corticosteroids can be painful. It is therefore better to use an association of corticosteroids and anesthetics from the outset.
Product: Methylprednisolone or methylprednisolone lidocaïne.
Amount: 0.20–0.50 ml.

1.1.2 Periarticular Shoulder

Tendon of the Musculus Supraspinatus (Fig. 11.3).
SUBDELTOID SEROSA BURSA
Technique: The patient sits down with the shoulder hanging down. One marks with the finger the external board of the acromion. The needle should be inserted horizontally just beneath, to a depth of 2–3 cm.
Material: Needle 0.80 × 40 mm or 0.55 × 25 mm. Local anesthesia is sometimes necessary.
Product: Methylprednisolone or methylprednisolone lidocaïne.
Amount: 0.50–1 ml.

Tendon of the Musculus Biceps Longus (Fig. 11.4).
Technique: This is a difficult injection that has to be given with precision extratendinously in order to avoid rupture. The sick tendon is localized and isolated in the sulcus bicipitalis when the patient is in a sitting position. The needle is inserted perpendicularly toward the tendon and when it's in the tendon sheet directed horizontally toward above over a length of 1-2 cm.

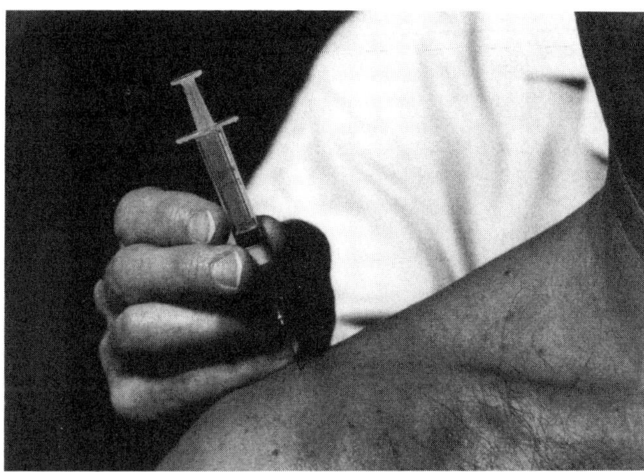

(a)

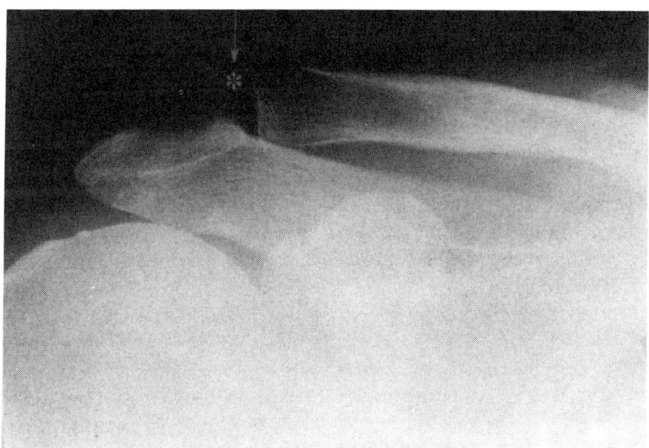

(b)

Figure 11.2 (a) Intraarticular injection acromioclavicular joint; (b) corresponding injection location on X-ray.

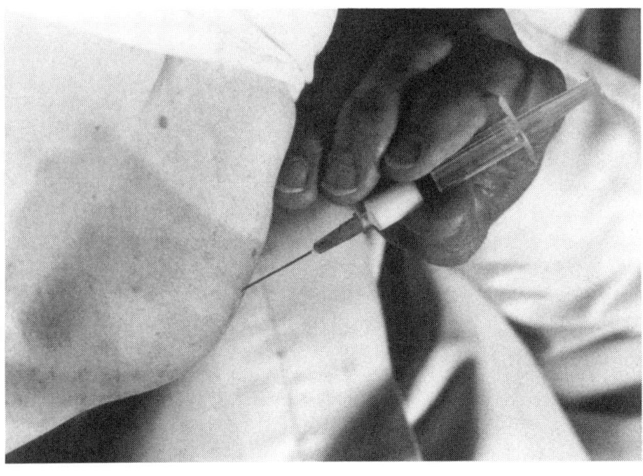

(a)

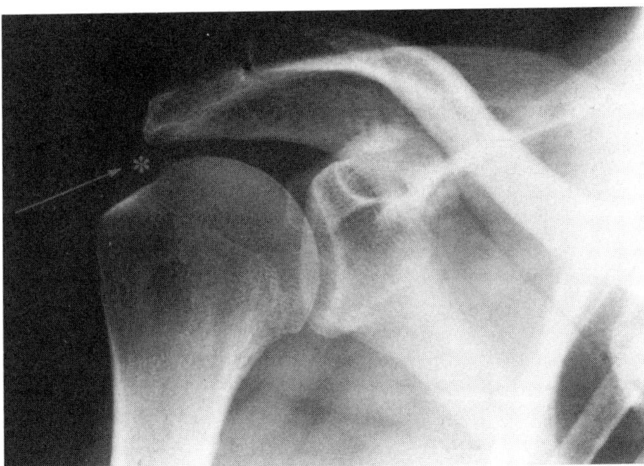

(b)

Figure 11.3 (a) Periarticular infiltration supraspinatus tendon and bursa subdeltoidea; (b) corresponding injection location on X-ray.

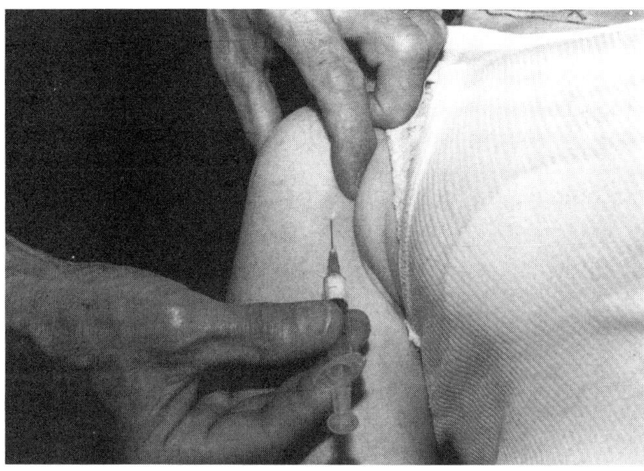

(a)

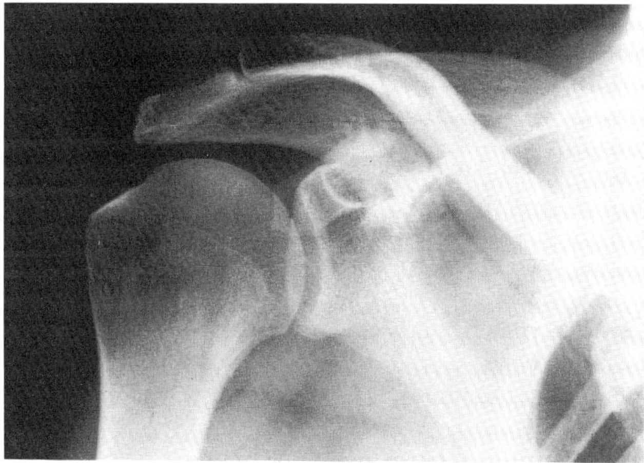

(b)

Figure 11.4   (a) Periarticular infiltration biceps longus tendon; (b) corresponding injection location on X-ray.

Material: Needle 0.80 × 40 mm or 0.55 × 25 mm. Local anesthesia
   is not necessary.
Product: Methylprednisolone.
Amount: 0.50–1 ml.

1.2   The Elbow

Depending on the pathology, the injection will be intraarticular or — and
this is most often the case — periarticular.

1.2.1   Intraarticular Elbow

There are two approaches.

Port of Entry Under the Olecranon or Posterior (Fig. 11.5).
Technique: The patient sits down with the elbow in flexion and supported by, say, the back of a chair. The top of the epicondylus is
   localized and a prick perpendicular in the direction of the upper
   point of the olecranon is given, followed by an inclined move inward and backward. The presence of intraarticular fluid will facilitate this technique.
Material: Needle 0.80 × 40 mm. Local anesthesia is not necessary.
Product: Methylprednisolone, triamcinolone, paramethasone.
Amount: 1 ml.

Radiohumeral or External Approach (Fig. 11.6).
Technique: When intraarticular fluid is present, which is often the
   case in rheumatoid arthritis patients, the fluid will accumulate
   around the radial head. The joint is then easily approachable. The
   patient places his elbow in a right angle (90°) on the couch. The
   needle is inserted perpendicularly under the epicondylus in the direction of the radial head.
Material: Needle 0.80 × 40 mm or 0.55 × 25 mm. Local anesthesia
   is not necessary.
Product: Methylprednisolone, triamcinolone, paramethasone.
Amount: 1 ml.

1.2.2   Periarticular Elbow

Epicondylitis (Tennis Elbow) (Fig. 11.7).
Technique: In this case, the injection is at the level of the epicondylus
   at the site of elective pain on pressure. As a rule, this position is
   situated at the anterior site of the epicondylus. The needle is inserted slightly inclined in the flexed elbow. The needle should come
   just in contact with the bone and then be slightly withdrawn before
   injection.

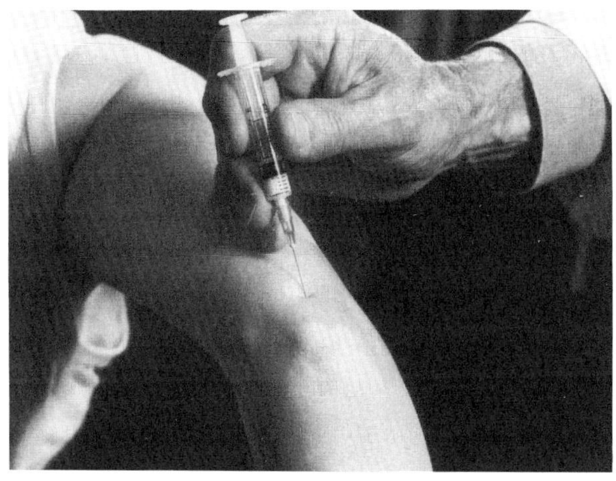

(a)

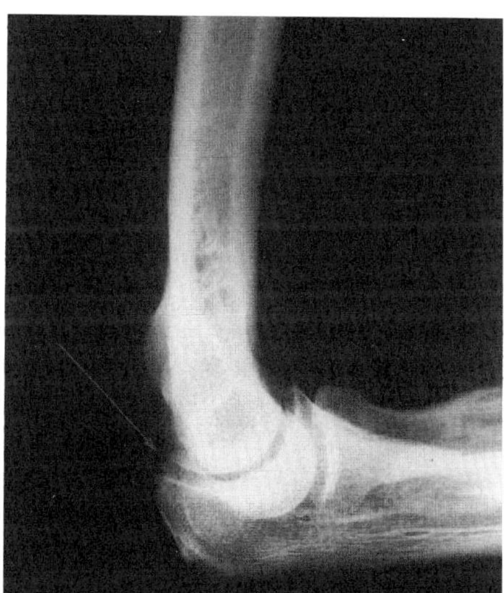

(b)

Figure 11.5 (a) Intraarticular injection elbow at the posterior site of the olecranon; (b) corresponding injection location on X-ray.

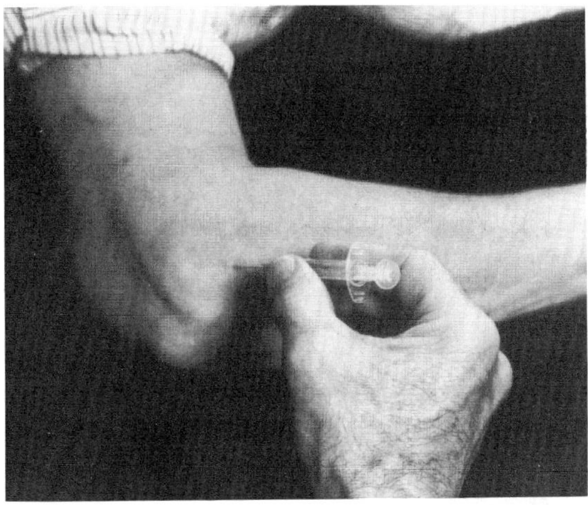

(a)

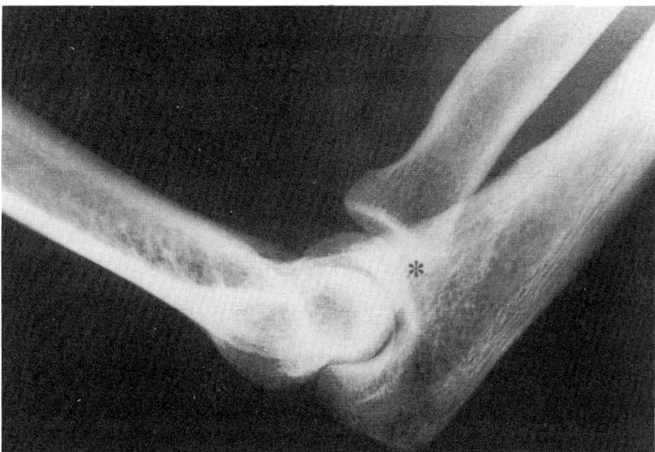

(b)

Figure 11.6 (a) Intraarticular injection elbow at the radiohumeral external site; (b) corresponding injection location on X-ray.

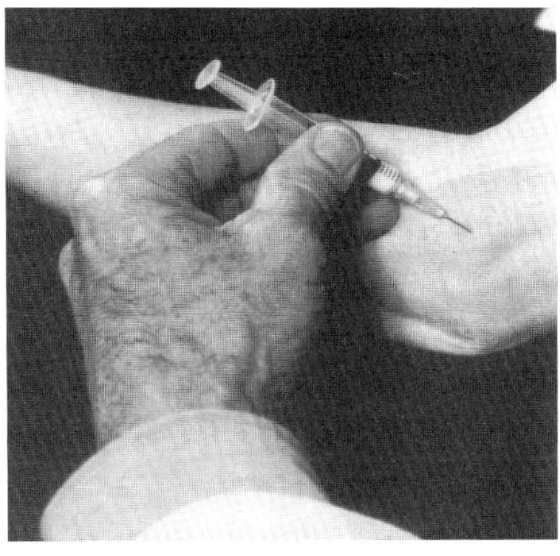

(a)

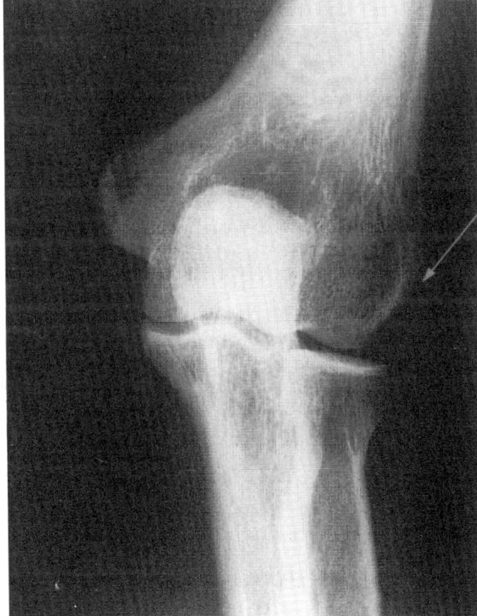

(b)

Figure 11.7 (a) Periarticular infiltration elbow for epicondylitis lateralis (tennis elbow); (b) corresponding injection location on X-ray.

Material: Needle 0.50 × 16 mm.

Product: Methylprednisolone at the lowest dosage. Avoid using fluor derivatives because of the risk of cutaneous or subcutaneous atrophy.

Amount: 0.20–0.30 ml.

Medial Humeral Epicondylus (Golfer's Elbow) (Fig. 11.8).

Technique: The technique is very similar to the one described above for epicondylitis. The elbow is supported by the couch in semiflexion and the arm is in exorotation. The needle is inserted until the bone structure is felt. Cubital nerve should not be touched (patients will feel typical pain).

Material and product: See epicondylitis.

1.3   The Wrist

Radiocarpal Joint (Fig. 11.9).

Technique: The injection of the wrist is performed via the dorsal approach. The patient sits down with the palm of the hand laying in extension on the couch. The processus styloideus is localized as well as the joint space. The needle is placed perpendicularly on the skin and inserted one finger width medially from the top of the processus styloideus at the radiocarpal joint space.

Material: Needle 0.55 × 25 mm. Anesthesia is not necessary.

Product: Methylprednisolone, triamcinolone, paramethasone.

Dosage: 0.50–1 ml.

Trapezometacarpal Joint (Fig. 11.10).

Technique: Hand in pronation; the joint approached from the posterior way. The basis of the first metacarpal is localized just under the anatomic snuff box. The needle is inserted perpendicularly to the bone. Trapezometacarpal osteoarthritis, osteophytes, subluxations, or chondrolysis may make the intraarticular injection difficult and painful. Experience has taught that juxtaarticular injections often give satisfactory results. Therefore it is not necessary to take an intraarticular approach when difficulties may arise.

Material: Needle 0.50 × 16 mm.

Product: Methylprednisolone, triamcinolone, paramethasone.

Dosage: 0.30–0.50 ml.

Carpal Tunnel (Fig. 11.11).

Technique: Hand in extension and supination. The medial palmar fold or, in case this is absent, the most proximal fold has to be localized. The tendon of the musculus palmaris brevis has to be

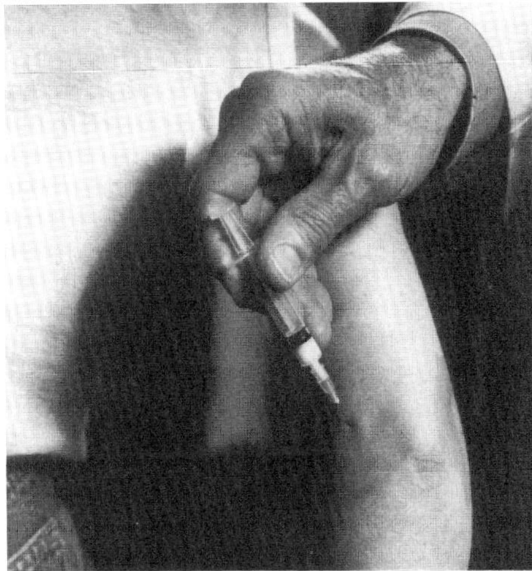

(a)

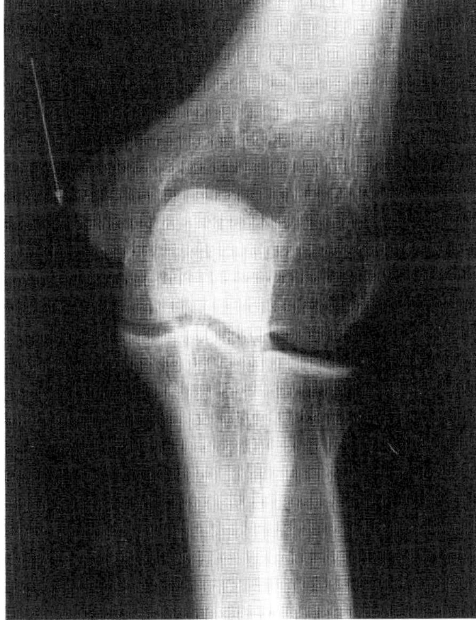

(b)

Figure 11.8 (a) Periarticular infiltration elbow for epicondylitis medialis (golfer's elbow); (b) corresponding injection location on X-ray.

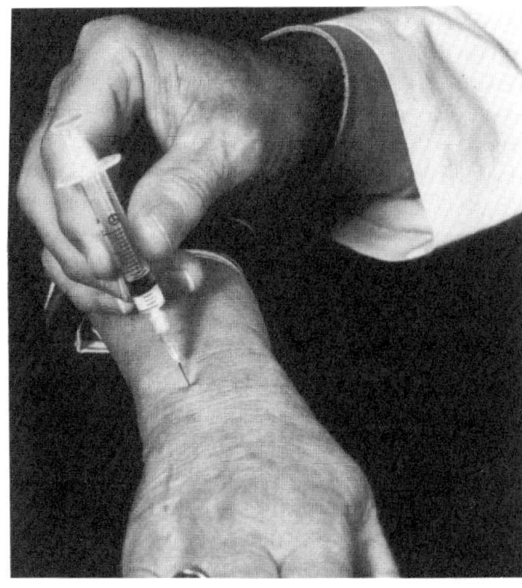

(a)

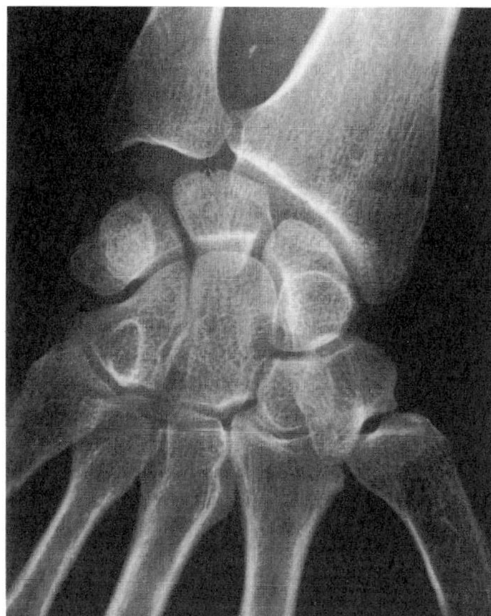

(b)

Figure 11.9 (a) Intraarticular injection wrist at radiocarpal joint; (b) corresponding injection location on X-ray.

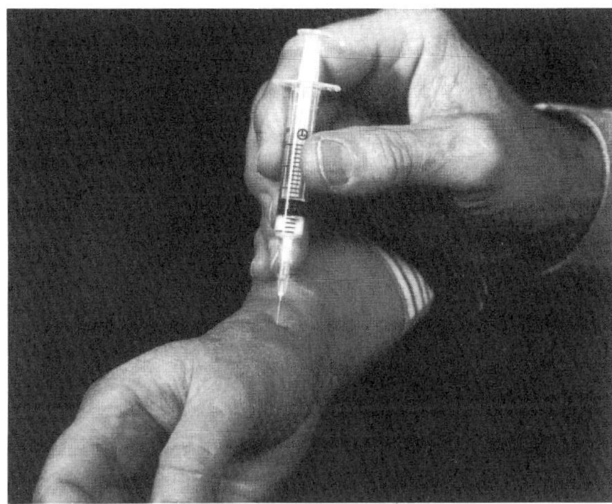

(a)

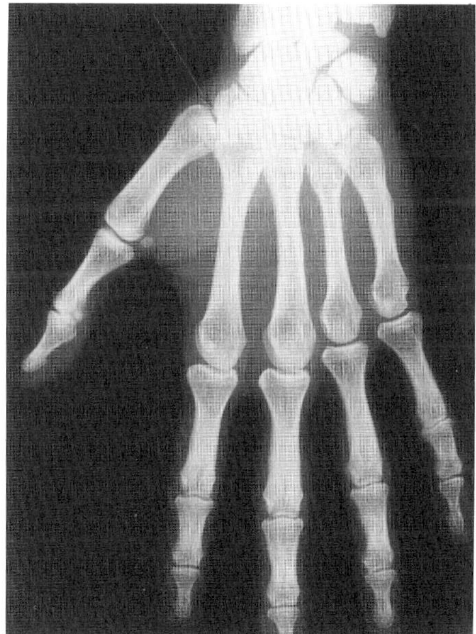

(b)

Figure 11.10 (a) Intraarticular injection wrist at trapezometacarpal joint; (b) corresponding injection location on X-ray.

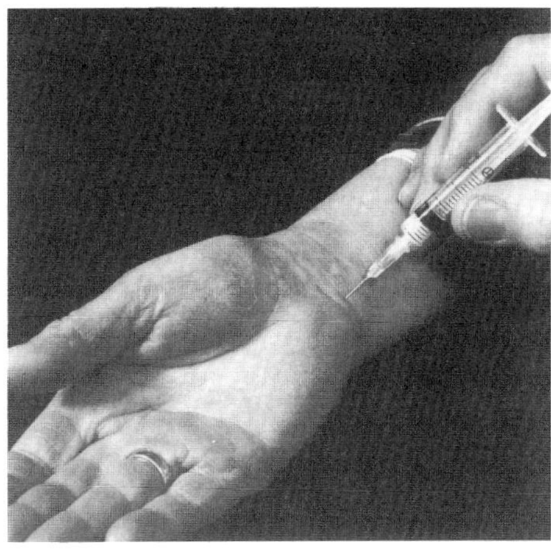

(a)

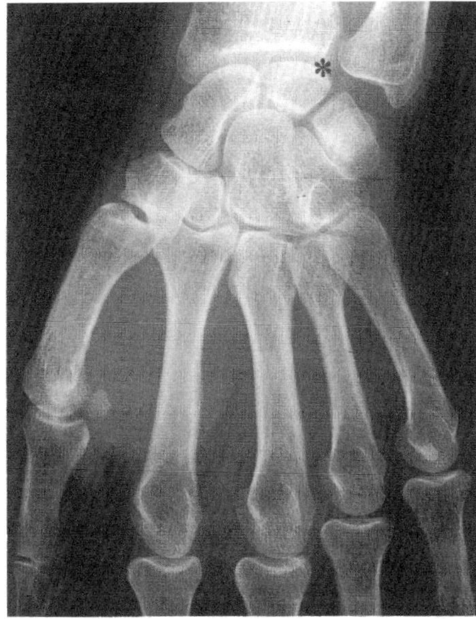

(b)

Figure 11.11 (a) Intraarticular injection wrist for carpal tunnel syndrome; (b) corresponding injection location on X-ray.

localized medial to the tendon of the musculus palmaris longus. The needle has to be inserted inclined in the direction of the crossing of the medial palmar fold and the internal part of the tendon of the musculus palmaris brevis. The ligamentum anulare anterior of the carpus is perforated. Now we are in the carpal tunnel. It is not necessary to go to the bottom. This external approach permits you to avoid contact with the nervus medianus.

Material: Fine needle 0.50 × 16 mm.

Product: Methylprednisolone, triamcinolone, or paramethasone.

Dosage: 0.20–0.30 ml.

1.4 The Hand

1.4.1 Metacarpophalangal and Proximal Interphalangeal Joints (Fig. 11.12)

Technique: It's easy to inject when there is a hydrops in the joints. When there is no fluid in the joint it's needless trying to give these injections. The approach should be on the lateral external or internal part of the joint where fluctuation is maximum. The hand is in pronation. The needle pricks the skin and consequently the joint capsule. The fine needle does not permit the investigator to see if there is any fluid present in the joint.

Material: Fine needle 0.50 × 16 mm.

Product: Methylpredinosolone, triamcinolone, paramethasone.

Dosage: 0.20–0.30 ml.

2 LOWER LIMBS

2.1 The Hip

The intraarticular injection of the hip is difficult and should not be done in routine practice. In contrast, infiltration of the major trochanter in case of periarthritis of the hip is easy and gives good results.

2.1.1 Periartritis of the Hip (Fig. 11.13)

Technique: The patient is laying in lateral decubitus on the nonpainful side. It's easy to palpate the upper board of the major trochanter. The needle is inserted perpendicular to the skin, until a depth where there is no longer resistance.

Material: Needle 0.90 × 50 mm. A longer needle is necessary in obese women.

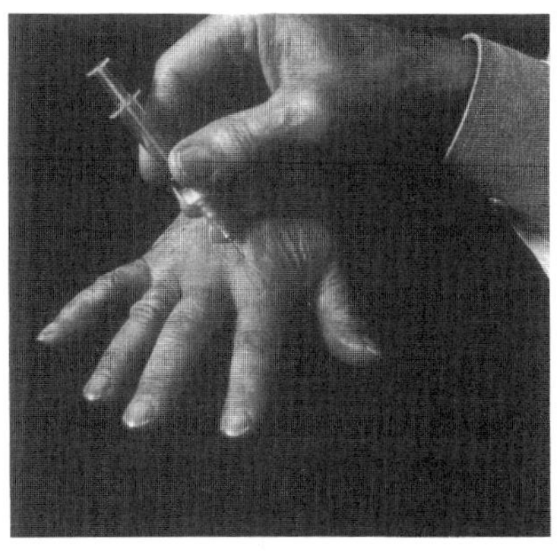 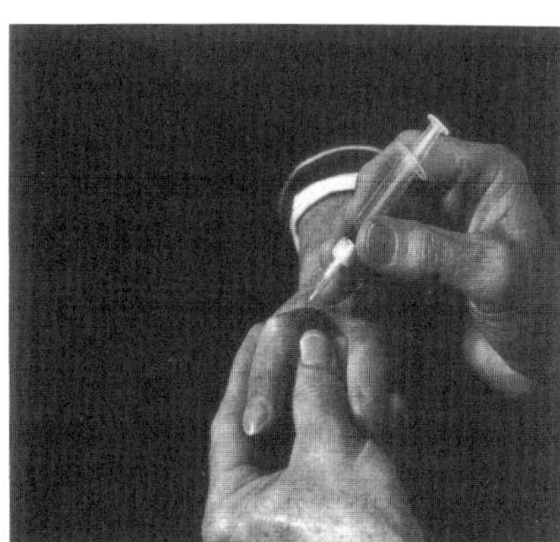

(a)

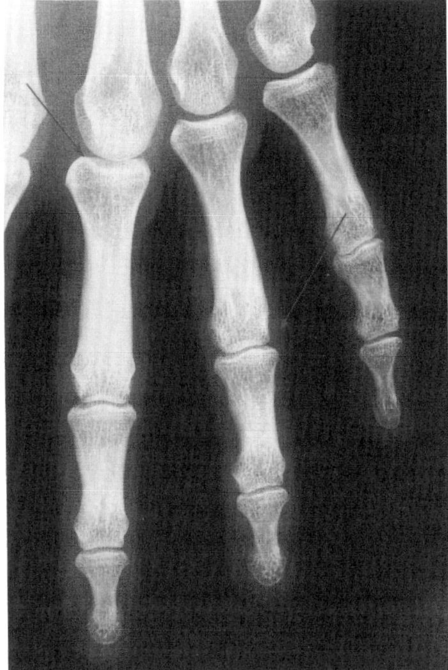

(b)

Figure 11.12 (a) Intraarticular injection metacarpophalangeal joints; (b) corresponding injection location on X-ray.

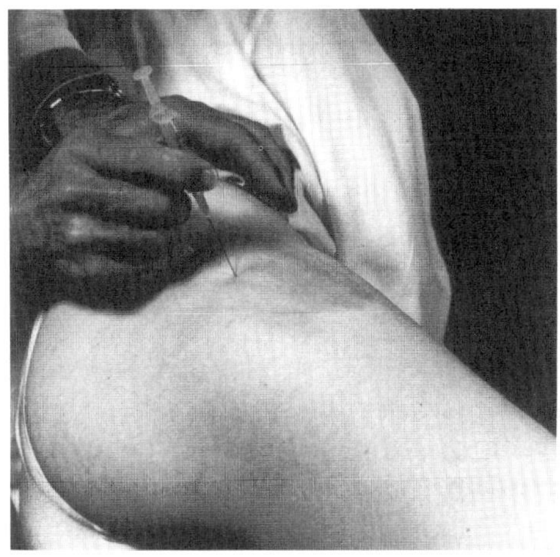

(a)

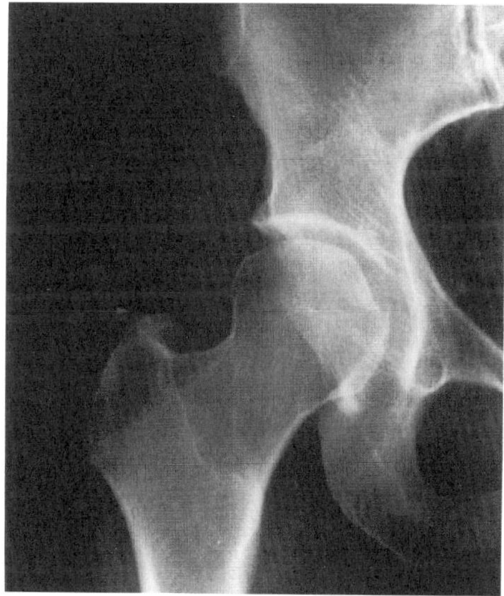

(b)

Figure 11.13 (a) Periarticular infiltration at the hip for trochanteritis; (b) corresponding injection location on X-ray.

Product: Methylprednisolone, triamcinolone, or paramethasone; sometimes an anesthetic can be useful.
Dosage: 1–2 ml.

2.2   The Knee

2.2.1   Intraarticular Knee

With Intraarticular Hydrops (Fig. 11.14).
Technique: There are several approaches, but the high lateral external way on the external side of the bursa suprapatellaris is the simplest and the least painful. The patient is laying in dorsal decubitus with the leg in extension. First localize the bursa suprapatellaris. One can move this bursa by giving a pressure on the internal part of it. The needle is inserted horizontally. As soon as one feels resistance, in particular when synovial fluid is present in the syringe after aspiration, one can be sure that the needle is intraarticular.
Material: Syringe of 20 ml for aspiration. Needle 0.90 × 50 mm.
Product: Methylprednisolone, triamcinolone, paramethasone.
Dosage: 1–2 ml.

Without Hydrops (Fig. 11.15).
Technique: When there is no fluid present in the articular space, then it is better and simpler to use the anterior way for giving the injection. The knee is then flexed 90°. One localizes the point of the patella. The injection site is situated 1 cm below and 1 cm medial of this mark. The needle is inserted perpendicularly up to a depth of 2–3 cm. As soon as one arrives in the joint, one feels a slight resistance.
Material: Needle 0.80 × 40 mm.
Product: Methylprednisolone, triamcinolone, paramethasone.
Dosage: 1 ml.

2.2.2   Periarticular Knee (Fig. 11.16)

Technique: The knee is placed in full extension. By palpation one localizes the tendon group, which is usually swollen and painful. One places the needle inclined to above and advances until the tendons are touched. One infiltrates paratendinously. The injection should not be given against resistance.
Material: Needle 0.90 × 50 mm or 0.80 × 40 mm.
Product: Preferentially methylprednisolone is used, associated with

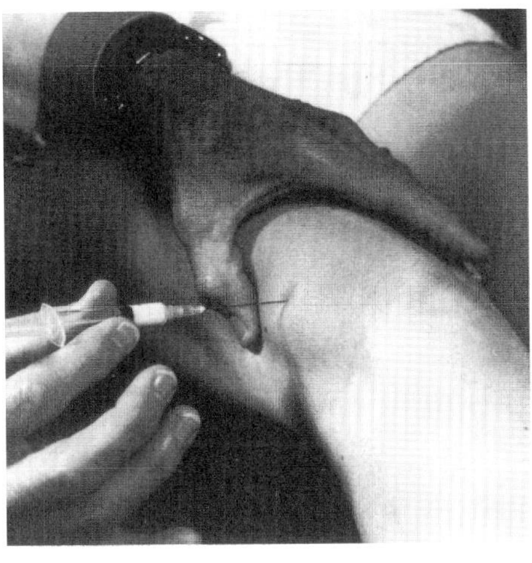

(a)

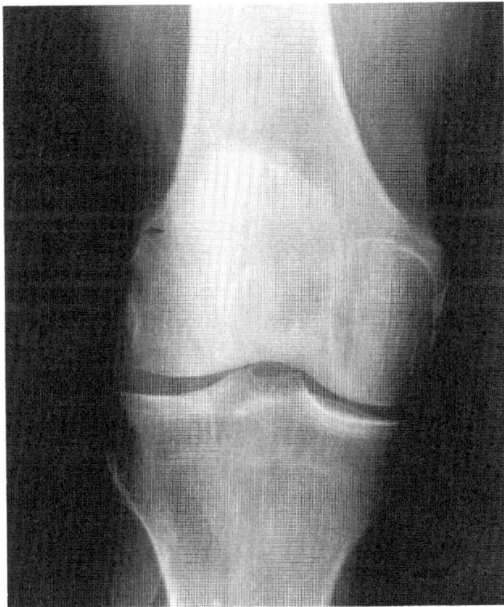

(b)

Figure 11.14 (a) Intraarticular injection in the knee joint with hydrops; (b) corresponding injection location on X-ray.

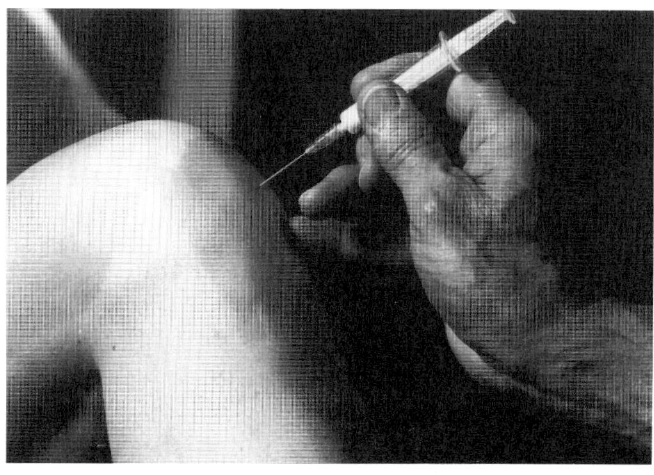

(a)

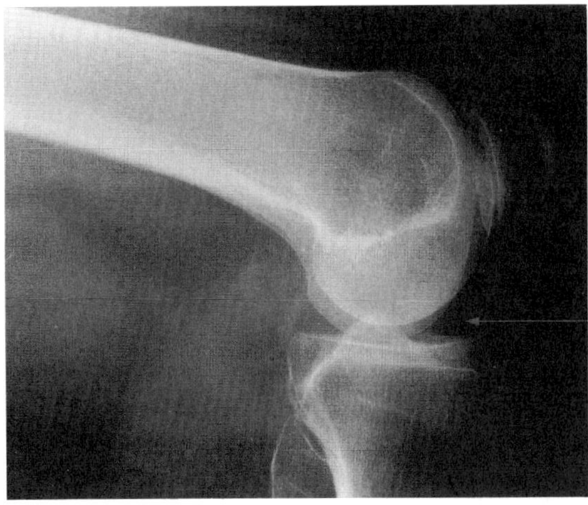

(b)

Figure 11.15   (a) Intraarticular injection in the knee joint without hydrops; (b) corresponding injection location on X-ray.

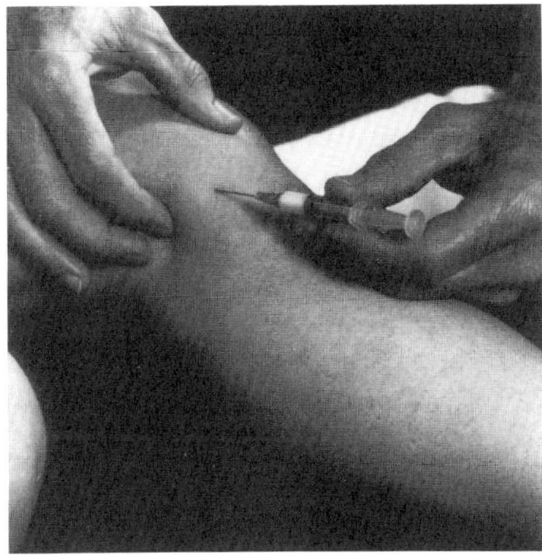

(a)

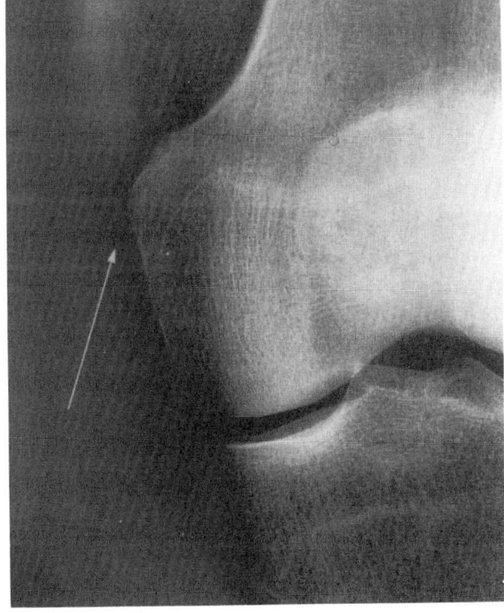

(b)

Figure 11.16 (a) Periarticular infiltration of the knee; (b) corresponding injection location on X-ray.

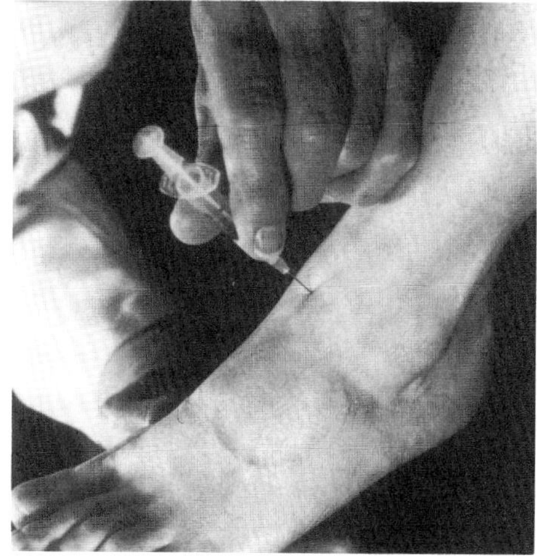

(a)

(b)

Figure 11.17 (a) Intraarticular injection at the ankle joint; (b) corresponding injection location on X-ray.

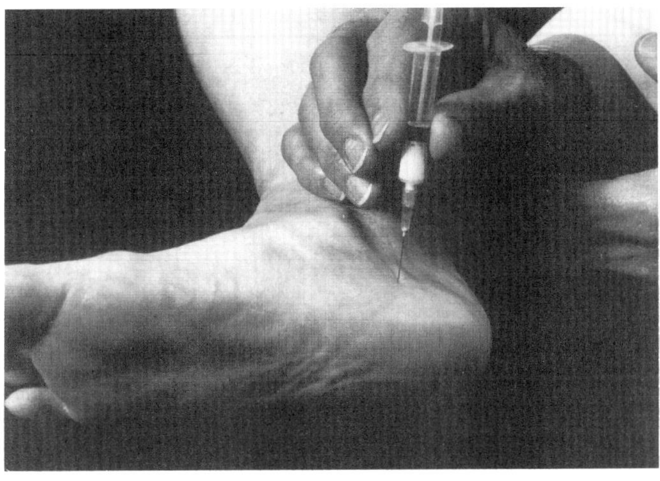

(a)

(b)

Figure 11.18 (a) Infiltration aponeurosis plantaris of the heel; (b) corresponding injection location on X-ray.

an anesthetic. The immediate effect of the anesthetic confirms the periarticular etiology of the knee pain.
Dosage: 1–2 ml.

2.3   The Ankle (Fig. 11.17)

Technique: The anterior way is the simplest and least painful. The foot is placed in slight plantar flexion. One takes the bimalleolar line as a reference. The injection point is situated between the tendon of the musculus tibialis anterior and the tendon of the musculus extensor hallucis longus, which is situated more laterally. The needle is inserted perpendicularly in the direction of the heel. The intraarticular penetration is usually felt.
Material: Needle 0.80 × 40 mm or 0.55 × 25 mm.
Product: Methylprednisolone, triamcinolone, or paramethasone.
Dosage: 1 ml.

2.4   The Foot

The intraarticular injections in the feet are difficult. They should not be done in daily practice. In contrast, the infiltration of the aponeurosis plantaris is easy and helpful.

2.4.1   Aponeurosis Plantaris (Calcaneus Spur) (Fig. 11.18)

Technique: The patient lays in lateral decubitus and presents the internal side of the heel. One localizes lateral the place of maximal sensibility which is usually in the anterior inferior part of the calcaneum. The needle is inserted near the calcaneum where the tendon enters the bone. This technique is often painful and necessitates the association of corticosteroids and an anesthetic. Eventually one can give the anesthetic first in the rami calcanei mediales.
Material: Needle 0.80 × 40 mm or 0.55 × 25 mm.
Product: Methylprednisolone lidocaïne.
Dosage: 0.75–1 ml.

Index

About the Authors

JAN DEQUEKER is Professor of Rheumatology and Director of the Arthritis and Metabolic Bone Disease Research Unit, Division of Rheumatology, University Hospitals, Katholieke Universiteit Leuven, Leuven, Belgium. The author or coauthor of numerous journal publications, he is the president of the International League of Associations for Rheumatism (ILAR) and a member of the American Society for Bone and Mineral Research, the Osteoarthritis Research Society, and the Royal Belgian Rheumatology Society. Dr. Dequeker received the M.D. (1961) and Ph.D. (1972) degrees from Katholieke Universiteit Leuven, Leuven, Belgium.

GABRIEL PANAYI is Arthritis and Rheumatism Council Professor of Rheumatology, United Medical and Dental Schools of Guy's and St. Thomas' Hospitals, Guy's Hospital, London, England. The author or coauthor of numerous scientific publications, he received the B.A. (1962), M.B. (1965), M.D. (1971), and D.Sc. (1991) degrees from Cambridge University, England.

THEODORE PINCUS is Professor of Medicine and Microbiology in the Division of Rheumatology and Immunology, Department of Medicine, Vanderbilt University School of Medicine, Nashville, Tennessee. The author or coauthor of numerous publications concerning basic microbiology, clinical serology, and long-term disease outcomes, and the coeditor of *Rheumatoid Arthritis: Pathogenesis, Assessment, Outcome, and Treatment* (Marcel Dekker, Inc.), he received the A.B. degree (1961) from Columbia College, New York, New York, and the M.D. degree (1966) from Harvard Medical School, Boston, Massachusetts.

RODNEY GRAHAME is Consultant Rheumatologist Emeritus, Guy's Hospital, London, England, Emeritus Professor of Clinical Rheumatology, University of London, England, as well as Senior Medical Advisor, Medicines Control Agency, Department of Health, London, England. He is a Fellow of the American College of Physicians and an honorary member of the Société Française de Rheumatologie, the Czech Rheumatology Society, and the former All-Union Society of Soviet Scientific Rheumatologists. Dr. Grahame received the M.B. (1955) and M.D. (1969) degrees from the University of London, England.